Families &
Life-Threatening
Illness

Maureen Leahey, RN, PhD
Team Director, Mental Health Services
Holy Cross Hospital
Adjunct Associate Professor
Faculty of Nursing, University of Calgary
Calgary, Alberta, Canada

Lorraine M. Wright, RN, PhD
Director, Family Nursing Unit
Professor, Faculty of Nursing
University of Calgary
Calgary, Alberta, Canada

D0877477

Springhouse Corporation
Springhouse, Pennsylvania

Publisher: Keith Lassner
Senior Acquisitions Editor: Susan L. Taddei
Art Director: John Hubbard
Editorial Services Manager: David Moreau
Senior Production Manager: Deborah C. Meiris
Special thanks to the following, who assisted in preparation of this volume: Carol Robertson, Bernadette Glenn, and Jean Robinson.

CHAPTER 7
The author wishes to acknowledge the Special Awards Grant from the California Division of the American Cancer Society for funding the research for this chapter. The contents of this publication do not necessarily represent the policies or views of the Society. Additional acknowledgments are made to the families and staff affiliated with the Children's Cancer Research Institute of San Francisco, especially the pediatric nurses at Presbyterian Medical Center.

CHAPTER 8
Some of the material contained in this chapter originally appeared in the author's book, *Coping When Life Is Threatened.* (Regina, Canada: Weigl, 1984).

CHAPTER 11
The author would like to acknowledge the Baltimore Regional Burn Center and the Department of Social Work, Baltimore City Hospitals, Baltimore, Maryland, under whose auspices the assessment described in this chapter was conducted.

CHAPTER 13
The author wishes to thank Ariella Lang, RN, BScN, Apnea Clinic, Montreal Children's Hospital, Montreal, Quebec, Canada, for her interest and assistance, and to acknowledge the contribution of the families who so willingly shared their experiences.

The clinical procedures described and recommended in this publication are based on research and consultation with nursing, medical, and legal authorities. To the best of our knowledge, these procedures reflect currently accepted practice; nevertheless, they can't be considered absolute and universal recommendations. For individual application, all recommendations must be considered in light of the patient's clinical condition and, before administration of new or infrequently used drugs, in light of latest package-insert information. The authors and the publisher disclaim responsibility for any adverse effects resulting directly or indirectly from the suggested procedures, from any undetected errors, or from the reader's misunderstanding of the text.

Printed in the United States of America.

Library of Congress Cataloging-in-Publication Data
Families and life-threatening illness.

(Family nursing series)
Includes bibliographies and index.
1. Intensive care nursing. 2. Critically ill—Family relationships. I. Leahey, Marueen, 1944-   . II. Wright, Lorraine M., 1943-
. III. Series.
[DNLM: 1. Acute Disease—psychology—nurses' instruction. 2. Attitude to Death—nurses' instruction. 3. Chronic Disease—psychology—nurses' instruction. 4. Crisis Intervention—nurses' instruction. 5. Family—nurses' instruction. 6. Nursing Process. WY 100 F1978]
RT120.I5F36 1987   362.1'042   87-10201
ISBN 0-87434-089-6

To my mother, Nora Neus, and in memory of my father, Harry Neus, for their encouragement of the pursuit of excellence.

Maureen Leahey

To my mother and father, Hazel and Jim Wright, for valuing health and the care of their elderly parents.

Lorraine M. Wright

ABOUT THE EDITORS

MAUREEN LEAHEY, RN, PhD, is a nurse/family therapist specializing in work with children/adolescents and families with health problems. Dr. Leahey is a chartered psychologist. She is a Team Director and Director of the Family Therapy Institute, Mental Health Services, Holy Cross Hospital; Adjunct Assistant Professor, Department of Psychiatry, Faculty of Medicine; and Adjunct Associate Professor, Faculty of Nursing, University of Calgary. Dr. Leahey maintains a part-time private practice in strategic marital and family therapy and is a consultant. She is a Member of the Commission on Accreditation of the American Association for Marriage and Family Therapy.

LORRAINE M. WRIGHT, RN, PhD, is Director, Family Nursing Unit, and Professor, Faculty of Nursing, University of Calgary. Dr. Wright's clinical and research interests include family somatics and systemic therapy; training and supervision of family clinical nurse specialists and family therapists; and split-opinion interventions. She maintains a part-time private practice in systemic marital and family therapy and is also a family therapy consultant. Dr. Wright is on the Board of the Alberta Foundation for Nursing Research and is a Member of the Research Committee of the American Association for Marriage and Family Therapy. She also serves on the editorial board of Contemporary Family Therapy—An International Journal.

Both editors have taught family nursing and family therapy to nursing and medical students, psychologists, social workers, and residents in family practice, pediatrics, and psychiatry. They have presented papers at national and international conferences in the United States, Canada, Israel, and Europe and have published their work in several journals. They are the co-authors of *Nurses and Families: A Guide to Family Assessment and Intervention* (Philadelphia: F.A. Davis Co., 1984).

CONTENTS

SECTION I: OVERVIEW OF FAMILIES AND LIFE-THREATENING ILLNESS

SECTION II: ASSESSING FAMILIES WITH LIFE-THREATENING ILLNESS

SECTION III: INTERVENING WITH FAMILIES WITH LIFE-THREATENING ILLNESS

PREFACE

Family Nursing Series

Although nurses have always interacted with the families of their patients, today's nurses are not only being encouraged but are also seeking ways to actively help families with health problems.

The Family Nursing Series, which consists of three volumes, focuses on clinically important family health issues. Titles include *Families and Life-Threatening Illness, Families and Chronic Illness,* and *Families and Psychosocial Problems.* Each volume provides an overview of family nursing with assessment and intervention sections on various health problems. Families at various stages of the developmental life cycle (for example, families with young children, families with adolescents, middle-aged families, and aging families) as well as various family forms (for example, single-parent, step-parent, and gay and lesbian families) are presented. Each chapter combines theory, research, and clinical examples to offer practical *how-tos* for assessment and intervention. Additionally, each chapter is organized according to the nursing process with direct access to information about assessment, planning, intervention, and evaluation.

Written for nursing students as well as practicing nurses, the Family Nursing Series provides current clinical information in a practical format. Essential theory is always presented in the context of clinical material, with the emphasis on sound family assessment and intervention. Descriptive case studies illustrate normal and dysfunctional families coping with health issues. Family Nursing Series contributors are authoritative clinicians and educators from a variety of distinguished nursing centers across North America.

Families and Life-Threatening Illness

This volume offers an in-depth clinical guide to assessment and intervention with families with life-threatening illness. It offers specific, clear instructions on *how to* assess and intervene effectively.

The first section provides the conceptual base for working with families. To interview families and accurately identify their strengths and problems a nurse must first have a sound conceptual framework. The chapters in this section deal with different aspects of family nursing and life-threatening illness. Reciprocity issues between the family and the illness are considered, as well as the nurse's assumptions about the family's ways to cope with the life-threatening illness. Intercultural issues are dealt with in a chapter on ethnicity.

The second section tells *how to* assess families with such specific life-threatening illnesses as biliary atresia, cancer, central nervous system trauma, open-heart surgery, and burns. Each chapter offers specific questions to use in interviewing families.

The third section goes into depth about the issues involved in intervening with families with specific illnesses. It considers various family forms, such as gay and lesbian couples and single-parent families. It focuses on families in various health care settings, for example, the intensive care unit, medical unit, patient's home, hospice center, and outpatient clinic. Each chapter in this section is organized according to the nursing process and includes detailed case studies of families at all stages of the developmental life cycle. Intervention chapters focus on families of infants with apnea, families of school-aged children with cancer, families of young adults with AIDS, and aging families and stroke. The chapter "Intervening with Families of Adolescents with Burns" also offers specific suggestions for dealing with conflicts between the patient, family, and nursing staff.

The major difference between this book and other books on families with life-threatening illness is that it emphasizes the application of family assessment and intervention models to deal with *specific* illnesses in *specific* clinical settings with families in *specific* family developmental stages.

ACKNOWLEDGMENTS

We are grateful to our many colleagues and friends who have helped in countless ways to make the Family Nursing Series a reality. They stood by us through the moments of exhilaration and exasperation over the two and a half years of this project.

In particular, we are indebted to:

Susan Taddei, Senior Acquisitions Editor at Springhouse Corporation, who first thought of the idea of the series and inspired us to undertake it.

Bernadette Glenn and the staff at Springhouse Corporation for their helpfulness in overseeing the technical aspects of the Family Nursing Series.

The 76 authors who contributed 65 chapters in the Family Nursing Series and who have shared their expertise and vision of family nursing.

The secretaries who have graciously assisted us: Lynda Gourlie, Louise Hamilton, Ilona Schiedrowski, and Evy Stadey.

Douglas Leahey, who had confidence in our ability throughout the project. He encouraged and supported us in numerous ways, not least of which was transporting chapters to the courier.

Fabie Duhamel, who patiently listened to the many tales of the various stages of the Family Nursing Series and provided steady support. She was also a very willing, efficient "courier" who transported chapters between us.

Laura Crealy, who graciously took in all our packages from Federal Express.

In the process of editing these books, we have remained friends as well as colleagues and have discovered new dimensions to our friendship. We learned to hone our negotiating skills, oscillate in inspiring and supporting each other, and enjoy punctuating our progress through mini-celebrations.

M.L.
L.M.W.

GENOGRAM KEY

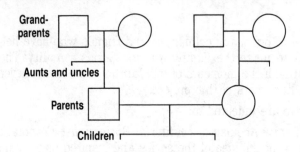

Grand-parents

Aunts and uncles

Parents

Children

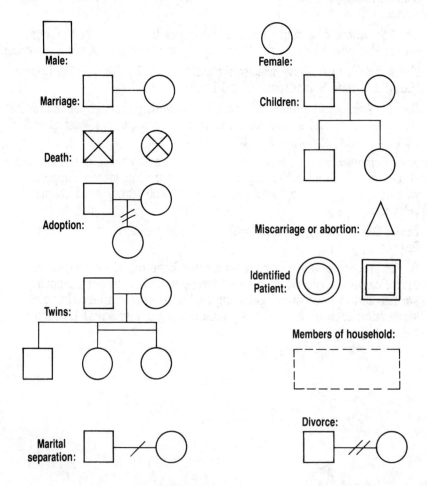

Male:

Female:

Marriage:

Children:

Death:

Adoption:

Miscarriage or abortion:

Identified Patient:

Members of household:

Twins:

Marital separation:

Divorce:

SECTION I

Overview of Families and Life-Threatening Illness

Family nursing and life-threatening illness

Frederick W. Bozett, RN, DNS
Professor, Graduate Program
College of Nursing
University of Oklahoma Health Sciences Center
Oklahoma City, Oklahoma

OVERVIEW

This chapter reviews the nursing care of families that include someone with a life-threatening illness. It discusses the history of family nursing, explores the education required for family nursing, and describes the theories the family nurse commonly uses. The chapter will stress the effective use of crisis and grief/loss theory. It will discuss family nursing diagnosis and will comment on trends and issues in the field. The chapter concludes by addressing the future of family nursing.

INTRODUCTION

The 1980s may go down in history as the "decade of the family." Many social changes have heightened public interest in families. During the 1960s and 1970s, blacks, gays, native Americans, and other minorities reclaimed their rights. Women, too, demanded equality. The number of working women soared, as did the divorce rate and the number of single-parent families. During this period, women won the right to remain childless or to have an abortion. Technological advances such as in vitro and in vivo fertilization, as well as the evolution of surrogate motherhood, reshaped the definition of "family." The tenor of the times was reflected in the emergence of communes, of gay life-styles, and of couples living together without the sanction of church or state. But this era has peaked. The divorce rate is declining, anti-abortion ("pro-life") campaigns are gaining momentum, and "pro-family" fundamentalists are acquiring a substantial following.

Although our society remains in a state of sociological and technological flux, the family now occupies the concern of our politicians and clergy. Not surprisingly, the family has also gained the attention of health care professionals. This chapter will discuss the role of nursing vis-à-vis families faced with life-threatening illness. The chapter is divided into four sections. Section one discusses family nursing, its historical evolution, and the education required for family nursing practice. The second section addresses the application of theories and models to this type of nursing. Section three focuses on the needs of the families of those with life-threatening illnesses and on family nursing diagnosis. The last section centers on trends and issues in family nursing, including ethical and legal concerns.

FAMILY NURSING

Evolution of Family Nursing

Family nursing is as old as nursing itself. Florence Nightingale, the founder of modern nursing, believed that nurses should teach families good health practices. Public health nursing was established in the United States during the last quarter of the nineteenth century. These nurses, the *first* nurses, visited homes to provide care, detect disease, and teach preventive health measures. Prominent among these early nurses was Lillian Wald, who in 1883 established Henry Street Settlement House in New York City, a community nursing service. Ms. Wald helped develop school nursing to detect communicable disease among children. School nurses also made home visits to teach hygiene to families (Benson and McDevitt, 1980).

Historically, midwifery has used a family-centered approach. Childbirth education classes now routinely include the woman's partner as an integral part of pregnancy, labor, and delivery. As the mentally ill have been deinstitutionalized, psychiatric nurses have expanded their practice to include patients' families. The family theory and therapy developed in the 1950s and 1960s was refined by Hill (1970), Broderick (1967), Jackson (1968), and by nursing theorists such as Orlando (1961), Wiedenbach (1964), Rogers (1970), King (1971), and Orem (1971).

Nurse practitioner roles emerged in the late 1960s and 1970s. Among them were the family nurse practitioner and family clinical nurse specialist. Both were trained to deal exclusively with the family. The family nurse practitioner "relates to the family in an interactional relationship offering continuous coordinated health care to the total family as a group...making complex multidimensional assessments and applying therapeutic interventions from autonomous interpretations of family interactional patterns" (Ford, 1979, p. 98).

Although nursing has moved toward a family-centered approach, it remains focused primarily on individuals. This holds true even for nurses who specialize in *family care* and for nurses who deliver care in the home. Hospital-based nursing has traditionally emphasized the individual patient, making it hard for nurses who sought employment in public health agencies to expand their concept of nursing to include the family. Today, factors that militate against family nursing include referral policies, health insurance coverage limitations, and private and governmental reimbursement policies (Ford, 1979). In short, nursing has a rich history of meeting the health care needs of families through many different specialties. However, there are still many constraints that deter full implementation of family nursing.

Family Defined

"Society is rapidly differentiating—becoming more diversified...we are experiencing profound changes in the structure of family life..." (Toffler, 1983, p. 226). As society becomes more diversified, it becomes increasingly difficult to define "family." In the past, a family has usually been thought of as a household in which the man worked and the woman stayed home as wife and mother. But, in the United States, this "traditional" configuration now constitutes only about 13% of families. According to 1977 U.S. Bureau of Labor statistics, the remaining 87% consists of married couples with children in which both spouses work (16%), single parent families (16%), married couples with no children or other adults (23%), single person households (21%), households with extended families (6%), experimental family configurations (4%), and an "other" category (1%). Included in one or more of the above categories are couples who live together, gay and lesbian families, and blended or stepfamilies, all with or without children.

With these dramatic changes in the structure of the family, nurses must adopt a definition of family that can accommodate different family forms. For example, defining family as "two or more people joined together by bonds of sharing and intimacy" (Family Service America, 1984, p. 7) meets these requirements. This definition covers a wide array of family structures. Narrower definitions leave no room for sociocultural modifications. A broader definition is not only more accurate, it is also more practical.

Family may also be defined by its functions. A family:
• provides for the physical and health needs of its members
• serves as a locus of love, intimacy, and motivation
• provides sociologic and psychologic roots.

In addition there exists a commitment to a perceived interdependence and a shared history. In some families, the transmission of culture might be a primary function. The most workable definition may be this: "Family is who the patient says it is" (Bozett, 1985b). This definition helps remove the nurse's value judgments from the realm of her practice. For example, hospital policy may allow only immediate family members to visit patients in the intensive care unit. If the patient or his representative is allowed to determine who the "immediate family" is, then the nurse cannot impose the hospital's or her own definition of family upon the patient. Obviously, a narrow definition of family is no longer in the best interest of patients (or their families). Nurses who practice in institutions with policies based on an outmoded definition of family should try to change both the policy and the definition to ones that better reflect social reality.

Family Nursing Defined

Levels of family nursing practice. There are three levels of family nursing. The level depends on the proximity of the nurse to the family. First-level family nursing considers the patient in the context of the family. On this level, a nurse's interventions are determined primarily by the patient's immediate needs, with family members' needs secondary. For example, nurses in the operating room focus on patients' needs while simply acknowledging that patients also have families. On the *second level* of family nursing, the nurse spends intervals of time directly with one or more family members; she may or may not involve the patient. For example, the intensive care nurse may prepare the patient and his wife for the patient's post–cardiac bypass experience, or she may intervene solely with the wife to relieve her anxiety. Level two incorporates level one in that the nurse plans and implements the patient's care with the family in mind and includes, at times, one or more family members. Levels one and two can be thought of as family focused or family centered. The *third level* of family nursing practice is family care, in which a nurse's assessment and interventions are directed toward the family as a unit, with direct face-to-face interaction with every family member. The nurse contracts with the family and it is the family as a dynamic, interacting unit that is the nurse's client.

At all three levels, the nurse delivers holistic care and considers the family in all phases of the nursing process, although each level dictates a different emphasis on the family. It is important to stress that no level is "better" than another. Circumstances, context, and competence often dictate the level at which the nurse will function. Nurses who manage life-threatening illnesses usually function at levels one and two when practicing within acute care institutions; nurses in community and home health agencies have a greater opportunity to practice at level three. Furthermore, since family nursing is not restricted to any particular setting, all nurses should see themselves as family nurses. All settings are appropriate for the education of nurses for family health care.

Contexts for family nursing practice. All settings in which nurses practice are at times appropriate for family nursing care. Institutional

settings in which a family member's life is threatened are one example. These settings are located primarily in critical and coronary care areas of tertiary care institutions, as well as pediatric and neonatal intensive care units, and emergency rooms. In all of these settings the nurse should meet with the family members to:
- assess their functioning abilities
- assess their problems and needs
- make necessary referrals
- learn more about the hospitalized family member
- establish an individualized plan of family care.

The approach to each family will depend upon the circumstances. Interventions in neonatal intensive care may focus, for example, on assisting the parents through the grief process, helping them give up their dream of a perfect child, and promoting their attachment to the defective newborn. In emergency rooms, where unanticipated health crises including sudden death are common, the nurse needs to be trained in crisis intervention techniques and in working with families in crisis. Epperson (1977) estimates that about 5 hours of family intervention are necessary for the family to recover from the crisis state.

Families with adult members in intensive care units need to be assessed early in the patient's hospitalization (within the first 24 hours) and regularly thereafter. It is best if the patient's nurse spends a specified amount of time with the family every day at a predetermined hour, in addition to prearranged times for telephone contact. Furthermore, the nurse should stress to the family that these regular conferences benefit them and the patient and are standard practice.

While it is easy to identify the need for family-centered care in intensive care settings, such care is often difficult to implement because of time restrictions, emergencies, and lack of understanding by others involved in patient care. These are the greatest impediments to family-centered care. However, there are several remedies. First, and most importantly, the department of nursing's philosophy must be family focused. The chief nurse officer and her staff, as well as all nursing personnel including nonlicensed assistants, should have a family-centered approach to patients.

A philosophy that encourages family nursing can be translated into practice in several ways. Staffing must be sufficient to make family conferences possible. Family clinical nurse specialists and psychiatric/mental health nurse practitioners can carry out this role if necessary. The institution should also provide inservice education. While nurses obtain a basic understanding of family intervention in their generic undergraduate program, continuing education is necessary for nurses to gain sufficient skill in this area. This education must be an ongoing program, not just a one-time event. In summary, patients who face life-theatening problems are cared for in multiple contexts. Therefore, nurses who practice in these various settings need to view the family as client and develop skill in managing families who face potential or actual loss.

Education for Family Nursing

Education for family nursing begins at the baccalaureate level. Undergraduate courses in sociology, psychology, and human development give the nurse a basic understanding of the family concept and the family's cultural significance. Although many schools do not require a specific course on the family, it is recommended. These introductory courses are prerequisite to the nursing courses, most of which are at the upper division level. It is preferable for nursing-centered family content to be included throughout the curriculum rather than be taught as a separate nursing course. Students also need practical experience in caring for families, given under the guidance of nurse faculty members. The types of families to whom students are assigned will depend upon the students' level in the program and the objectives of the particular course.

Early in their course of study it is preferable for students to interact with healthy families in order to learn about family structure, function, roles, strengths, and health values. Later, they should care for families with multiple problems—physical, mental, or social. In addition to formal classroom and clinical instruction, small group seminars are helpful. They assist the student in applying theory to the real world of practice, identifing the family's strengths and coping patterns, determining strategies for intervention in problem areas, and enhancing the family's health.

Lack of space limits full discussion of specific course content. Briefly, however, the concept of family should be investigated and students asked to arrive at their own definition of family. The relationship between family structure and function should also be explored. The family life cycle and family developmental tasks need to be addressed. A nurse should study various types of families. For example, the expectant family with its maturational crisis of parenthood should be examined. Its problems include preparing for parenthood, caring for the newborn infant, and learning to mother and to father—as well as defining the roles of men and women in family planning. Families with school-aged and adolescent children, as well as middle-aged and older families, also need to be considered. The effects of chronic illness, aging, and nursing home care, as well as the impact of death and dying should also be placed within a family context. Likewise, the provision of nursing care must be considered within the context of the family's cultural and social milieu.

Moreover, the special nursing needs of nontraditional families such as single-parent, gay, step, or communal families should also be studied, because they are becoming much more common. Education for family nursing practice at levels one and two, as discussed earlier, is taught primarily within the institutional setting. However, education for level three, family care, is most reasonably taught in the last year of study, when students most commonly have experience in the community and home setting. Family care focuses primarily on health maintenance and health promotion of the family as a unit.

The current trend is to educate nurses in family-centered care. In practice, however, this is difficult to do because most faculty are not family oriented, and they often resist changing the focus of their teaching from the individual to the family. In fact, most of the health professionals who serve as role models for students have an individual orientation to health care delivery. This problem is also found within community and home health agencies. It is infinitely easier for the nurse to manage a dyadic situation—the nurse and patient—than it is to manage a group. This is a problem that nurse educators and practitioners must resolve if families are to receive the care they need and deserve.

At the master's degree level, there are a wide variety of family-centered programs. The most common programs are those for family nurse practitioners and family clinical nurse specialists. Other courses that often have a strong family orientation are pediatric and maternal-child nursing. Gerontological, community, and psychosocial nursing specialties may also be family centered, depending upon the philosophy of the particular faculty and school.

Many graduate schools offer one or more core courses for all family nursing majors regardless of subspecialty. These courses often focus on the understanding and application of family process, theory, and research to nursing practice. Core courses may also focus on family stress and coping. Both healthy and ill families are studied. In addition to core courses, specialty family courses are offered. These courses cover health assessment of persons of all ages, health promotion and maintenance, acute and chronic illness, decision making, and collaboration and leadership. Growth and development across the life span, counseling, human sexuality, and research are also commonly covered.

Some universities offer doctoral programs in nursing (doctor of nursing science or doctor of philosophy) in which the student may major in family health care. The focus of these programs is conceptual and theoretical, rather than practical. The purpose of any experiential component is to test a new or evolving theory to determine its usefulness in the practice setting. In addition to course work in family nursing, courses in theory building, research, and issues in health care are required. Courses in other areas may also be required, in addition to a dissertation (Bozett, 1985a). While graduates of master's degree programs are prepared for advanced practice roles and may also be prepared to be teachers or administrators, nurses at the doctoral level are primarily prepared to work as researchers, administrators, and/or teachers.

THEORIES AND MODELS USED IN FAMILY NURSING AND LIFE-THREATENING ILLNESS

Family nursing theories and models

There are at least 20 published conceptual nursing models (Jacobson, 1984). Theories such as the ones proposed by King (1971), Orem (1971), Roy (1976), and Rogers (1970) are broad theoretical models that attempt to encompass the whole of nursing practice. Whichever model a nurse uses in her practice depends upon many factors, including her education, her familiarity with different theory models, and her own philosophy of human nature and nursing. Hence, it is unlikely that one nursing model will be more useful than another for practice with families with life-threatening illnesses. For a quantitative comparison of nursing models, refer to the study by Jacobson (1984), who conducted an external comparison of five conceptual nursing models. While the value of such quantification has been questioned (Nicholl et al., 1985), it may help determine which models are best suited, for example, to family nursing practice and which to individual care. Because families are complex systems, a single explanatory model that shows relationships among variables can be useful (Miller, 1980).

Theoretical models that attempt to encompass the whole of practice are referred to as "grand" theories. Examples of nonnursing grand theories applicable to the nursing care of families are family developmental theory (Duvall, 1977) and communication theory (Satir, 1967), among others. Moreover, professionals in the field of family study commonly incorporate family systems theory (Miller, 1980) into their practice.

Of equal importance are "middle-range" theories, which often help explain particular components of the nursing practice. For example, theories of pain transmission, such as the gate-control mechanism, are useful in the management of patients in pain, regardless of other factors. Likewise, many middle-range theories apply to the nursing care of families in specific circumstances. Two theories most useful for the management of families in life-threatening situations are crisis theory and loss/grief theory.

Crisis theory

"A crisis is a state of psychological emergency rendering one's usually effective problem-solving skills useless or greatly diminished" (Kus, 1985, p. 277). A crisis, it is important to understand, is created not only by an immediate problem but also by the inability of a family to solve that problem, combined with the emotional distress that this inability to cope creates. The two most common types of crisis are maturational and situational (Hoff, 1978; Riley, 1980; Wilson, 1979). A family with a critically ill member is in a situational crisis. Crisis theory is based upon the work of Lindeman (1944) and Caplan (1964). According to Caplan, crises are self-limiting, usually lasting no longer than 6 weeks, during which time the individual or family is vulnerable. Because of this the family is more receptive to suggestions and more amenable to nursing interventions. The nurse must always be alert to clients' "teachable moments" (Duvall, 1977), and a period of crisis is one of them.

Caplan has identified the following four phases of crisis:
• A person's basic needs are threatened by a situation or event. He uses his normal methods of problem solving to regain emotional balance.
• The usual methods fail, and his level of tension rises. He tries trial-and-error problem-solving approaches.
• If these problem-solving techniques fail, his tension continues to rise and he may try to redefine the problem using different means to solutions.
• If these measures fail, his tension peaks to a dangerously high level; major system disorganization occurs.

As previously stated, crises seldom last for long. The person usually resolves his problem and the crisis subsides. If he cannot find a solution, he experiences increasing disequilibrium until some form of mental or physical disorganization occurs, such as severe family disruption (for example, marital dissolution), or a breakdown in a family member's physical or mental health.

Basic tenets of crisis intervention are the following:
• The nurse should consider the family facing a life-threatening crisis situation as healthy but unable to cope temporarily because of the overwhelming nature of the stress.
• The nurse's assessment should focus on the problem that precipitated the family's crisis and on related problems, such as the care of children or support systems.
• The time frame for nursing intervention is limited because crises are self-limiting.
• The nurse should be assertive. Because of the family's vulnerability, a nurse's assertiveness facilitates the family's acceptance and implementation of her interventions.

• The nurse needs to be flexible and assume the role that will benefit the family most. The nurse may be a teacher or consultant or may take on other roles. She may intercede between the family and the physician, or she may refer a distraught family to a social worker.

• The goal of crisis intervention is always the same: to help the family return to a level of functioning that is at least equivalent to the pre-crisis level (Kus, 1985).

The method of crisis intervention should help families confront their problem in manageable pieces so they are not overwhelmed. It should take place as follows: first, the nurse helps the family to identify and describe the problem. Second, the nurse helps the family explore possible solutions. The nurse may suggest alternatives based on her experience. The consequences of each suggested solution should be discussed with the family. The family members choose a solution, knowing that they will have the nurse's support. Last, the family implements the decision and later evaluates its effect. Resolution of the problem may require change in the situation, change in the behavior of family members, or both. A change in family roles, temporary or permanent, may be required. Also, the nurse may help the family members identify role changes that are needed to solve their problem and restore the family's integrity.

Loss/grief theory

The theory of loss and grief is highly utilitarian in the management of families who have a member with a life-threatening illness. Loss is the state of being deprived of or being without a valued object. This may include the loss of a valued person, of a part of the self, or of external objects, or development losses (Peretz, 1970). Grief is the intense emotional suffering a person experiences as a result of a significant loss (Simos, 1979). Kübler-Ross (1969) identified five stages of the grief process, beginning with denial and isolation, and progressing to anger, bargaining, depression, and ultimately to acceptance. Engle (1962), on the other hand, identified three stages of grief and mourning: shock and disbelief, awareness of the loss, and restitution. Regardless of the theory one subscribes to, there are predictable, identifiable stages one must go through to regain equilibrium after a significant loss. While all family members will experience the threat of losing or the actual loss of a family member equally, each will proceed through the stages at a different pace and intensity. How they proceed depends upon their age, their relationship with the afflicted family member, and other factors.

Shock and disbelief. Immediately after the loss, confusion reigns. The family may be stunned and unable to accept or comprehend their loss, especially if it was unanticipated. The death may tear into the life of the family, disrupting its normal functional pattern. While making necessary arrangements, the family may be out of contact with reality. This activity itself may help protect the family from overwhelming or paralyzing emotions. Another reaction, one of stoicism and detachment, may be interpreted as unusual strength, coldness, or indifference. This reaction, seen more often in men than women, is protective and allows the person time to make necessary decisions and plans (Wiener, 1970).

Developing awareness of the loss. The stage of shock and disbelief is relatively short, and the loss gradually becomes a reality. Each family member, in his own distinct way, will experience pain, anguish, sadness, anger, and even denial. The family may feel helpless and hopeless. One or more family members may blame themselves for the death and suffer guilt. A family member may even feel angry at the loved one for dying and thus depriving him of needed love and companionship. Or anger may be directed at health care personnel because they were unable to save the victim's life. The family's need to cry during this phase is intense. Inability to cry may reflect an ambivalent relationship with the deceased. This could have serious implications; it often indicates guilt, which may seriously hamper the normal grieving process (Carlson, 1970).

Restitution. This phase of the loss/grief process begins after the family leaves the institutional setting. Funerals and religious beliefs help families accept the reality of their loss. During restitution, the family begins to cope with the absence of the loved one. Physical symptoms, often similar to those of the deceased, may develop but are usually short lived. There may be repetitive talk about the loved one, and he may be idealized. Feelings of guilt, as well as idealization, gradually disappear as detachment occurs and intellectual reasoning takes over. Eventually, family members become less preoccupied with the deceased. The structure of the family is reconstituted so that the roles formerly assumed by the deceased member are assumed by others. Family equilibrium is restored.

Anticipatory grief. The prior discussion describes loss/grief theory as it applies to unexpected loss of a loved one. If the life-threatening situation provides the family time to prepare for the loss, then anticipatory grief may occur. This form of grief may be experienced by families in situations that are *potentially* life-threatening (for example, surgery in which a favorable outcome is unlikely) or in situations in which loss is inevitable (for example, cases in which no life-saving measures are known) (Aldrich, 1974). Rehearsing the loss in fantasy many times over can assist the individual and the family to better cope with the loss and its accompanying distress. Whether it actually serves this function, however, is uncertain (Arkin, 1974).

FAMILY NURSING AND LIFE-THREATENING ILLNESS

Needs of Families Facing Life-Threatening Illness

Most patients with life-threatening illness are found in emergency departments and intensive care units. Each of these patients has one or more others who are concerned about his well-being. These others constitute family, whether they are related biologically, legally, or by other strong bonds. Nurses within institutional settings need to conceive of the entire family as client. According to Craven and Sharp (1972):

> If the nurse expands her concept of the patient from that of an individual in a bed to that of a participating member of a family, then she will expand her role to assist relatives to cope with the patient's illness while simultaneously maintaining the family functions (p. 191).

Total patient care must by definition include the family, since illness is experienced not individually but collectively (Gaglione, 1984; Molter, 1979). In the acute care setting, it is easier for the nurse to care for the hospitalized patient's family if she considers herself a family nurse. The nurse's role in the family-centered approach should be the same, whether or not she is treating the identified client (level one) or one or more of his family members (level two). Level three is rarely practiced within the hospital setting.

Hospitalization of a family member alone is stressful to families, but admission to intensive care units, whether planned or not, causes acute anxiety. Hospitalization in an intensive care unit threatens the integrity of the family system, not only because it separates family members but also because it restricts the visits of children, the number of visitors permitted at one time, and the length of each visit, and enforces a lack of privacy. Separation may also be heightened by the patient's physiological deficits, such as neurological handicaps, the effects of drugs, or other conditions that may cause the patient's responses to be inappropriate or uncharacteristic (Mathis, 1984).

Caring for the family as well as the hospitalized patient carries certain benefits:
- The patient will have fewer concerns, thus enhancing his physical recovery.
- The family is likely to be more supportive of the hospitalized member, which speeds his recovery.
- The family system is less likely to be disrupted.
- Family members will communicate less anxiety to the patient, thus directing positive energies toward the patient (Gaglione, 1984).

Doerr and Jones's (1979) study demonstrated that preparation of coronary care patients' relatives significantly reduced their anxiety. Research has shown that family members' attitudes are contagious and that they affect the patient's reaction to his treatment and his emotional adjustment to the illness and to his rehabilitation (Chatham, 1978; Schwartz and Brenner, 1979; Wishnie et al., 1971). Therefore, identification of family needs is imperative if the nurse is to effectively intervene in intensive care settings.

Data for determining how a family nurse should intervene can be derived from multiple sources. The patient's record provides useful data. The patient himself may offer valuable information about his family, how each of them copes with illness or other crises, and how they are coping now. He may also mention any family problems resulting from his hospitalization and thereby help the nurse comprehend the family's reaction. The patient may even give clues as to how the family will react, such as "My children have never seen me sick before." The behavior of family members is an important source of data on how the family is coping. Their facial expressions, degree of physical control, free expression of emotions, frequency of visits, the presence or absence of specific members, and length of their visits are all key (Gaglione, 1984).

Another major source of potential nursing interventions is the medical literature. A number of reports on families in intensive care settings have been published. They should be of use to nurses working with families who have members with life-threatening illnesses (Bedsworth and Nolen, 1982; Bouman, 1984; Bozett and Gibbons, 1983; Breu and Dracup, 1978; Craven and Sharp, 1972; Daley, 1984; Doerr and Jones, 1979; Epperson, 1977; Gaglione, 1984; Gardner and Stewart, 1978; Geary, 1979; Hampe, 1975; Hodovanic et al., 1984; Lust, 1984; Mathis, 1984; Molter, 1979; Rogers, 1983; Stillwell, 1984).

Molter (1979) identified 45 needs of relatives of critically ill patients. None of these needs varied in importance as a function of socioeconomic status or age of the family member. The 10 highest ranked needs in order were:
• hope
• caring hospital personnel
• a waiting room near the patient
• frequent calls at home about changes in the patient's condition
• knowing the patient's prognosis
• receiving honest answers to their questions
• knowing specifics concerning the patient's progress
• receiving updated information about the patient once a day
• receiving explanations they can understand
• frequent visits with the patient.

In a study of grieving spouses, Hampe (1975) identified eight needs:
- to be with the dying person
- to be helpful to the dying person
- to be assured that the dying person is as comfortable as possible
- to be informed of the spouse's condition
- to be told when death is imminent
- to be allowed to ventilate emotions
- to receive comfort and support from family members
- to feel acceptance, support, and comfort from health professionals.

These needs were also confirmed in a study by Breu and Dracup (1978), who also identified a ninth need—the need for relief from anxiety. These authors consolidated these nine needs into five basic needs of grieving spouses:
- relief of initial anxiety
- information
- time with the patient
- need to help the patient
- support and expression of feelings.

In two studies of families with relatives in intensive care settings, their needs were classified into categories. Daley (1984) developed six categories from highest to lowest significance:
- relief of anxiety
- information
- time with the patient
- need to help the patient
- support and expression of feelings
- need to meet personal needs.

Families' primary needs were to be informed of their relative's condition, for the information to be as honest as possible, to be able to speak with the physician, and to know that the relative is receiving the best possible care. Ranked the least important were being alone, having friends or children visit, and having amenities such as coffee or food available.

Bouman (1984) developed three categories of needs: cognitive, emotional, and physical. Although the needs of family members may vary according to factors such as age, ethnic background, language, and diagnosis and prognosis of the hospitalized patient, these studies provide the nurse with useful beginning knowledge upon which to base interventions. Since the average length of stay in an intensive care unit is 4 days, anything that assists rapid assessment and intervention is especially useful.

Family Nursing Diagnosis and Life-Threatening Situations

It is uncommon for nurses in institutional settings to write family nursing diagnoses. However, nurses who work with clients in life-threatening situations commonly identify signs of family disruption that require a diagnosis followed by interventions. The nurse interprets cues given off by the family and places it in one or more diagnostic categories (Gordon, 1976). It behooves nurses in intensive care settings to diagnose family as well as patient problems, so that the whole family's needs will be met.

No taxonomy of family problems or diagnoses has yet been developed. Smoyak (1977) divides family problems into external and internal stressors. External stressors are those arising from jobs, welfare agencies, legal systems, school systems, and religious institutions. Internal stressors relate to a structural change in the family, stemming from the addition of a family member or from a conflict over rules of organization, such as division of household labor. According to Lamberton (1980), family diagnoses should reveal dysfunction or anticipated dysfunctions, with the goal of maintaining positive practices. The duration of the problem (intermittent, chronic, acute-situational) and its etiology should also be specified in the diagnosis. Two examples of family diagnosis are:
• anticipating the acute grief related to the potential death of a newborn infant
• anticipating the difficulty in reassigning family roles because of a critically ill husband/father's hospitalization.

A taxonomy of family nursing diagnoses related to life-threatening situations probably could be developed. For example, three elements of a taxonomy for families experiencing a life-threatening illness could be disruption in roles, economic hardship, and geographic separation. The development of such a taxonomy is recommended.

Family Psychological Autopsy

Weisman and Kastenbaum (1968) conceived of the psychological autopsy as a reconstruction of the "final days and weeks of the patient's life by bringing together every available observation, fact, and opinion about the recently deceased person in an effort to understand the psychosocial components of death" (p. 1). Weisman and Kastenbaum propose that conducting a psychological autopsy by means of a "retrospective reconstruction and coordination of information" (p. 2) will improve management and treatment of terminally ill patients and contribute to basic research. They outline a detailed procedure for conducting the psychological autopsy that includes conferring with hospital personnel who were responsible for the care of the deceased. Based upon the psychological autopsies they conducted, they make suggestions for improving the conditions under which the terminally ill live out the remainder of their lives.

This author recommends that a similar procedure be developed and implemented in intensive care settings for families in which the patient survived and was later transferred, *and* for families in which the patient died. A procedure similar to the one described by Weisman and Kastenbaum could be followed. The sessions would include nurses, physicians, and others who cared for the patient and/or his family. In addition, the families, and the patient if he survived, could be asked to participate. The group leader would be the nurse or other specialist who was primarily responsible for the family's care. The psychological autopsy would focus on the retrospective reconstruction of the care of the family as a unit including the hospitalized member. Its purpose would be to improve subsequent care of families with members in life-threatening situations.

ISSUES AND TRENDS IN FAMILY NURSING AND LIFE-THREATENING ILLNESS

Changes in Health Care Delivery

The single most powerful influence on the future of the practice of family nursing was the introduction in 1983 by the federal government of a prospective system of reimbursement to hospitals in the form of diagnostic related groupings (DRGs). Although the system applies only to Medicare recipients (primarily persons 65 years of age and older), the number of these persons receiving hospital care is a significant portion of the total. Some private insurers have also adopted a similar system for all their members regardless of age, and more are likely to follow suit. The effect of this system is to reduce the cost of health care by reducing the length of hospital stay. For example, between 1982 and 1984 the national average length of stay for hospital patients declined 13% (Selby, 1985). As a result, patients are being discharged earlier and often in less stable condition. It is assumed that these patients will have their continuing health care needs met when they are discharged to their own home, to a long-term nursing care facility, to a city shelter, or to some other facility.

The ramifications of these changes for the practice of family nursing are enormous. As patients are discharged earlier to their own homes, nurses must begin to view the family as the unit of service; serving only the individual patient at home will never suffice. Nurses must become expert at teaching family members care techniques that are complex and were once reserved for professional practitioners, such as those in the areas of tracheostomy care and peritoneal dialysis. It is

imperative that nurses develop skills for ascertaining each family
member's readiness and ability to learn and gradually incorporate them
into the nursing care plan. In addition, determining the family's social
and emotional needs and meeting them or providing referrals is essential. Everything must be done to help the family members provide
quality care to the patient with the least stress possible.

The health and well-being of all family members must also be the
nurse's concern. Assessment and intervention by teaching prevention
and promoting good health to all family members constitutes a major
nursing objective. However, as mentioned previously, several factors
militate against this approach. Governmental and private insurance
companies reimburse for services to individuals, not families. Moreover,
wellness care is often not reimbursable. The nurse's case load may
not allow sufficient time for a family-centered approach, and her accessibility to the family may be limited (Johnson, 1984). Family nurses,
as well as home health agency administrators and others, need to
become more vocal advocates of family health care so that these, or
other, inhibiting factors are reduced or eliminated.

Early discharge has further ramifications for the continuing education
of the family nurse. A large percentage of the nurse's patients will be
older; the average life span is now 75 years, with 12% of the population
65 years of age or older (Halamandaris, 1985). Hence, the nurse must
have a sound knowledge of gerontological nursing and psychogerontol-
ogy. Also, some states have implemented early maternity discharge
programs. Nurses who provide follow-up home care for these patients
need to be well versed in postpartum and neonatal care. They must
also have expertise in breast-feeding management and in infant care,
growth, and development. The nurse must also understand the transition to parenthood (Hanson and Bozett, 1985) if her care is to be truly
family centered.

Thus, the scope of practice of nurses employed outside of institutional
settings will need to be critically examined. In the past, public health
nurses have cared for patients in the home, regardless of diagnosis.
More recently, limited specialization in the community has developed,
with respiratory care nurses being employed by some visiting nurses
associations, and with pediatric nurse practitioners working within public health departments. The trend will be toward increased specialization within community agencies. The nurse must be aware that caring
for a patient at home requires skills not required in the hospital setting. Thus, nurses who move from hospital to home care practice need
further education in order to satisfy the requirements and needs of
individual families. In the future, home health nurses will not care for
patients in all diagnostic categories. One nurse cannot be expected

to teach breast-feeding, manage home dialysis, and assist the family adjusting to a child with Down's syndrome. Thus, additional education through formal degree-granting tracks, or by means of continuing education programs, will be necessary. Specialization will undoubtedly increase among nurses based in community agencies.

Changes in Nursing Roles

As a result of the implementation of prospective reimbursement through DRGs, the work place, and thus the role, of many nurses will also change. Because health maintenance organizations (HMOs) and home health agencies are more oriented toward family-centered care, more nurses whose philosophy of care is family focused will seek employment in those agencies. Similarly, as more terminally ill patients seek hospice care, the number of hospice agencies will increase, with a concomitant increase in the number of nurses staffing them. The use of outpatient departments of acute care facilities will also increase. This trend has special significance for family nursing, since outpatient clinics are probably the least family oriented of all health services. More nurses will also be providing services in long-term care facilities and city shelters. Others may develop innovative care centers, such as Medi-Kid, Inc., in Jacksonville, Fla., which provides day care to infants and young children who need long-term care for such disorders as gastrostomies and seizures. Moreover, the family health care nurse may serve as a hospital discharge planner, working with the nursing staff, physician, and family to locate the best facility for the patient after discharge—whether it be at home or elsewhere—and to ease his transition to it.

Assessment of each family member's willingness and ability to provide home care is a crucial component of this role. In this regard, the nurse needs to remove her cultural and sociological blinders. For example, it would be easy to overlook the contribution that an 8-year-old child might provide, yet he might be the most motivated, available, and appropriate family member. Similarly, a handicapped member may be able to provide selected aspects of care. The employment opportunities for the nurse who has academic preparation in family theory and family nursing, as well as practical experience, will increase as less medically stable patients are discharged into the community and fewer qualified home care nurses are assigned to care for them. Furthermore, there will be a market for the entrepreneurial nurse to own and manage her own consulting firm or home health care agency.

Family nursing within acute care hospitals will also change drastically as a result of current cost containment measures. As the hospital census declines, so will the number of nurses. This is already a reality. Only those nursing services considered to be essential will be retained.

Thus, the number of family clinical nurse specialists will be reduced
or eliminated entirely, with their functions subsumed by staff nurses.
Those who are retained will have an increased case load and may
be expected to assume traditional staff nurse activities. They may also
be placed in supervisory positions. In addition, staff nurses, whether
or not they are prepared to do so, will be expected to teach family
members the physical and technical aspects of care, such as drug and
diet regimens, before each patient's discharge. Moreover, this teaching
will need to be done in less time than in the past. This author foresees
that, due to time constraints and the reduction of personnel, the family's preparation for home care by hospital nurses will be of lesser
quality, and the job satisfaction and morale of staff nurses will deteriorate. Creative measures must be sought to prevent erosion of family-
centered inpatient care which, to begin with, has been less than com-
mendable. The immediate future of family-centered nursing within
the acute care setting is bleak. The distant future depends upon a
notable improvement in health care economics. No antidotes to the
current situation have yet appeared (although the implementation of
primary nursing offers some hope), but an increase in family-focused
care in basic nursing curricula would enable future nurses to provide
higher quality family care and better prepare them to teach families
how to assume home health care responsibilities.

Legal and Ethical Considerations

The increasing social and technological complexity of our world inevita-
bly leads to difficult choices. What should I do? What is the right
thing to do? Moral claims of what is "good" may conflict with what is
"right" (Davis and Aroskar, 1984). What may be considered "good,"
such as discontinuing life-support systems on a patient who is legally
dead, may not be within the nurse's rights. Thus, care of the patient
must continue until others who have the right to discontinue support
systems do so. Conflicts between "right" and "good" may arise between
the nurse and patient. For example, family members may consider
certain aspects of treatment a violation of their right to free choice,
while the nurse may claim that care is justified by its value to the
family. The question is one of the right of family autonomy vs. the right
of the nurse to limit that autonomy. In one instance, it may be in the
family's best interest to reduce its autonomy; in the same instance,
reducing its decision-making ability might be considered paternalistic.

There are many situations in which family nurses will find that
moral claims conflict with one another or in which the choice is between
equally unsatisfactory alternatives. The nurse may disapprove of surrogate parenting, believing that it is nothing but the wholesale profiteering
of infants, yet the alternative may be for a couple to remain childless.

Women's right to abortion is yet another common dilemma. The right of a gay male couple to adopt children or to serve as foster parents, as opposed to remaining childless, may present a moral conflict for some nurses. The list is endless, and as society and technology increase in complexity, the situations that nurses and other health care workers encounter will also become more complex.

It will become increasingly important for agencies to provide their staffs with access to an ethicist, preferably someone not directly involved in providing patient care. One person within the agency might be selected for formal course work, so that he or she can act as ethicist. This person would be available for private consultations, as well as for unstructured and structured ethics conferences.

Many institutions, especially large teaching hospitals, already have such personnel available. However, smaller hospitals, home health agencies, long-term care institutions, and other health care facilities in both urban and rural areas are not so fortunate, despite the need. Likewise, a lawyer should be available to deal with the staff's legal concerns. Helping the health care staff to analyze the legal and ethical ramifications of medical practice will help to ensure quality care. In addition, such analysis will assure the staff that their actions are legal and within the guidelines set forth in the American Nurses Association Code of Ethics, or the code of ethics of the country in which the nurse practices. As a result, nurses will also know that they are executing their professional responsibilities in a manner that is consistent with their own moral beliefs.

CONCLUSIONS

Nursing is becoming more concerned with the health of the individual and family as a unit. A sociocultural shift is occurring; the state is reducing its responsibilities for social welfare and expecting families to increase their participation. As the family regains some of the functions previously assumed by society, deinstitutionalization of much of health care naturally will occur. The responsibility for the care of family members is being placed back onto the family.

In the future, nurses face a number of exciting challenges. One is the further development of a theoretical base for family nursing practice—a base that cuts across all definitions of family and meets the needs of all types of families without moral judgments. This is not to discount past research but rather to encourage further work.

Another challenge relates to the basic and advanced education of nurses. Schools of nursing must develop conceptual frameworks in which the family is central to the curriculum. Without the development of family-centered nursing curricula, nursing practice at the individual level will remain the predominant mode of practice.

Yet another challenge is for nursing education and practice to become interdisciplinary. No health profession has a history of devotion to families greater than that of nursing, and nursing leaders need to develop collaborative relationships with other health and family professionals for the promotion of joint practice, education, and research. Nursing is now sufficiently sophisticated in these three domains to make significant contributions. Advances in these areas of family health care will occur much more rapidly if nurses work both inter- and intraprofessionally.

Finally, the challenge is to create our own future. We can merely react to societal changes, or we can put ourselves on the cutting edge of society. We can create the context of family health care that we believe is best for society. It will require the will, the commitment, and the belief that it is possible.

REFERENCES

Aldrich, C.F. "Some Dynamics of Anticipatory Grief," in *Anticipatory Grief.* Edited by Schoenberg, B., et al. New York: Columbia University, 1974.

Arkin, A.M. "Notes on Anticipatory Grief," in *Anticipatory Grief.* Edited by Schoenberg, B., et al. New York: Columbia University, 1974.

Bedsworth, J.A., and Nolen, M.T. "Psychological Stress in Spouses of Patients with Myocardial Infarction," *Heart & Lung* 11:450–56, 1982.

Benson, E.R., and McDevitt, J.W. *Community Health and Nursing Practice.* Englewood Cliffs, N.J.: Prentice-Hall, 1980.

Bouman, C.C. "Identifying Priority Concerns of Families of ICU Patients," *Dimensions of Critical Care Nursing* 3:313–19, 1984.

Bozett, F.W. "The Education of Nurses for Family Health Care," in *Family Systems and Health: Focus on Prevention.* Edited by Patterson, J.M., and McCubbin, H.I. Symposium conducted at the meeting of the National Council on Family Relations Pre-Conference Workshop, San Francisco, 1985a.

Bozett, F.W. *Family Centered Care—Who Is Family?* Paper presented at the High Tech/Intensive Caring Conference of MCN, The American Journal of Maternal/Child Nursing, Baltimore, 1985b.

Bozett, F.W., and Gibbons, R. "The Nursing Management of Families in the Critical Care Setting," *Critical Care Update* 10:22–27, 1983.

Breu, C., and Dracup, K. "Helping the Spouses of Critically Ill Patients," *American Journal of Nursing* 78:50–53, 1978.

Broderick, C.B. "Reaction to Familial Development, Selective Needs, and Predictive Theory," *Journal of Marriage and the Family* 29:237–40, 1967.

Caplan, G. *Principles of Preventive Psychiatry.* New York: Basic Books, 1964.

Carlson, C.E. "Grief and Mourning," in *Behavioral Concepts and Nursing Intervention.* Edited by Carlson, C.E. Philadelphia: J.B. Lippincott Co., 1970.

Chatham, M. "The Effect of Family Involvement on Patients' Manifestations of Postcardiotomy Psychosis," *Heart & Lung* 7:995-99, 1978.

Craven, R.F., and Sharp, B.H. "The Effects of Illness on Family Functions," *Nursing Forum* 11:187–93, 1972.

Daley, L. "The Perceived Immediate Needs of Families with Relatives in the Intensive Care Setting," *Heart & Lung* 13:231–37, 1984.

Davis, A.J., and Aroskar, M.A. "Health Care Ethics and Ethical Dilemmas," in *The Nation's Health.* Edited by Lee, P.R., et al. San Francisco: Boyd & Fraser, 1984.

Doerr, B.C., and Jones, J.W. "Effect of Family Preparation on the Stated Anxiety Level of the CCU Patient," *Nursing Research* 28:315–16, 1979.

Duvall, E.M. *Marriage and Family Development.* Philadelphia: J.B. Lippincott Co., 1977.

Engle, G.L. *Psychological Development in Health and Disease.* Philadelphia: W.B. Saunders Co., 1962.

Epperson, M.M. "Families in Sudden Crisis: Process and Intervention in a Critical Care Center," *Social Work in Health Care* 2:265–73, 1977.

Family Service America, *The State of Families, 1984–85.* New York: Family Service America, 1984.

Ford, L. "The Development of Family Nursing," in *Family Health Care*. Edited by Hymovich, D.P., and Barnard, M.U. New York: McGraw-Hill Book Co., 1979.

Gaglione, K.M. "Assessing and Intervening with Families of CCU Patients," *Nursing Clinics of North America* 19:427–32, 1984.

Gardner, D., and Stewart, N. "Staff Involvement with Families of Patients in Critical-Care Units," *Heart & Lung* 7:105–10, 1978.

Geary, M.C. "Supporting Family Coping," *Supervisor Nurse* 10:520–59, 1979.

Gordon, M. "Nursing Diagnosis and the Diagnosis Process," *American Journal of Nursing* 76:1298–1300, 1976.

Halamandaris, V.J. "The Future of Home Care," *Caring* 4(10):4–11, 1985.

Hampe, S.C. "Needs of the Grieving Spouse in a Hospital Setting," *Nursing Research* 24:113–20, 1975.

Hanson, S.M.H., and Bozett, F.W. *Dimensions of Fatherhood*. Beverly Hills, Calif.: Sage Pubns., 1985.

Hill, R. *Family Development in Three Generations*. Cambridge, Mass.: Schenkman Books, 1970.

Hodovanic, B.H., et al. "Family Crisis Intervention Program in the Medical Intensive Care Unit, *Heart & Lung* 13:243–49, 1984.

Hoff, L.A. *People in Crisis: Understanding and Helping*. Menlo Park, Calif.: Addison-Wesley Publishing Co., 1978.

Jackson, D., ed. *Communication, Family, and Marriage*. Palo Alto, Calif.: Science and Behavior Books, 1968.

Jacobson, S.F. "A Sematic Differential for External Comparison of Conceptual Nursing Models," *Advances in Nursing Science* 6:58–70, 1984.

Johnson, R. "Promoting the Health of Families in the Community," in *Community Health Nursing*. Edited by Stanhope, M., and Lancaster, J. St. Louis: C.V. Mosby Co., 1984.

King, I.M. *Toward a Theory for Nursing: General Concepts of Human Behavior*. New York: John Wiley & Sons, 1971.

Kübler-Ross, E. *On Death and Dying*. New York: Macmillan Publishing Co., 1969.

Kus, R.J. "Crisis Intervention," in *Nursing Interventions: Treatments for Nursing Diagnoses*. Edited by Bulechek, G.M., and McCloskey, J.C. Philadelphia: W.B. Saunders Co., 1985.

Lamberton, M.M. "Alterations in Family Dynamics," in *Introduction to Nursing Practice*. Edited by Shortridge, L.M., and Lee, E.J. New York: McGraw-Hill Book Co., 1980.

Lindeman, E. "Symptomology and Management of Acute Grief," *American Journal of Psychiatry* 101:101–48, 1944.

Lust, B.L. "The Patient in the ICU: A Family Experience," *Critical Care Quarterly* 6:49–57, 1984.

Mathis, M. "Personal Needs of Family Members of Critically Ill Patients with and without Acute Brain Injury," *Journal of Neurosurgical Nursing* 16:36–44, 1984.

Miller, J.R. "The Family as a System," in *Family-Focused Care*. Edited by Miller, J.R., and Janosic, E.H. New York: McGraw-Hill Book Co., 1980.

Minuchin, S. *Families and Family Therapy*. Cambridge, Mass.: Harvard University, 1974.

Molter, N.C. "Needs of Relatives of Critically Ill Patients: A Descriptive Study," *Heart & Lung* 8:332–39, 1979.

Nicholl, L.H., et al. "Critique: External Comparison of Conceptual Nursing Models," *Advances in Nursing Science* 7(4):1–9, 1985.

Orem, D.E. *Nursing: Concepts of Practice.* New York: McGraw-Hill Book Co., 1971.

Orlando, I.J. *The Dynamic Nurse Patient Relationship.* New York: G.P. Putnam Pub. Group, 1961.

Peretz, D. "Development, Object-Relationships, and Loss," in *Loss and Grief: Psychological Management in Medical Practice.* Edited by Schoenberg, B., et al. New York: Columbia University, 1970.

Riley, B. "Crisis Intervention," in *Adult Psychiatric Nursing.* Edited by Lancaster, J. Garden City, N.Y.: Medical Examination Pub. Co., 1980.

Rogers, C.D. "Needs of Relatives of Cardiac Surgery Patients During the Critical Care Phase," *Focus on Critical Care* 10:50–55, 1983.

Rogers, M.E. *An Introduction to the Theoretical Basis of Nursing.* Philadelphia: F.A. Davis Co., 1970.

Roy, C. *Introduction to Nursing: An Adaptation Model.* Englewood Cliffs, N.J.: Prentice-Hall, 1976.

Satir, V. *Conjoint Family Therapy.* Palo Alto, Calif.: Science and Behavior Books, 1967.

Schwartz, L., and Brenner, Z. "Critical Care Unit Transfer: Reducing Patient Stress Through Nursing Interventions," *Heart & Lung* 8:540–46, 1979.

Selby, T.L. "Nurses Meet Challenges as Cost Cuts Take Toll," *The American Nurse* 1, 10, 13, 14, 16, 18: November/December 1985.

Simos, B.G. *A Time to Grieve: Loss as a Universal Human Experience.* New York: Family Service Association of America, 1979.

Smoyak, S.A. *Family Therapy: A Systems Perspective to Answer Referral Questions.* Paper presented at Chautauqua "77", Vail, Colo., August 1977.

Stillwell, S.B. "Importance of Visiting Needs as Perceived by Family Members of Patients in the Intensive Care Unit," *Heart & Lung* 13:238–42, 1984.

Toffler, A. *Previews and Premises.* New York: William Morrow, 1983.

Weisman, D.D., and Kastenbaum, R. *The Psychological Autopsy.* New York: Behavioral Publications, 1968.

Wiedenbach, E. *Clinical Nursing a Helping Art.* New York: Springer Publishing Co., 1964.

Wiener, J.M. "Reaction of the Family to the Fatal Illness of a Child," in *Loss and Grief: Psychological Management in Medical Practice.* Edited by Schoenberg, B., et al. New York: Columbia University, 1970.

Wilson, H., and Kneisel, C. *Psychiatric Nursing.* Menlo Park, Calif.: Addison-Wesley Publishing Co., 1979.

Wishnie, H., et al. "Psychological Hazards of Convalescence Following Myocardial Infarction," *Journal of the American Medical Association* 215:1292–96, 1971.

2 The impact of life-threatening illness on the family and the impact of the family on illness: An overview

Claus Bahne Bahnson, PhD

Clinical Professor of Family Medicine and
  Psychiatry
University of California, San Francisco
  Medical School
Fresno, California

President
The Nordische University
Flensburg, West Germany

INTRODUCTION

As the title of this chapter indicates, life-threatening illness profoundly
affects the patient and his family; the behavior of family members
significantly influences the course of the patient's disease. These facts
are recognized by any nurse or other health professional. The family
may also contribute to the development of life-threatening illness
through destructive emotional conflicts and unresolved tensions, or by
isolation of the patient.

The patient participates in these premorbid conflicts as well. Research by Holmes and Rahe (1967) shows that even benign life
changes—marriage, birth of a child—that are perceived as positive can
trigger physical disease.

Life-threatening illness places a family under unusual stress. As a
result, interpersonal problems that might have been resolved often
escalate into full-blown conflicts. This "uncovering effect" is only one
consequence of serious illness. The realization that an expected future
may not happen or that family stability may be destroyed can interrupt
the homeostatic family process. Serious illness can ruin fiscal, emotional, educational, as well as individual plans. Illness-related discontinuity is particularly disturbing when young individuals are affected,
although life-threatening illness in geriatric patients can also produce
guilt and anxiety that may keep families out of balance. In an age

where biology and psychology have come to understand the importance of thinking systemically, caretakers should think of patients as parts of family systems, just as they think of a diseased organ as part of a complex biological organism. Patients must be treated within the contexts of their families, as well as within the context of their psychophysiological makeup.

PSYCHOPHYSIOLOGICAL CONSIDERATIONS IN LIFE-THREATENING DISEASE

In the systems interaction approach, neither disease nor treatment can be thought of as unrelated to the patient's psychological state—his emotions, coping style, degree of denial, anxiety level, and so forth— any more than he can be said to function independent of family and medical staff. This psychosomatic understanding began with Sigmund Freud's ([1896] 1959) concept of conversion in hysterical disorders and was followed by the studies of his students, such as Franz Alexander (1950), Felix Deutsch (1959), Lawrence Kubie (1953), and others, who demonstrated the impact of emotional conflicts on such somatic illnesses as asthma, colitis, duodenal ulcer, dermatoses, hypertension, and migraine headaches. During the mid-twentieth century, diseases once considered "purely somatic" were recognized as having strong psychological components that emerged under specific psychosocial conditions, usually in patients with specific personality features (for example, the so-called "Type A" personality of the stereotypic heart patient) (Friedman and Rosenman, 1974).

Current research is changing traditional concepts about such autoimmune diseases as multiple sclerosis and systemic lupus erythematosis, as well as arthritis and many malignancies (Solomon, 1970; Bahnson, 1980, 1981). A new concept, "psychoneuroimmunology" (Locke and Rohan, 1983; Ader, 1981), refers to the interaction of emotional/ experiential, nervous, and immune system phenomena, which are directed largely by the brain. More advanced studies have shown how the nervous system (that which is linked to human experience) communicates with the immune system, for example with the T4 lymphocyte cells. Clearly, the immune system can be influenced, via the nervous system, by emotional factors (Schleifer et al., 1985).

The psychophysiological relationships that guide interactions between mind and illness reflect general conditions that determine all human, and possibly animal, existence. But there may be a large difference between individuals who go through life experiencing only minor brushes with illness and those who struggle with major disease. Freud (1959a) hypothesized that repression leads to somatization of conflicting drive and affect. His concept of conversion hysteria posited that the individual's inability or unwillingness to perceive, experience, or act on a difficult or threatening emotion would lead to its repression and somatization in a way that would symbolize simultaneously the forbidden and repressed wish or drive and the defense against it. By denying the wish and its associated anxiety, the patient would be able to function *interpersonally* without disturbing effects, but would "pay" for that comfort by a somatic conversion symptom that would combine symbolic wish or need fulfillment with punishment. In other words, the patient would "trade in" anxiety for a so-called conversion symptom. Freud contended that, since basic biologic or derived drives can be ignored only with difficulty, they must be released pathologically, through such functional illnesses as paralysis, paresthesias, partial blindness, and inexplicable pain. His main tenet was that physical expression of the repressed drive or wish and its associated anxiety allow the patient's conscious psyche to remain undisturbed.

Freud's theory of drive and affect repression was continued and expanded by Franz Alexander (Freud, 1959b) to include autonomic nervous system (ANS) manifestations. Alexander and others expanded the concept of repression to include diseases that could be influenced by ANS disequilibria that could, in turn, upset the endocrinologic and autonomic balances that guide many vegetative functions. This condition, they argued, could lead to colonic dysfunction and spasms that favor the development of colitis, or respiratory disturbances that favor asthma.

One common thread runs through psychosomatic studies—the concept that repression of an emotional problem can result in "translation" of this problem to a somatic level of expression, creating havoc in endocrine or other somatic balances. In recent years this concept has been reformulated as "alexithymia" (Nemiah et al., 1976), which refers to the inability of patients with somatic diseases to contact, monitor, and express their underlying emotional states. In other words, alexithymia refers to the effect of repression. Studies by Kissen (1966), Bahnson (1969), Greene (1966), Greer and Morris (1975), and Derogatis et al. (1979) have illustrated this concept by indicating that patients suffering from malignancies of different types (lung, breast, colon, cervix, etc.) are characterized by a repressive coping style and that those cancer patients who repress the most fare the worst.

These psychophysiological relationships are not only of theoretical interest and importance; they provide crucial insights into the care of any affected patient. The caretaking staff should not reinforce repressive attitudes that can exacerbate a patient's somatic condition, even when the patient may seem better off unaware, with his "head in the sand." The linkage of denial and repression to poor prognosis is an important consideration in choosing a psychological treatment style and plan.

THE IMPORTANCE OF THE PATIENT'S FAMILY

Although the nursing staff's focus is on the patient and his welfare, it is also important to consider his family members, whose reactions are intensely interwoven with his fate. The patient arrives at the hospital *from* the context of family togetherness and he goes home to that same psychological environment. There are special cases, where patients live alone or in a nursing home, in which the focus must be broadened to include friends or professionals, but even there the subjective family— perhaps memories of significant others, or siblings or other relatives living far away—is of extreme emotional importance.

While the treating physician and psychotherapist are intensely involved in the family dynamics of serious illness, so is the nursing staff. Nurses are confronted with family reactions to the patient's condition and must cope with very difficult reactions to different phases of the illness, particularly when intensive care is required or the patient is terminally ill.

As discussed above, serious illness develops more frequently in members of repressive somatizing (also referred to as "centrifugal") (Bahnson, 1982) or alexithymic families (Sifneos, 1973). Moreover, the timing of serious illness, which commonly appears in more than one family member, is often linked to a family situation in which one or more members' development has been arrested and the family (particularly the patient) has arrived at an existential dilemma from which there seems to be no escape. One such situation involves the changing family structure as teenaged family members grow up and leave. The translation of familywide unhappiness and tension into somatic disturbance often prevents feared or unwanted change by prolonging the interpersonal status quo and blocking development.

The sequelae of serious illness affect both patient and family. Without treatment of both parties, psychosomatic and behavioral symptoms can occur. Otherwise healthy family members may show the stress of the patient's illness through their own somatization or through such "acting-out" or destructive behavior as substance abuse or juvenile delinquency. Adequate, balanced care, on the other hand, can help patient and family "grow" as a result of the health crisis. It can refocus and reframe relationships and goals that may have fallen by the wayside. In some happy instances, serious illness has been a beacon for families that had gone astray, enabling them to rethink their priorities and life-styles.

Obviously, the weight of serious illness is carried not by the patient alone, but by the entire family. What remains is to consider how specific

illnesses, in specific sites and family members, create their own specialized family problems.

THE TREATMENT TEAM AS "FAMILY"

Medical and nursing staffs carry enormous responsibility for seriously
ill patients. Life and death are often in their hands, and their specialized knowledge makes them "magical" providers and "rescuers" in
their patients' eyes. This situation often promotes regressive adaptation
in patients—regression often supported by institutional rituals—until
caretakers are perceived as parental figures with power to support,
help, or punish. As Elizabeth Kübler-Ross (1969) pointed out, this
regression can result in childlike pleading, rebellion, or bargaining with
the medical staff as patients try to get well. Thus, the "treatment
family" is endowed with powers and controls that even overshadow
parental omnipotence during early childhood.

There is some validity to the notion that the treatment staff becomes
the patient's "family." During prolonged hospitalization, the patient
interacts more closely and intimately with the care staff than with a
family that might appear only irregularly and that may even tend to
stay away. Considering the anxiety related to many medical procedures,
the discomfort, pain, and danger of impending mutilation and death, it
is no wonder that patients turn to the nursing staff for emotional
reassurance and help.

Patients' reactions to hospital anxiety can differ widely, from the
angry executive's tendency to order the "nursing family" around like
secretaries to the panicked young patient's attempts to enlist the
"nurse/parent's" empathy, assistance, and perhaps pity. In such cases,
it is important to understand that the objective conditions perceived
by the nursing staff may be totally at odds with the patient's subjective,
anxious view. As von Uexkull (1981) describes it, people walk around
with "bubbles" around their heads, constructed from their own biases,
feelings, and expectations, making them perceive the world differently
from those around them. This condition is exaggerated in seriously
ill patients, who may have regressed and distorted views of themselves
and their environment. The "bubble of bias" is pertinent in cases of
frank psychosis, as is sometimes seen in postsurgical patients, but it
also affects patients' everyday perceptions, making them seem "difficult," "unreasonable," or "inappropriate."

The "treatment family" has its own structure and function and is of
utmost importance to the patient. Often the physician is the "father"
and the nurse the "mother," although role reversals are common when
the patient has female physicians and male nurses. Whatever their
distribution, the care team's leading members are perceived as "par-

ents," and it is important that they work together well. Poor coordination between nursing and medical staff, especially where competition or disagreement thrives, can cause the patient to suffer in many subtle ways that are difficult to untangle and are manifested primarily through health status. Strife in the treatment team can produce anxiety, which might cause the patient to "act out" or try to play the warring authorities against each other. The patient may complain to one authority and play up to another. It is important for the treatment team to maintain open internal communication and hold frequent meetings about, and sometimes with, the patient. An uncoordinated approach, in which one team member does not know which communications are given or received by another, can be destructive emotionally, medically, and interpersonally for all concerned. It can affect disease outcomes and family relationships for years to come. The secondary effects can include treatment noncompliance, "physician shopping," or plain patient disillusionment with their physicians and overall treatment. Such negative reactions may even trigger malpractice suits and other legal actions. Thus, the treatment "family" must show the same maturity, creativity, and communication required in the patient's own family in order to prevent deterioration and poor results.

The treatment climate can be improved in many ways, including case conferences, Balint groups, joint nurse/physician training in key areas, and promotion of personal maturity and integrity, for instance, through personal psychotherapy. This is not the place to delineate all the details of team training, but it is important to mention that the "treatment family" is a neglected mental health area. We often hear about person "burnout," but not about systemic problems and interactional successes or failures.

FACTORS CONTRIBUTING TO ILLNESS ONSET OR EXACERBATION

Research has identified at least four general circumstances which, separately or in combination, seem to constitute premorbid conditions. They are:
- stress
- unresolved family conflict
- retirement
- personal loss and depression.

Stress

Selye (1956) defined the concept of stress in his description of the general adaptation syndrome—a characteristic, sequential organismic response to a severe stressor, such as a burn. Selye pointed out that an organism usually responds to a major stressor in three phases—alarm and mobilization, resistance and restructuring, and finally, exhaustion of available resources, or death. While the stressor itself may not kill, he said, the organism's reaction to it can.

It is important to discriminate between a stressor, the external challenge, and stress, the organism's response to that challenge. The concept of stress and stress response is a popular topic and is associated with many illnesses, including coronary heart disease (myocardial infarction) (Arlow, 1945; Wolf, 1958; Wardwell and Bahnson, 1973). As Selye found with burns, it may not be the stressor so much as the patient's perception of it (the stress response) that is most significant in heart attack etiology. The studies mentioned document that, compared to control subjects, coronary patients do not have more objective life stressors; they merely perceive their lives as more stressful than those of their brethren. Underlying—perhaps even pervasive—anxieties may result in chronically high levels of discomfort for which the individual overcompensates through competition. Bruhn et al. (1969) labeled the subjective feelings of stress and strain that anxious people experience when they are in competitive situations "the Avis syndrome (we try harder)." Research (Bahnson and Wardwell, 1966) also indicates that the childhood family and the circumstances of leaving home (in the case of coronary patients, usually much later than the average age) can affect the stress associated with launching one's own children into the world, perhaps representing a multigenerational cycle of premorbidity.

Unresolved Family Conflicts

Family conflicts, as related to disease vulnerability, can be multigenerational in the sense that reactions to one's current family circumstances may echo relationships in one's family of origin. Frequent somatic illness indicates still-unresolved conflict(s) with the family of origin. Examples of this multigenerational etiology can be found in such psychosomatic diseases as bronchial asthma, colitis, or the dermatoses. In asthma, for example, many research projects (for example, Knapp and Bahnson, 1963) have indicated that maternal overprotectiveness can lead to a complex, conflicting emotional reaction in the child, with yearnings for protection and love offset on a less conscious level by rage and fantasies of destruction of the intrusive maternal figure. Such ambivalence and difficulty in a key relationship may color the individual's relationships to other persons, for example, the spouse, later in life. The fact that people often select spouses who resemble a parent, often the mother, or someone the exact opposite, helps carry over emotional attitudes and responses from parent to spouse. Thus, interactions between adult spouses may reflect regressive and infantile responses and may exacerbate, for instance, a childhood respiratory difficulty. Unresolved family conflict, for instance, between mother and child, may be carried two and sometimes three generations through repeated physiologic "communications" between family members, indicating that the unresolved conflict is being carried over.

In colitis (Engel, 1950) the main issue seems not to be an overprotective doting, but rather severe conflicts about maternal control over the child's digestive functions. Rather clear-cut symbiosis between mother and child has been noted in such cases, in the sense that the mother's symptoms often disappear when the child's appear and vice versa. When the adult patient with a functional colitis syndrome interacts with a new "significant other" who provokes previous conflicts about control and mastery over one's own life, the old digestive symptoms often reappear. In this way, unresolved family conflict can be transmitted from generation to generation.

A third example may be the male coronary heart patient who lost his father at an early age, or whose father was uninvolved in the home routine, and who also had a dominant, controlling mother with whom he lived for longer than most control patients. Many such individuals later have serious marital problems, perceiving spouses as dominant and destructive—much as they saw their beloved but domineering mothers (Bahnson and Wardwell, 1962).

Although there may be exceptions, the general impression is that any conflict that characterizes patients' development and handling of illness has multigenerational roots involving parents and grandparents as well as current families. A nurse should not forget that the patient's subjective memory and perception of, for example, a grandmother, may be quite different from her own perceptions of the same person. Where the nurse might see a nice little old lady entering the room, the quivering patient might see a dragon.

Retirement

Retirement is dangerous to health. Both morbidity and mortality skyrocket within 1 or 2 years of retirement from active work. Forced retirement may be perceived as a rejection by society, particularly in cultures such as ours, with a strong work ethic, in which an individual's worth is measured by productivity and earning capacity. Were it not so, retirement might not be so widely perceived as a major stressor but might, instead, serve as a watershed between socially demanding activities and the individual's central interests. Social reality, however, is that retirement brings a loss of self-esteem and family respect and a sense of being discarded as useless or burdensome. Strong parental figures may experience a transition from being feared and respected to being pitied and humored. Aggression that may have been suppressed for years is often released against the retiring person on whom one is no longer dependent. No wonder that in this situation many people develop serious illness or exacerbations of illnesses they may have handled well for some time. The treatment staff can help such patients to retain some self-respect and to carve out meaningful, new family roles. A hardworking father or mother, for instance, may become the wise judicial figure from whom younger relatives seek advice and insight. Or a mother preoccupied with orchestrating and organizing her family may at retirement become their creative mentor, inspiring artistic or self-expressive pursuits in younger family members.

Loss and Depression

For centuries, it has been known that severe loss and resultant depression can usher in deadly illness. Classical Greek literature, as well as Greek medicine, reflected a keen understanding of the role of emotion in health. Cousins (1983) rediscovered this phenomenon in modern times through a sophisticated analysis of and mastery over his own illnesses and those of others.

The specific relationship between depression and immune incompetence has been highlighted in empirical research by Locke (1983), Stein et al. (1976), Ader (1981), Solomon et al. (1974), and others. Greene (1966) and Schmale and Iker (1966) studied loss and depression patients with lymphomas and leukemias, and uterine malignancies, respectively, and concluded that severe loss or separation, with concomitant depression, helplessness, and hopelessness, were characteristic antecedents of both types of malignancy. Greene (1969) also reported that, in monozygotic twin pairs discordant for leukemia, the twin subjected to the greatest individual frustration or misfortune developed leukemia while the more fortunate twin remained well. Greene's and Schmale and Iker's work has been replicated by others; Spence (1979), for instance, demonstrated the power of depression in the prediction of illness. Prospective population studies in Europe (Hagnell, 1966) and in the United States (Bieliauskas et al., 1979) have indicated that otherwise healthy individuals suffering depression were much more likely to develop cancer within 15 to 20 years than were their nondepressed peers.

Depressed persons seem to have a choice of responses to their emotional state—physical disturbance, frank neurotic, or depressive withdrawing states. This author (1969) related this choice to the individual's own coping style or ego-defensive choice, proposing that those who deny and repress unwelcome emotions are more vulnerable to physical illness than those who use such coping mechanisms as projection, displacement, or acting out.

This choice leads back to the childhood family in which each individual learns to cope. Key predictors of the physiological response are marked emotional coldness in the family of origin or early loss of significant family members through death, separation, or fragmentation. These experiences discourage investment in and closeness to other family members and predispose the extension of this reserve into later relationships.

Obviously, health professionals cannot change a patient's past. But the most devastating coping mechanisms might be counteracted through the presentation of new options for dealing with emotional conflicts. This is primarily a task for psychotherapists, but nursing and medical staffs can help such patients face their illnesses and associated emotional problems in a more mature, less destructive manner. By allowing discussion and ventilation of difficult and perhaps long-suppressed emotions, they can help the patient find new solutions. This therapeutic process may revolve around the illness itself and the patient's and others' reactions to it. Often this presents a welcome change from the patient's morbid or depressive patterns, leading to improvement and effective adaptation.

PATIENT AND FAMILY IN SERIOUS ILLNESS

Serious illness often develops in an individual when his entire family finds itself in an apparently inescapable emotional dilemma. A sense of hopeless entanglement may develop in the face of unresolvable ambivalence. His or his family's progress may be hindered by anxiety, fear of others' hostility, or uncertainty. These difficult emotional circumstances can force a patient into what might be called "somatic loneliness"—a situation characterized by regressive self-preoccupation in which frustrated wishes and hopes from childhood and youth reemerge without any immediate possibility of gratification.

A serious illness may nearly always be seen as the patient's last alarm reaction, indicating, for both him and his family, that life under the present circumstances is intolerable. Health professionals should therefore be cautious about advising the patient to return to a life situation that may have contributed to the illness in the first place. Yet efforts at "rehabilitation" and reconstitution of patients' lives make exactly this mistake, thereby enhancing rather than reducing vulnerability. The therapeutic team must always attempt to find *new* solutions that integrate the patient's needs into a new life constellation or family context.

Giving up old patterns and daring to look for new and untried solutions usually produces anxiety. The therapeutic team must support both patient and family by allaying anxiety and permitting new resolutions—resolutions that may take the pressure off the family, allow improvement in the patient's health, and minimize the destructive process.

Regardless of the patient's functional role within the family, the fact that the "family body" is ailing has a profound effect on every family member. Any attack on the undisturbed family structure can carry the seed of profound anxiety to each person. Disturbances in one part of the network are noticeable throughout. Disease in one family member constitutes an attack on the unconscious expectations of the existing family structure. The effects can last a lifetime. This threat is more potent when the ill member is a young adult with considerable family responsibility rather than a grandparent or small child. Ill grandparents do not threaten the long-term security of the family, and if a child is lost, restitution always is possible so the *system* may survive.

Whether the patient is young or old, serious or terminal illness introduces a confrontation with the unknown, as well as a threat to the myth of the current structure's eternal survival. In short, the uncertain survival of a given family member is not the only important consideration. Uncertainty about systemic order and predictability tends to shatter long-held and comfortable expectations of constancy and safety.

Even healthy families have difficulty with developmental transitions—the addition of new members, teenagers or young adults leaving home, and geographic or other external changes. Unexpected threats to family integrity are even more upsetting because they alter family decisions and relationships. Families in many instances ask health professionals about the consequences of their relative's illness, as if looking for new, workable, and secure structures.

Even successful medical intervention can compound family difficulties. For instance, new cancer therapies that take the patient in and out of the family, sometimes with unpredictable results, can create serious problems for families who need a psychological closure concerning the life or death of a sick member in order to function properly. Patients in remission may even be seen as "overstaying their welcome" at home. This quest for clear family structure can make patients in the "twilight zone" between remission and near death, and their families, one of the nurse's greatest challenges. Families must be helped to support the patient even during fragile and short-lived remissions at home. Rejection of the sick member (the "Lazarus syndrome") may cause the patient's condition to deteriorate dramatically and may lead to death even when optimal treatment is administered.

When Parents Fall Ill

Whenever an ill parent slides out of close family relationships, the system tries to reestablish balance by redistributing positive and/or hostile affective charges. Remaining family members become the ailing person's "delegates." Redistributed charges become "homeless" when the parent dies. Those who gave or took affection from him must begin to discharge or receive such emotions elsewhere. This often creates problems. It is usually not safe, for instance, for a daughter to receive a father's or son's affections for an ailing or dead mother; at the same time, family members "substituting" emotionally for an ill or deceased relative cannot always fill the void. And no matter how well the new affective object fulfills the family's function, relatives can rarely rearrange such bonds without experiencing guilt and defensive retaliation against the self (or projecting it to others) related to preoedipal or oedipal dangers. Intrasystemic punitive behavior of one type or another usually follows.

Affection is not the only impulse "orphaned" by the loss of a relative. The hostility, aggressiveness, and ambivalence associated with strong affective ties also become "homeless." One family member may even perceive that his hostility has been discharged when another falls ill, because he has, in his mind, caused the illness or killed the relative. This is one reason why the ill or departed person is usually described with affection and glorification; consciously hostile feelings have been discharged, and only affective or positive perceptions remain. However, unresolved, bound hostility may remain, directed toward other family members, producing sudden, unaccountable anger against a sibling or parent.

The family often perceives a member's illness or death as either an excretion or rejection of the individual from the system *or* rejection or destruction of the system by the ill or departed member. Nurses often hear children describe a parent's terminal illness as a "cop-out," as if that parent deliberately deserted them—on a very subtle level, there may even be some truth to this.

The disturbance in family equilibrium during one member's hopeless illness, or after a death, may also be expressed as illness elsewhere in the family; indeed, other members often develop diseases like those of their terminal relatives. Statistics show that spouses demonstrate multiple health problems after their partner's death. This is but one destructive way of recreating equilibrium and combating the guilt associated with a death. Another unfortunate resolution involves narcissistic reinvestment of the affectionate charges originally centered around the sick or dying family member. As separation from the dying patient increases, the remaining individuals become more self-absorbed, reversing *their* developmental progress to childlike narcissism. Although Freud's description of mourning includes a brief period of narcissistic reinvestment, it mandates a return to externalization as grief is resolved. This phenomenon (narcissistic reinvestment) may block the therapist's efforts to reestablish emotional equilibrium and reopen communication within the family, and may inhibit relations with the terminal patient. The terminal diagnosis itself changes the interpersonal process, as the surviving relatives prepare for the separation that comes with death. At this time, the patient needs increased communication with his family, and nurses should try to facilitate it for the reasons mentioned above. Narcissistic withdrawal and the family's attempts to reinvest its "homeless" affects make the task difficult, however.

Certain affects and reactions relate directly to the stricken individual's role within the family. When fathers fall ill, for example, they and their families often feel they have "failed" as providers and guides, a perception that generates guilt in the patient and anger in the rest of the family. Anger at a sick father cannot be expressed openly; often it is thoroughly repressed, creating further guilt. The treatment staff should carefully uncover these feelings before they lead to psychosomatic and behavioral pathology, which may create more unconscious guilt in the sick father and start a spiral of anger and guilt.

Although parental roles today are less differentiated than they were generations ago, a mother's terminal illness still has different implications than a father's. Disturbance of archetypal nurturance and security relationships with the mother creates deep anxiety about future satisfaction and care in the family. Frustrated dependency needs often have a strong regressive pull—even stronger than those associated with loss of the father. The sick mother, in turn, often feels despair at not being able to nurture her children. She may verbalize the need to see her smaller children grow up, meaning that if she could care for them until adulthood, they might succeed in life and not be left without a source of nurturance. Families with terminally ill mothers should develop alternative nurturant resources not only because the mother cannot fill that role, but because she herself needs care—or "mothering." The displaced nurturing functions are best assumed by older members of the extended family, such as aunts and grandmothers, but any constellation of relatives, including the father, can provide support. Such shifts are easier to bring about in less traditional households, but each family provides its own unique solution.

Younger children need the stability of older nurturant family members in order to prevent "parentification" or assumption of responsibility incommensurate with their years. Consciously or not, children are often enraged at the parent who "deserts" them or withdraws care. They often perceive the loss as a result of their own inadequacy or hostility and feel guilty and anxious over their imagined power to "create pain for their parents." Similarly, terminally ill parents feel guilty about depriving their offspring of a solid and protected childhood; the healthy parent might feel unconscious bitterness against the ill spouse for deserting and leaving all the burdens behind. The family therapist and nursing staff should help relatives communicate these feelings to each other and relieve the burden of repression that may reinforce family members' regressive somatization and thereby exacerbate disease. Clinically, it is known that mood and disease progression are more benign after guided communication of these difficult issues.

When Children Fall Ill

Serious illness in a child gives rise to additional family problems. When older individuals die, there are younger ones to fill the gap. But to have the roots cut away under the family is disquieting and upsetting. Childhood illness generates a great deal of guilt because of the unconscious suggestion of poor or insufficient parenting. The guilt can, in extreme cases, destroy a family; it is known, for instance, that exacerbations in childhood leukemia and Hodgkin's disease often coincide with family disintegration and strife. What is unclear is whether the strain of the child's illness and death were more than the relationship could handle, or if the parents were somehow inadequate. The nurse must address any parental problems that may be associated with the exacerbation of the child's illness, and take the pressure off the child as the parents' mediator or "mentor." Under no circumstances should parental guilt be increased. On the contrary, the therapist should help the family deal with issues not related to the child or the illness. In some cases resolution of the parents' conflict, along with reintegration of the family system, can take enough pressure off the sick child to bring about remission. If the parents no longer need the child's mediation to maintain the family structure and can master any covert hostility arising from their ambivalence about the child, a fresh reorganization can take place. In both young and old patients, the nurse should prevent the ill person's return to a premorbid situation—in the case of a child, perhaps a demanding school schedule, athletics, or any other counterphobic forced activity. In sessions with the family, a new role for the child should be defined—one directed more closely to his needs and responsive to his developmental stage. Unfortunately, family, medical, and social pressure can push ill children into inappropriate competition, forcing them to function "like other healthy children." This misunderstanding of the ill child's needs can cause serious mental health problems and exacerbate his physical condition.

The Deserted Patient

Young and old terminal patients often feel deserted and shunned, even when people around them show superficial interest and care. The terminal patient, as a reminder of even the healthiest individual's mortality, is never welcome and may even become a phobic object. Since isolation and disease feed on each other, the nursing staff should build interfamily contacts, rip down barriers, increase communication, and facilitate cathartic expression in order to counteract the emotional isolation of the seriously ill. To feel like a member of the family again helps these patients tremendously, and they often find new roles for themselves—roles that not only help them regain their self-respect and sense of purpose, but also represent true helpfulness within the system itself.

One family member who may be particularly traumatized by illness-related isolation is the traditional father. A loss of personal authority within the family generally produces high anxiety, and although responsibilities must necessarily be shifted when he is ailing, there are many ways he can maintain a helpful consulting role to the benefit of the family. This principle applies to mothers and other authority figures in the family as well, especially at a time when roles are becoming less rigidly defined and sometimes even reversed.

At some point in the course of a serious illness the question ceases to be how to mobilize the patient and family *against* the disease, and becomes how to best complete the patient's *disengagement* and prepare for death. In families with terminally ill patients who have frequent contact with health care personnel and who have waxing and waning hopes of remission, support and general energizing must alternate with periods of natural disengagement. The longer the illness prevails, the more the treatment staff must focus on the pain of the family's impending loss. These periods will not and need not be sharply defined; indeed, patient and family will often discuss their current situation and their ultimate parting in the same conversation.

Patient and family reactions to the threat of death can also occur on several levels simultaneously. At such times, the nurse must accept the fact that no simple, logical approach can ensure successful intervention. The single most important nursing goal must be to help members of the family overcome their fear of the unknown, so they can support the patient and alleviate the despair that comes with the knowledge of impending death.

CONCLUSIONS

Nursing the seriously or terminally ill patient requires empathy, wisdom, and unlimited kindness. Such cases are professionally very demanding. They call for both human and psychological sensitivity, tolerance of difficult patients and their families' reactions under stress, and an understanding of the patients' and families' varied and often irrational reactions to life-threatening illness.

Nurses providing care in terminal illness must be thoroughly aware of their patients' conscious and unconscious emotional lives and must be able to decipher nonverbal and other covert messages. They must be sophisticated about family relationships and managing families under stress, ready to tolerate extreme stress themselves, and able to maintain empathy and a willingness to help even in the face of extreme irrationality or provocation.

The success of this humanistic treatment strategy relies on true team care in the hospital or clinic. Open communication among members of the treatment team and a democratic approach to care delivery are essential, not only from the point of view of the patient, who fares better under coordinated and harmoniously integrated treatment efforts, but also from that of participating professionals in all disciplines. Territorial disputes between physicians and nurses benefit no one, and only make it certain that everyone, including the patient, will suffer. To avoid this counterproductive scenario, regular team meetings should be held; in such forums not only can patient and family problems be studied, but interdisciplinary problems among professionals can be resolved.

A modern systems approach is also necessary in solving such difficult patient problems as choice of therapy (for example, chemotherapy vs. surgery) and interpersonal conflicts between the nurses and the patient's family. Staff, patient, and family should meet together and work out any differences that might hinder treatment or serve as an obstacle to the patient's ultimate return home. Nurses must be particularly sensitive to the problems within the patient-family system as well as to any tensions and conflicts between the "treatment family" and the patient's own family. Unless such issues are addressed, even the best therapeutic intentions will encounter a disintegration of the treatment process.

REFERENCES

Ader, R., ed. *Psychoneuroimmunology.* New York: Academic Press, 1981.

Alexander, F. *Psychosomatic Medicine.* New York: W.W. Norton & Co., 1950.

Arlow, J.A. "Identification Mechanisms in Coronary Occlusion," *Psychosomatic Medicine* 7:195–209, 1945.

Bahnson, C.B. "Psychological Complementarity in Malignancies: Past Work and Future Vistas," in *Annals of the New York Academy of Science NYAS* 164(2):319–34, 1969.

Bahnson, C.B. "Stress and Cancer: The State of the Art, Part 1," *Psychosomatics* 21(12):975–81, December 1980.

Bahnson, C.B. "Stress and Cancer: The State of the Art, Part 2," *Psychosomatics* 22(3):207–20, 1981.

Bahnson, C.B. "Systems Concepts in Group and Family Therapy," in *The Individual and the Group,* vol 1. Edited by Pines, M., and Rafaelson, L. New York: Plenum Press, 1982.

Bahnson, C.B., and Wardwell, W.I. "Parent Constellation and Psychosexual Identification in Male Patients with Myocardial Infarction," *Psychological Reports* 10(3):831–52, 1962.

Bahnson, C.B., and Wardwell, W.I. "Personality Factors Predisposing to Myocardial Infarction," in *Psychosomatic Medicine, Proceedings of the First International Conference of Academy of Psychosomatic Medicine, Exc. Med.,* 134:249–256, 1966.

Bieliauskas, L., et al. *Prospective Studies of Psychological Depression and Cancer.* New York: Paper presented at meeting of the American Psychological Association, 1979.

Bruhn, J.G., et al. "A Psychological Study of Survivors and Nonsurvivors of Myocardial Infarction," *Psychosomatic Medicine* 31:8–19, 1969.

Cousins, N. *The Healing Heart.* New York: W.W. Norton & Co., 1983.

Derogatis, L.R., et al. "Psychological Coping Mechanisms and Survival Time in Metastatic Breast Cancer," *Journal of the American Medical Association* 242:1504–08, 1979.

Deutsch, F., ed. *On the Mysterious Leap from Mind to Body.* New York: International University Press, 1959.

Engel, G.L. "Studies of Ulcerative Colitis, V., Psychological Aspects and Their Implications for Treatment," *American Journal of Digestive Diseases* 3:315–37, 1950.

Freud, S. *The Aetiology of Hysteria, Collected Papers,* vol. 1. New York: Basic Books, 1959.

Freud, S. *Repression, Collected Papers,* vol. 4. New York: Basic Books, 1959.

Friedman, M., and Rosenman, R.H. *Type A Behavior and Your Heart.* New York: Alfred A. Knopf, 1974.

Greene, W.A. "The Psychosocial Setting of the Development of Leukemia and Lymphoma," *Annals of the New York Academy of Science* 125(3):794-801, 1966.

Greene, W.A., and Swisher, S.N. "Psychological and Somatic Variables Associated with the Development and Course of Monozygotic Twins Discordant for

Leukemia," *Annals of the New York Academy of Science* 164(2):394–408, 1969.

Greer, S., and Morris, T. "Psychological Attributes of Women Who Develop Breast Cancer: A Controlled Study," *Journal of Psychosomatic Research* 19:147–53, 1975.

Hagnell, O. "The Premorbid Personality of Persons Who Develop Cancer in a Total Population Investigated in 1947 and 1957," *Annals of the New York Academy of Science* 125(3):846–55, 1966.

Holmes, T.H., and Rahe, R.H. "The Social Readjustment Rating Scale," *Journal of Psychosomatic Research* 11:213–18, 1967.

Kissen, D.M. "The Significance of Personality in Lung Cancer in Men," *Annals of the New York Academy of Science* 125(3):820–26, 1966.

Knapp, P.H., and Bahnson, C.B. "The Emotional Field—a Sequential Study of Mood and Fantasy in Asthmatic Subjects," *Psychosomatic Medicine* 25:460–83, 1963.

Kubie, L. "The Central Representation of the Symbolic Process in Relation to Psychosomatic Disorders," *Psychosomatic Medicine* 15:1–7, 1953.

Kübler-Ross, E. *On Death and Dying.* New York: Macmillan Publishing Co., 1969.

Locke, S.E., and Rohan, M.H. *Mind and Immunity: Behavioral Immunology.* New York: Praeger Pubs., 1983.

Nemiah, J., et al. "Alexithymia: A View of the Psychosomatic Process," in *Modern Trends in Psychosomatic Medicine 3.* Edited by Hill, O. Woburn, Mass.: Butterworth Pubs., 1976.

Parsons, T. *The Social System.* Glencoe, Ill.: Free Press, 1951.

Schleifer, S.J., et al. "Depression and Immunity: Lymphocyte Function in Ambulatory Depressed Patients, Hospitalized Schizophrenic Patients, and Patients Hospitalized for Herniography," *Archives of General Psychiatry* 42:129–33, 1985.

Schmale, A.H., Jr., and Iker, H.P. "The Psychological Setting of Uterine Cervical Cancer," *Annals of the New York Academy of Science* 125(3):807–13, 1966.

Selye, H. *The Stress of Life.* New York: McGraw-Hill Book Co., 1956.

Sifneos, P.E. "The Prevalence of 'Alexithymic' Characteristics in Psychosomatic Patients," *Psychotherapy and Psychosomatics* 22:255–63, 1973.

Solomon, G.F. "Psychophysiological Aspects of Rheumatoid Arthritis and Autoimmune Disease," in *Modern Trends in Psychosomatic Medicine.* Edited by Hill, O.W. Woburn, Mass.: Butterworth Pubs., 1970.

Solomon, G.F., et al. "Immunity, Emotions and Stress," *Psychotherapy and Psychosomatics* 23:209–17, 1974.

Spence, D. *Somato-Psychic Signs of Cervical Cancer.* New York: Paper presented at 87th Annual American Psychological Conventions, 1979.

Stein, M., et al. "Influence of Brain and Behavior on the Immune System. The Effect of Hypothalamic Lesions on Immune Processes," *Science* 191(4226):435–40, 1976.

Vidich, A.J., and Stein, M.R. "The Dissolved Identity in Military Life," in *Identity and Anxiety.* Edited by Stein, M.R., et al. Glencoe, Ill.: Free Press, 1960.

von Uexkull, T. *Textbook of Psychosomatic Medicine.* Munich: Urban & Schwarzenberg, 1981.

Wardwell, W.J., and Bahnson, C.B. "Behavioral Variables and Myocardial Infarction in the Southeastern Connecticut Heart Study," *Journal of Chronic Disease* 26:447–61, 1973.

Wolf, S. "Cardiovascular Reactions to Symbolic Stimuli," *Circulation* 18:287–92, 1958.

3 Families and life-threatening illness: Assumptions, assessment, and intervention

Lorraine M. Wright, RN, PhD
Director, Family Nursing Unit
Professor, Faculty of Nursing
University of Calgary
Calgary, Alberta, Canada

Maureen Leahey, RN, PhD
Team Director, Mental Health Services
Holy Cross Hospital
Adjunct Associate Professor, Faculty of Nursing
University of Calgary
Calgary, Alberta, Canada

OVERVIEW

This chapter presents basic assumptions about families with life-threatening illness. Guidelines for a systemic family assessment are outlined and examples of circular questions are given. To help nurses maximize change, specific interventions are described.

INTRODUCTION

Nursing assessments of and interventions with family systems are most often derived from beliefs, premises, and assumptions about human nature, the nature of human illness, and the nature and creation of therapeutic change. These beliefs enable nurses to determine the impact of life-threatening illness on the family and the influence of the family on the illness. Family responses during the assessment and intervention process perturb our beliefs, however, and modify our thoughts about the way families experience serious illness. Thus, the assumptions described in this chapter are based on research and clinical experience with families experiencing life-threatening illness. Ideas for assessment and intervention are also presented.

BASIC ASSUMPTIONS ABOUT FAMILIES WITH LIFE-THREATENING ILLNESS

Life-threatening illness challenges family stability, adaptability, resources, and, most intensely, beliefs and assumptions. It also challenges health professionals' beliefs about their ability to alleviate suffering and to cure. As a result, in both the family and treatment systems the "meaning" assigned to disease becomes paramount. The assumptions listed below are perhaps the most salient in this situation.

Assumption #1: The Diagnosis of Life-Threatening Illness Is a Social Contract

Diagnosis of a life-threatening condition combines clinical expertise, medical science, and intuition; however, it becomes meaningful only when placed in an interactional context. Diagnosis is a social event that occurs when one person (the medical or nursing expert) affixes a classification to another (the identified patient) (Glenn, 1984). At this point, the patient, family, and health care system enter into a contract regarding the problems. The diagnosis implies that a cluster of signs and/or symptoms exists, places those manifestations in context, gives them meaning, and suggests treatments. However, as nurses are only too aware, it is difficult to have all parties in the contract agree on all aspects of the diagnosis. Thus, a life-threatening diagnosis is subjected to "negotiations." Initially, the patient may accept a diagnosis of myocardial infarction, but other family members may not; the patient, while accepting the label of the illness, may not agree with the proposed treatment. Not even the health care system presents a united front regarding management of the illness. The diagnosis is scrutinized by all parties involved.

Among the most powerful implications of any diagnosis are the patient's and family's conclusions about it. They will spend much time thinking about the origins of the illness and its implications. Complicating matters is the illness's profound effects on those around the patient. Thus, families can experience confusion, anger, pleasure, or relief. Health care professionals who understand this broader context will be more sensitive to their anxiety and guilt and can better involve them in the management process.

Nurses need to review the circumstances surrounding the life-threatening diagnosis to help the family integrate the new information into their lives. Most families vividly remember how they received the diagnosis: who told them, what they were doing at the time, and how they reacted. Families are, of course, unique and complex, responding to life-threatening incidents or diagnoses differently. But all families need to discuss the circumstances and details of the diagnosis.

Assumption #2: A Life-Threatening Diagnosis Changes the Family's Life Trajectory

Before middle adulthood, few people think about their own deaths. Pattison (1977) suggests that serious consideration of that subject constitutes projection of "a trajectory of our life." A life-threatening diagnosis, a "crisis knowledge of death," changes the family life trajectory. Often, family members' reactions to the diagnosis are influenced by the type of dying trajectory the patient faces. Glaser and Straus (1968) identified four types of dying trajectories:
- certain death at a known time
- certain death at an unknown time
- uncertain death but a known time when the questions will be resolved
- uncertain death and an unknown time when questions will be resolved.

Wright (1985) emphasizes that nurses are obligated to help patients and their families experience the crisis knowledge of death.

Assumption #3: Families Need to Review a Life-Threatening Event

When a family experiences a life-threatening event (for example, a member's coronary or cranial injury), that event becomes a kind of videotape that needs to be played, viewed, and discussed repeatedly, not unlike the circumstances surrounding a death. Many nurses have noted families' spontaneous references to tragic incidents during family nursing interviews. Further questioning revealed that they would almost be relieved to be able to describe the incident, regardless of how painful it might be. Life-threatening events impinge so deeply upon family members' cognitive and affective functioning that one method of regaining stability and reducing sensitivity to the event is to relive it through detailed description.

Assumption #4: Family Members' Reactions Influence the Course of a Life-Threatening Illness

Nurses and other health care professionals know that individuals' responses to life-threatening illness vary (for example, denial, anger). However, some family clinicians (Palazzoli, 1985) now propose that patients respond more to their family's responses to the illness than to the condition itself. This interactional phenomenon has seldom entered into previous efforts to understand the reciprocity between illness and family dynamics. The research of Reiss et al. (1986) suggests that affected families who are too emotionally close may precipitate death in the sick member. Death represents an "arrangement" between the family and the patient—the patient dies so that "the family may live." This is often an extreme but perhaps the only "reasonable" patient response to the family's feelings of grief and burden. Rolland (1984) states that "some families' hope to resume a 'normal' life might only come through the death of their ill member" (p. 255).

In recognition of this, various studies have examined family outcomes when support interventions have been provided. For example, Morisky et al. (1983) offered impressive support for the efficacy of family interventions in individual hypertension. A five-year mortality survey demonstrated 57% lower mortality in groups receiving intervention, compared with control groups. One significant finding was that brief family intervention had as strong an effect as combined individual-plus-family interventions in terms of treatment compliance.

Family (typically spousal) support also affects the course of an illness. Barbarin and Tirado (1985) contributed greatly to family support research by discovering that a spouse's support works only in the context of a cohesive marriage.

Therefore, family reactions can significantly influence the decision to initiate or delay treatment, the perceptions of symptom or disease seriousness, compliance, and satisfaction with the treatment outcome (Weakland and Fisch, 1984). In extreme cases, the family may even influence the patient's will to live.

Assumption #5: Family Function is Often Altered by Life-Threatening Illness

Dealing with a life-threatening illness within a family commonly alters usual family functioning. Koch's (1985) study of 32 families of children with newly diagnosed cancer revealed these changes within families: increased negative affect, prohibition of emotional expression, new or exacerbated health and behavior problems following diagnosis, role changes, and increased emotional closeness among family members. Giaquinta (1980) specified 10 functional phases for families facing cancer. These phases (functional disruption, search for meaning, informing others) can be useful if health care professionals do not reify the particular phases as was done with Kübler-Ross's (1969) five stages of facing death. The effect an individual's life-threatening illness has on the family differs in *intensity* depending on the nature of the illness itself, the timing of the illness in the family life cycle, the openness of the family system, and the family position of the patient (Herz, 1980; Brown et al., 1982). However, in the Brown et al. study of patients with serious coronary problems, there was little evidence of any correlation between severity of illness and impairment of the patient's family functioning. Therefore, the nurse should actively investigate critical variables and then draw a conclusion.

When nurses assume particular models of family functioning to be "true" rather than simply the observer's (nurse's) assumptions, they reduce their receptiveness to other possibilities or assumptions. Care providers must behave more like anthropologists, viewing the study of changes in families facing illness as a study of unmapped territory, rather than as an area to be explored using a preexisting map. Even after assessment, the territory is *still* not a map, nor the map the territory. Nurses can only behave as if that is so.

Assumption #6: Family Members' Beliefs about a Life-Threatening Illness Influence How They and the Patient Cope with the Situation

Beliefs about the cause of a life-threatening illness can profoundly affect the ways a family copes with and responds to the crisis. Borhek and Curtis (1975) define a belief system as a set of related ideas (learned and shared) which are more or less permanent and to which individuals exhibit commitment. The authors' experience has been that families are powerfully attached to their beliefs, and display more commitment to beliefs about life-threatening illness than about chronic illness because grave illness confronts beliefs about mortality. Therefore, some families perceive illness as a challenge, while others consider it a punishment or perceive it as a threat. One family whose adolescent had a life-threatening illness explained their ability to cope by saying "God knew that our family could handle it—other families would have fallen apart."

Family beliefs significantly determine the impact of illness, the choice of coping patterns used, and ultimately physical and behavioral reactions (Wright and Bell, 1981). Sometimes these beliefs are held so strongly that family members appear more willing to invalidate data than to invalidate perceptions (Dell, 1986). This provides an additional challenge for family nurses.

FAMILY NURSING ASSESSMENT

The nurse must consider whether an assumption about families facing life-threatening illness applies to a given client. If it does apply, is the effect negative or positive? Rather than focus on particular assessment models, many of which are described elsewhere in this volume, to answer these questions, this chapter presents procedural ideas applicable to many assessment styles.

Guidelines for Systemic Assessment

The assessment process is predominantly based on a systemic model of interviewing (Palazzoli et al., 1980) developed by four Italian psychiatrists known as the Milan Associates. The model was originally developed through their work with families with psychosocial problems (for example, anorexia nervosa), but it has proven useful in interviewing families with grave or chronic illness. This model proposes three guidelines: hypothesizing, circularity, and neutrality. Recently, Tomm (1987) has proposed a fourth guideline, strategizing. All four of these principles are interrelated.

In a systemic family interview, the nurse must be aware of personal assumptions about families and serious illness and remain open to feedback that might modify them. It is important to apply these assumptions individually, in the form of hypotheses, to each family. These unconfirmed hypotheses help organize information; they are affirmed or disaffirmed with information obtained through assessment. Generally, these hypotheses are the parameters or variables associated with specific family assessment models. The behavioral or actual executive skills necessary to explore them require the selection of linear or circular questions.

Circular questioning involves obtaining information about relationships (Palazzoli et al., 1980). The nurse must be able to respond to the elicited descriptions without judgment or blame. For example, if a family sees a connection between illness and punishment from God, the nurse's response must be neutral; this does *not* mean that the nurse must accept the family's reasoning. Information obtained by circular questioning will greatly assist the intervening nurse. Intervention is only necessary, however, if a particular belief interferes with the family's ability to solve problems or care for the ill member.

Strategizing refers to clinical decision making: evaluating the effects of past nursing actions, constructing new plans, anticipating possible consequences of various alternatives, and deciding how to proceed on the basis of ultimate therapeutic utility (Tomm, 1987).

Assessment Questions

Lineal descriptive vs. circular descriptive. Regardless of the particular model(s) chosen by the nurses, certain questions may create a recursive loop between nurse and family. There is also ongoing interaction between family functioning and illness (Weakland, 1977). Some questions aid understanding of the family system while others serve to effect change (Tomm, 1985; Tomm, 1987). The questions are usually lineal descriptive, such as problem-oriented questions. For example, when a family reviews a life-threatening event (Assumption #3), the nurse could ask: "How did the family learn about John's motorcycle accident? How were other family members informed? Where was John taken in the ambulance? How long was he in Emergency? What was explained to you at the time about John's condition? What do you now understand happened in the accident?" Such questions inform the nurse of the circumstances of a life-threatening accident and establish a therapeutic context for further review. The authors have found that many details need to be sifted in order for all to arrive at a "common crisis story."

To reduce the family's sensitivity to the tragic event and thus to effect change, the nurse should move from lineal descriptive to circular descriptive questions. For example, the nurse could ask, "Who in the family worried the most while John was in the emergency room?" ("Mother did because she didn't think he'd live.") "How did she show that she was the one worrying the most?" ("She kept asking the doctors and nurses 'He's going to be all right, isn't he?'") "What did your father do while your mother was so worried?" ("He stayed in the hospital cafeteria and drank gallons of coffee—he can't be around sick people.") Circular descriptive questions are directed more toward *explanation*, whereas lineal descriptive questions are more *investigative*. Both types are useful. Remember, though, that the *effect* on families of these two types of questions differs: lineal questions can have a moderate effect, whereas circular questions tend to have a liberating effect (Tomm, in press).

The primary distinction between circular questions and lineal questions lies in the notion that information reveals differences in relationships (Bateson, 1979). With circular questions, a relationship or connection is always sought between individuals, events, ideas, or beliefs.

Some questions are more difficult for nurses to ask because they confront the professionals' own beliefs and philosophies. Nevertheless, it is important to assess each family's ability to adjust to the change in their trajectory (Assumption #2). To sensitively assess the family systems, the nurse should begin with lineal descriptive questions about the circumstances surrounding the diagnosis. For example, "Who told your father about his diagnosis of cancer of the lung? How did your mother learn of the diagnosis?" By asking such questions, the nurse can assess not only how the medical system informed the family but also how the family shares "crisis information." Next it is important to assess each family member's reaction to the diagnosis. This can be done through such circular descriptive questions as: "Who in the family was most surprised by the diagnosis? Who in the family was most upset by the news? Who between your mother and father is the most optimistic about the future? How do you explain that *your* family has to cope with this situation while other families do not?" This helps the nurse target the family's beliefs about illness.

Family members' beliefs about the illness or event may be *the* most important factor to assess; their implications for nursing intervention are enormous. A family who believes a father's lung cancer is due to smoking and who concludes that he caused his own illness will need dramatically different interventions than a family who attributes the cancer to an occupational hazard and blames an employer. In the former case, a family's reaction could be resentment and blame directed towards the ill relative. In the latter case, family reactions could be sorrow and sympathy and a projection of blame and anger onto the employer.

Circular descriptive questions such as the following are also useful in the evaluation of advice given to the family by relatives, friends, and community resources: "What is the worst advice that friends have given you? What is the best advice? What advice have you acted on?" These questions yield significant information about the types and sources of advice that the family values; they also give the nurse clues about what advice to avoid.

Once assessment through lineal and circular descriptive questions has been completed, the nurse can begin making critical clinical decisions regarding interventions. If assessment indicates that family functioning and/or problem solving is blocked (for example, if members blame themselves for the life-threatening illness), then family intervention is indicated.

FAMILY NURSING INTERVENTION

Nurses who provide family health care should target interventions at health promotion, treatment, management, and resolution of biopsychosocial problems. A myriad of helpful family interventions are available for families experiencing difficulties with a serious illness. This chapter presents those interventions that, based on research and the authors' own clinical practice, seem most critical in such situations. Unfortunately, despite the large quantity of family and health care research, there are few studies of family interventions (Doherty, 1985).

Interventive Questions

One of the simplest but most powerful nursing interventions for families coping with life-threatening illness is the use of interventive questions.

Lineal strategic vs. circular reflexive questions. Questions that serve as interventions are primarily of two types: lineal strategic and circular reflexive (Tomm, in press). The two types have vastly different effects on families: strategic questions tend to be constraining, while reflexive inquiries are generative—that is, they introduce new cognitive connections, creating the potential for behavioral change.

The following two interventive questions could be used in a situation where a young adult has been in a serious motorcycle accident with resultant head and spinal cord injuries:
- "Don't you think that your continual blaming of your son for the

accident might discourage him from the rigorous physiotherapy he has to endure?" This question is lineal strategic. It takes a harsh, blaming, confrontational stance and gives a strong message or directive for change to the parents. The implication is that the nurse knows what is best for the family.

• "If you became even more critical of your son's reckless motorcycle driving, do you think it would be more or less likely that he would continue with his rigorous physiotherapy exercises?" This question is more reflexive and is intended to facilitate change by mobilizing the parents to *reflect* on their actions. It allows the parents to choose their own position and thus respects family autonomy more. Strategic questions often imply a corrective intent while reflexive questions imply a facilitative intent.

One type of reflexive question, the *future-oriented question*, is particularly useful for work with families experiencing catastrophic illness. Families with serious health problems find it difficult to speculate on the future because they are so preoccupied with *present* difficulties and so fearful of the future. This attitude inhibits problem-solving efforts. Reflexive questions about the future can encourage a family to consider the future (Tomm, in press); questions to a family with a young son with serious burns might include: "What are you worried will happen if these skin grafts continue to be so painful for your son? What's the worst thing that could happen?" To a father diagnosed with terminal lung cancer, the powerful and penetrating question was asked: "When you die, do you think it is more or less likely that your wife and son will fight as much as they do now?" Such questions help families discuss catastrophic expectations, which they can then affirm or disaffirm. They help establish awareness of important connections between family functioning and illness. In the above example, the father had always mediated between his wife and son and the nurse hypothesized that the father believed their fighting would worsen after he died. To the father's surprise and delight, the son answered that he would not fight as much with his mother because that was his way of getting his father involved in decision making. While his father was ill, the son stated he was fighting more because he wanted his father involved in decisions.

In one family that seemed to conspire against mentioning the life-threatening diagnosis, members were asked a question focusing on outcome: "If things continue going the way they are now, what do you expect will become of your family in 6 months to a year?"

And finally, future-oriented questions—"What changes would you like to see in a month from now with regard to your mother's care? And what about other family members?"—were used to open discussion about family goals with respect to the illness.

In the authors' clinical experience, interventive questions alone have often been sufficient to effect change within families that have difficulty dealing with their crisis.

Provide Information

The context in which a nurse encounters a patient with a grave illness will help determine the amount of involvement with family members. However, family research and clinical experience in family nursing both indicate that families, regardless of setting, desire more information from nursing and medical personnel than is offered spontaneously. Families with a member in an intensive care unit seem to express the highest need for regular and current information on the client's condition. The family has to be kept informed, especially when the patient's condition worsens or death is imminent. One useful strategy is for the nurse to initiate regular telephone contact. This punctuates the usual nurse-family interaction in a dramatically different way. Instead of having the family call and request information (and the nurse caring for the family member frequently being unavailable), the nurse calls the family. This reduces family members' anxiety and allows them to be absent from the hospital so they can meet other obligations and obtain rest (Bozett and Gibbons, 1983).

This strategy also helps reframe the family's need for the nurse. Instead of labeling particular family members as "bothersome" or a "nuisance," the nurse who initiates contact is more likely to perceive clients as appreciative and grateful. This reframe of family members' behavior occurs because the nurse has assumed control of the dissemination of information. It also allows her to feel competent. When phoned spontaneously by family members, without having a chance to organize the necessary information, the nurse may feel out of control and/or incompetent.

Nurses can also provide information to families during regular visiting times. Hampe (1975) found that relatives do not expect nurses to be concerned about *them;* rather, they think the nurse's responsibility is solely to the hospitalized patient. Ideally, the nurse should have short family meetings to assess their functioning and to explore the family's perceptions of the situation. Assessment and interventive questions appropriate to the nurse's chosen assessment model are helpful during these meetings.

Promote Family Involvement in Care of the Ill Family Member

Families with a member hospitalized due to a life-threatening illness or event often feel helpless. To reduce these negative feelings, the nurse needs to involve relatives in patient care. A few suggestions follow:
• Teach family members how to touch and hold the patient without

interfering with life support systems.
- Ask family members if they would like to feed the patient at scheduled mealtimes.
- Encourage different family members to adopt particular roles (for example, one to take daily calls from the nurse and one to prepare a favorite dish that is permissible on the patient's diet).
- Encourage younger children to make gifts.

The primary goal of this intervention is to reduce family stress. Just being with the patient can help. Many intensive care units have rigid visiting times that often magnify family members' anxiety by limiting the amount of time they can be with their loved one. The hospitalization of a family member makes many families feel powerless, out of control, and at the mercy of both the illness and health care personnel.

Provide Consistent Care

Ideally, primary nursing is provided for all hospitalized patients and their families. Family members should know the names of their primary nurses so they can call them in times of need. In some circumstances, however, someone other than the patient's nurse, such as a family clinical nurse specialist or a psychiatric liaison nurse, may be responsive to family needs. In these situations, the family should also know these nurses by name and know how to contact them.

Provide Opportunities to Discuss the Possibility of the Patient's Death

Families experiencing a catastrophic illness or event also have to face the possibility and eventual reality of the patient's death. It is often emotionally challenging for nurses to arrange appropriate and therapeutic discussions between family and patient about the impending loss. Just as each person's grief is unique, so is each person's anticipation of grief. Some family members will deny, others will be resentful or angry, others will accept the situation. The anticipation of loss is a functional response, usually related to how other family members are preparing for it. Thus one family member's denial may be more a relational than an intrapsychic phenomenon. Stein (1984) emphasizes this point when discussing the case of a patient with terminal metastatic cancer. He suggests asking the question: "In what context does the patient's denial make sense?"

Another important intervention is for nurse, family, and physician to discuss the use or nonuse of life support systems. Nurses need to anticipate that most families cannot make such a critical decision the first time it is discussed. Also, families commonly change their minds. This decision brings to bear the full spectrum of familial, cultural, and religious beliefs.

These recommended interventions are by no means inclusive. However, the authors believe them to be crucial considerations in nursing practice with families experiencing the upheaval of a life-threatening illness or event.

CONCLUSIONS

Family health care, particularly in the event of life-threatening illness, is shaped by assumptions, family research, and clinical practice that enhance compliance with treatment, provide social support, and sustain motivation for health-promoting behavior even in the absence of extrinsic reinforcement (Barbarin and Tirado, 1985). Nurses, because of the variety of contexts in which they encounter patients, because of their availability, and because of the involvement with families that has traditionally been a part of their profession, have an immense opportunity to alleviate the intense family stress and anxiety associated with tragic illness or events.

REFERENCES

Barbarin, O.A., and Tirado, M. "Enmeshment, Family Process, and Successful Treatment of Obesity," *Family Relations* 34:115–21, 1985.

Bateson, G. *Mind and Nature: A Necessary Unit.* New York: Dutton, 1979.

Borhek, J.T., and Curtis, R.F. *A Sociology of Belief.* Malabar, Fla.: Kreiger Publishing Co., 1975.

Bouman, C.C. "Identifying Priority Concerns of Families of ICU Patients," *Dimensions of Critical Care Nursing* 3(5):313–19, 1984.

Bozett, F.W., and Gibbons, R. "The Nursing Management of Families in the Critical Care Setting," *Critical Care Update* 10:22–27, 1983.

Brown, J.S., et al. "Family Functioning and Health Status," *Journal of Family Issues* 3:91-111, 1982.

Dell, P.F. "Why Do We Still Call Them 'Paradoxes'?" *Family Process* 25:223–34, 1986.

Doherty, W.J. "Family Interventions in Health Care," *Family Relations* 34:5–11, 1985.

Giaquinta, B. "Helping Families Face the Crisis of Cancer," in *Role of the Family in the Rehabilitation of the Physically Disabled.* Edited by Power, P.W., and Orto, A.E.D. Baltimore: University Park Press, 1980.

Glaser, B.G., and Straus, A.L. *Time for Dying.* Hawthorne, N.Y.: DeGruyter/Aldine Pubs., 1968.

Glenn, M.L. *On Diagnosis: A Systemic Approach.* New York: Brunner/Mazel, 1984.

Hampe, S.C. "Needs of the Grieving Spouse in a Hospital Setting," *Nursing Research* 24:113–20, 1975.

Herz, F. "The Impact of Death and Serious Illness on the Family Life Cycle," in *The Family Life Cycle: A Framework for Family Therapy.* Edited by Carter, E.S., and McGoldrick, M. New York: Gardner Press, 1980.

Koch, A. "'If Only It Could Be Me': The Families of Pediatric Cancer Patients," *Family Relations* 34:63–70, 1985.

Kübler-Ross, E. *On Death and Dying.* New York: Macmillan Publishing Co., 1969.

Morisky, D.E., et al. "Five-Year Blood Pressure Control and Mortality Following Health Education for Hypertensive Patients," *American Journal of Public Health* 73:153–62, 1983.

Palazzoli, M. Personal communication, Milan, Italy, 1985.

Palazzoli, M., et al. "Hypothesizing, Circularity, Neutrality: Three Guidelines for the Conductor of the Session," *Family Process* 19:3–12, 1980.

Pattison, E.M. *The Experience of Dying.* Englewood Cliffs, N.J.: Prentice-Hall, 1977.

Rasie, S.M. "Meeting Families' Needs Helps You Meet ICU Patients' Needs," *Nursing 80* 32–35, 1980.

Reiss, D., et al. "Family Process, Chronic Illness and Death: On the Weakness of Strong Bonds," *Archives of General Psychiatry* 43:795-804, 1986.

Rolland, J.S. "Toward a Psychosocial Typology of Chronic and Life-Threatening Illness," *Family Systems Medicine* 2:245–62, 1984.

Stein, H.F. "The Boundary of the Symptom: Whose Death and Dying?" *Family Systems Medicine* 2:188–94, 1984.

Tomm, K. "Circular Interviewing: A Multifaceted Clinical Tool," in *Applications of Systemic Family Therapy: The Milan Approach*. Edited by Campbell, D., and Draper, R. New York: Grune & Stratton, 1985.

Tomm, K. "Interventive Interviewing: Part I. Strategizing as a Fourth Guideline for the Therapist," *Journal of Marital and Family Therapy* 26:3-14, 1987.

Tomm, K. *Reflexive Questioning: A Generative Mode of Enquiry*. Calgary, Alberta: University of Calgary, 1985.

Weakland, J.H. "Family Somatics—a Neglected Edge," *Family Process* 16:263–72, 1977.

Weakland, J.H., and Fisch, R. "Cases That 'Don't Make Sense': Brief Strategic Treatment in Medical Practice," *Family Systems Medicine* 2:125–36, 1984.

Wright, L.K. "Life Threatening Illness," *Journal of Psychosocial Nursing* 23(9):7–11, 1985.

Wright, L.M., and Bell, J. "Nurses, Families and Illness: A New Combination," in *Treating Families with Special Needs*. Edited by Freeman, D., and Trute, B. Ottawa: The Canadian Association of Social Workers, 1981.

Wright, L.M., and Leahey, M. *Nurses and Families: A Guide to Family Assessment and Intervention*. Philadelphia: F.A. Davis Co., 1984.

4 Ethnicity, families, and life-threatening illness

Fredda Brown Herz, RN, PhD
Director of Training
Family Institute of Westchester
Private Practice
Mount Vernon, New York

OVERVIEW

This chapter provides a framework for understanding the impact of ethnicity on families' perceptions of, and methods for dealing with, life-threatening illness. The author considers the relationships between ethnicity, illness, and the perceptions of patients and health professionals. The chapter also looks at the impact of ethnicity and the health care subculture on varying approaches to illness. Clinical examples clarify each area.

THE CONCEPT OF ETHNICITY

Ethnicity, the characterization of historically unique subgroups as autonomous structures within a larger culture (McGoldrick, 1982), is a relatively new concept in the study of mental and physical health. The United States' traditional view of its culture as a "melting pot," which ignores individual and group differences, colored for generations the work of health professionals and scholars. In many respects, this attitude persists; the U.S. Census Bureau, for instance, does not record the specific ethnicity of anyone who is not foreign born or the child of foreign-born parents. Although ethnic values, perceptions, and traditions diminish with intermarriage and experience in another culture, such characteristics may be retained for many generations after immigration (Greely, 1978; McGoldrick et al., 1982).

Ethnicity and the Individual

McGoldrick (1982, p. 4) summarized the importance of ethnicity to the individual:

> Clinically, ethnicity is much more than race, religion, and national or geographic origin.... It involves conscious and unconscious processes that fulfill a deep psychological need for identity and a sense of historical continuity.

Ethnicity colors the way we perceive and experience life, death, emotions, health, and illness. It provides a framework, in both obvious and subtle ways, for thoughts, feelings, and behavior. Activities from family celebrations to child rearing are influenced by ethnic beliefs.

Ethnicity is transmitted primarily through family emotional processes, reinforced by the community at large (Giordano and Giordano, 1977). It establishes a sense of community and of historical continuity. Individuals tend to view their community's standards as universal unless they are confronted by differing values and characteristics. Ethnicity can be identified only in contrast to a separate ethnic identity.

Ethnicity and Family Care

Because of the family's importance in maintaining and transmitting ethnicity, family studies and family nursing must take this concept into consideration. However, such studies have been undertaken only recently (Boyd, 1980; Foley, 1980; McAdoo, 1977). Only with the publication of *Ethnicity and Family Therapy* (McGoldrick et al., 1982) did ethnicity become an active part of the family therapy knowledge base. Few family therapy models refer to ethnic influences. Little of the sparse body of family research considers family or clinician ethnicity in examining illness, pursuing treatment, or choosing interventions. One exception is Minuchin's (1974) work with inner-city black and Hispanic families.

ETHNICITY AND LIFE-THREATENING ILLNESS

Since there is no specific literature on the influence of ethnicity on the family's reaction to a life-threatening illness, this chapter examines the relationship between ethnicity and definitions of health and illness, patient and family perceptions of health care providers, and the professional health care subculture.

Ethnicity and Health/Illness

Definitions of health and illness dwell in the eye of the beholder—that is, in the ethnic "eye" of the affected persons. Therefore, effective nursing diagnosis and intervention depend upon an understanding of the client family's ethnic norms. As Kleinman (1978, p. 252), a prominent physician and researcher, has observed:

> How we communicate about our health problems, the manner in which we present our symptoms, when and to whom we go for care, are all affected by cultural beliefs. Illness behavior is a normative experience governed by cultural rules; we learn "approved" ways of being ill...and doctors' explanations and activities as those of their patients are culture specific.

Not only does ethnicity teach the acceptable ways of being ill, it may also determine whether or not a symptom is considered serious enough to require medical help. Some ethnic groups define most complaints as symptoms while others rarely complain. For example, the Irish seek help from the church before pursuing traditional medical and health assistance (McGoldrick, 1982). Eastern European Jews tend to seek help soon after symptoms appear (Herz and Rosen, 1982). Also, Jews notice symptoms quickly and consult as many professionals as necessary until they get satisfactory help (Herz and Rosen, 1982).

Some emergency department personnel have observed that specific ethnic groups have "target" organs or organ systems. For instance, Hispanics, especially young children, are often brought into emergency rooms with upper respiratory symptoms. Jews, on the other hand, often have gastrointestinal complaints.

Some ethnic groups' method of dealing with issues can generate major health difficulties. Jews, for instance, tend to be pessimistic, to notice symptoms earlier, and to see their treatment outcomes negatively (Herz and Rosen, 1982). Since traditional Jewish thought values a detailed analysis of multiple levels of meaning, many such patients view medical problems from so many angles that treatment for even serious illness is delayed. WASPs (white Anglo-Saxon Protestants), on the other hand, tend to be more cheerful and optimistic; indeed, their confidence and flexibility may be liabilities in the face of tragedy or mourning (McGill and Pearce, 1982).

Ethnicity also influences an individual's perceptions and expressions of illness and pain (Stoeckle et al., 1964). Health care professionals should know how a cultural group perceives pain; it will help them understand requests for medication and calls to the bedside. In Zborowski's (1969) classic study of physically ill Jews, Irish people, Italians, and WASPs, Jews and Italians complained more about pain than did Irish people and WASPs. Descriptions of pain also differed. Jews and WASPs described their discomfort more objectively, while the Irish denied their pain and the Italians exaggerated theirs.

Ethnicity also plays a role in pain expression. For instance, the intensive interaction between Italian, Jewish, and Greek family members offers a nurse valuable insights into a client's needs. WASP, Irish, and Scandinavian families interact less intensely and tend to deal with illness or crisis with stoic detachment. Such stoicism can hide urgent patient needs from health professionals. Cultural differences in expression can also lead to difficulties when people from two cultural groups intermarry (see case study below) or when a health care professional's ethnicity differs from that of the client family.

CASE STUDY

Carole and Bruce have been married 10 years. For the last 3, Bruce has had cancer. Carole, an Irish Midwesterner, found it difficult to take care of Bruce; no matter what she did, he always complained about how he felt and what he still needed her to do. After some exploration, it became clear that Bruce, who was Jewish and of eastern European ancestry, was just doing what he had been socialized to do when ill and in pain—complain. In fact, he thought it was therapeutic. Carole, on the other hand, had been raised to believe that one should be quiet about one's pain and considered complaining rude.

Ethnicity can also affect the degree to which individuals expect to suffer in life. Jews expect suffering to be a way of life, but differ from Irish Catholics in that the latter consider suffering to be punishment for one's sins. The Irish tend to be embarrassed by displays of physical or emotional pain; in the face of illness, they appear quiet or even stoic. On the opposite extreme is the Jewish idea of "participatory suffering," in which individual suffering becomes a group activity, one that has held the group together through a history of oppression. Suffering is done aloud, with others participating or observing.

Naturally, ethnic views of pain and suffering influence the way a group copes with death and serious illness. Both religion and sociocultural ethnicity help determine the attitudes and rituals associated with the end of life. Generally, the more rituals and prescriptions an ethnic group has for dealing with crisis, the better its people seem to cope. Some groups, in particular WASPs, have few rituals relating to death. Death is viewed simply as the end of life, another part of the "moving on" theme integral to that group: "You move on, not dealing with the past but focusing on the future." Jews, on the other hand, mark the ending of life and relationships with many rituals. While sitting "shiva," the 7-day mourning period, Jewish families frequently reminisce about the dead loved one. In a ritual called "cutting kvias," the rabbi cuts a piece of cloth or, in more orthodox groups, survivors rip their clothing to denote cutting ties with the deceased.

Expectations or prescriptions for family conduct during illness also differ with culture. Jewish American families tend to gather around the ill or dying individual to offer not only comfort, but advice on treatment and commiseration. Close family members are expected to be present if the patient is hospitalized; even extended relatives take pains to maintain contact with the patient and family. It would be unacceptable for a family member not to call or visit, as illustrated by the following example.

CASE STUDY

Joan was in Europe when her maternal aunt became seriously ill. She knew she should return home "because her mother would want her to" but she was busy with graduate work and called instead of going home. Her mother and her aunt's family were furious and threatened to "cut her off" unless she came home.

The Jewish family's intensive reaction to death and illness can lead to disproportionate anger among its members. The WASP reaction to illness contrasts sharply. The following is a common WASP response to the stress of serious illness.

CASE STUDY

Jean Lyons, 28, sought psychotherapy because of extreme depression and inability to sleep. The nursing history revealed that her depression had begun 3 months before, when her mother died of cancer. Jean's mother had lived across the country and had died and been buried several thousand miles from Ms. Lyons' home. Jean had seen her mother once during the fatal illness but had not been present when her mother died. She had flown in for the brief funeral her older brother had arranged, had stayed a few days to help clean out her mother's apartment, and had flown back to New York City. Ms. Lyons had denied any "unusual" upset about her mother's death and saw no connection between that and her own symptoms.

WASP families often have few rituals for dealing with illness or death. Families are not expected to visit frequently; individuality is the focus. Funerals are a way to bury the dead, something to go through so that one can move on. This response may lead to personal crises as family members try to simultaneously resolve their own distress and fulfill the cultural expectation of "moving on." It is the author's experience that such families display the most intensive reaction to death and the most rigid denial; many develop serious illness and require a nurse to help them discuss the illness or death.

Ethnicity and Therapeutic Choice

Perceptions of health care personnel and institutions can determine when and how people seek medical help. Italians tend to rely on family and turn to outsiders as a last resort (Gambino, 1974; Rotuno and McGoldrick, 1982; Zborowski, 1969). If an illness is life threatening, they may blame themselves for failing to treat it sooner. Black Americans, long distrusting the help available from traditional middle-class institutions, usually rely on church and family (nuclear and extended) (Hines and Boyd-Franklin, 1982; McAdoo, 1977). The more grave the illness, the more anxious the family, and the greater the animosity felt toward the white establishment. Black families view the treatment of their loved ones as inferior to that of other patients, and at times, in fact, it may be. The author has observed that the more "out" or "different" a patient from a particular ethnic group feels from society, the more likely he will be to judge society's assistance inadequate and to rely on more culturally relevant forms of treatment.

Puerto Rican (Preto, 1982) and Chinese families tend to somatize their problems and usually seek medical rather than emotional treatment. The Irish do not recognize illness readily, and when they do, they tend to postpone treatment (McGoldrick and Pearce, 1981). They often turn first to the church, speaking with the priest directly or in the confessional, before seeking medical or psychological help.

Ethnic traditions may discourage people from seeking traditional medical therapy, directing them instead toward religion, self-help, alcohol, chiropractors, spiritualists, yoga, acupuncturists, or other nontraditional remedies suggested by mothers, families, friends, or neighbors.

Studies of ethnic differences in expectations of treatment (Zborowski, 1969; Zola, 1966) have clear implications for nurses working with families facing a life-threatening illness. Part of Zborowski's study examines what patients from various backgrounds expected of those trying to help them. Because Italians worried about the immediate effects of their illness on their work, family, and finances, they wanted an immediate solution to their pain. Once the pain was relieved they forgot their illness; purely symptomatic treatment was enough. Jewish subjects, on the other hand, feared anything that might stop the pain without addressing the source of the problem. They worried about the implications of chosen therapies—for instance, about harmful drug side effects. They sought explanations of their pain or illness as well as solutions. Most Irish patients were fatalistic, not even expecting a cure. They did not even mention their pain, partially because they viewed discomfort as a result of their sins. On the other hand, WASP patients were confident of the curative ability of science. They sought to control their pain in whatever way the physician recommended. The value of this type of knowledge about ethnic differences is illustrated in the following case extract.

CASE STUDY

Mrs. Kaplan, a seriously ill 50-year-old, frequently refused her pain medication. The nurses were puzzled by this since the patient was clearly in a great deal of pain. When Mrs. Jones, the head nurse, talked with Mrs. Kaplan, it became clear that Mrs. Kaplan thought that as long as she took the medication, the physicians would not discover the source of her pain and would not be able to help her.

Other cultural groups may also refuse medication, but not for the same reason and not in the same way. For instance, the Irish often refuse pain medication because of their stoicism.

Ethnicity and the Health Care Subculture

Many ethnic groups' attitudes and expressive styles oppose those of health care professionals. "Americanized" health care personnel are taught to remain objective and professional, which an ethnic patient may interpret as detached and cold. Such professionals may distrust Jewish and Italian clients' uninhibited displays of suffering and dismiss them as exaggerations (Zborowski, 1969). For example, Zola (1966) found that physicians commonly diagnosed Italian patients' problems as psychiatric. In the author's experience, Jewish patients are viewed by health care personnel as "doctor shoppers" who search for a diagnosis that matches their own. Patients whose response to illness is similar to that of the health subculture are those most often labeled "normal"; Irish and WASP patients are generally so classified. By the same token, they might be less well understood by Jewish and Italian health personnel. An example follows.

CASE STUDY

A young man of Scottish-English descent was admitted to a hospital with a diagnosis of Hodgkin's disease. Although his family lived near the hospital and his parents visited each day after work, the young nurse who administered his care found herself angry and upset with them. Her nurses' notes indicated that the patient's family was not dealing well with the illness, as illustrated by their lack of expressiveness toward him. Upon questioning by her supervisor, the nurse's difficulty became obvious: in her own family, everyone would be at the bedside all the time. The supervisor stressed that although this was certainly one way to handle life-threatening illness, and one consistent with the nurse's Jewish heritage, it was not the only one. She suggested that the nurse spend some time with the patient's parents, discussing their son's illness and treatment and answering questions. The nursing supervisor further suggested that the nurse use her own ethnic skills to help parents and son deal with the issue of the young man's illness.

This example points out the pitfalls and strengths of an ethnic perspective. On the one hand, an ethnic bias can blind one to another's reaction to illness. On the other hand, it can enrich a nurse's ethnic perspective and her method of dealing with her own and her clients' crises.

REFERENCES

Boyd, N. "Family Therapy with Black Families," in *Minority Mental Health*. Edited by Corchin, S., and Jones, E. New York: Holt, Rinehart & Winston, 1980.

Foley, V.C. "Family Therapy with Black Disadvantaged Families: Some Observations on Roles, Communication, and Technique," *Journal of Marriage and Family Counseling* 1:57–65, 1980.

Gambino, R. *Blood of My Blood: The Dilemma of Italian-Americans*. New York: Doubleday, 1974.

Giordano, J., and Giordano, G.P. *The Ethno-Cultural Factor in Mental Health: A Literature Review and Bibliography*. New York: Institute on Plurism and Group Identity, 1977.

Greely, A.M. *The American Catholic*. New York: Basic Books, 1978.

Greely, A.M. "Creativity in the Irish Family: The Cost of Immigration," *International Journal of Family Therapy* 1:295–303, 1979.

Greely, A.M. *That Most Distressful Nation*. Chicago: Quadrangle, 1972.

Herz, F., and Rosen, E. "Family Therapy with Jewish Americans," in *Ethnicity and Family Therapy*. Edited by McGoldrick, M., et al. New York: Guilford Press, 1982.

Hines, P., and Boyd-Franklin, N. "The Black American Family," in *Ethnicity and Family Therapy*. Edited by McGoldrick, M., et al. New York: Guilford Press, 1982.

Kleinman, A., et al. "Culture, Illness and Care: Clinical Lessons from Anthropologic and Cross-Culture Research," *Annals of Internal Medicine* 88:251–58, 1978.

McAdoo, H. "Family Therapy in the Black Community," *American Journal of Orthopsychiatry* 47:75–79, 1977.

McGill, D., and Pearce, J.K. "Family Therapy with White, Anglo-Saxon Protestant Families," in *Ethnicity and Family Therapy*. Edited by McGoldrick, M., et al. New York: Guilford Press, 1982.

McGoldrick, M. "Ethnicity and Family Therapy: An Overview," in *Ethnicity and Family Therapy*. Edited by McGoldrick, M., et al. New York: Guilford Press, 1982.

McGoldrick, M., and Pearce, J.K. "Family Therapy with Irish Americans," *Family Process* 20:223–41, 1981.

McGoldrick, M., et al., eds. *Ethnicity and Family Therapy*. New York: Guilford Press, 1982.

Minuchin, S. *Families and Family Therapy*. Cambridge, Mass.: Harvard University Press, 1974.

Papajohn, J., and Spiegel, J. *Transactions in Families*. San Francisco: Jossey-Bass, 1975.

Preto, N.G. "Puerto Rican Families," in *Ethnicity and Family Therapy*. Edited by McGoldrick, M., et al. New York: Guilford Press, 1982.

Rotuno, M., and McGoldrick, M. "Family Therapy with Italian Americans," in *Ethnicity in Family Therapy*. Edited by McGoldrick, M., et al. New York: Guilford Press, 1982.

Stoeckle, J., et al. "The Quantity and Significance of Psychological Distress in Medical Patients," *Journal of Chronic Disease* 17:959–70, 1964.

Watzlawick, P. *How Real Is Real?* New York: Random House, 1976.

Zborowski, M. *People in Pain.* San Francisco: Jossey-Bass, 1969.

Zola, I. "Culture and Symptoms: An Analysis of Patients Presenting Complaints," *American Sociological Review* 5:141–55, 1966.

Zola, I.K. "Oh Where Oh Where Has Ethnicity Gone?" in *Ethnicity and Aging.* Edited by Gelfand, D.E., and Kutzik, A.J. New York: Springer Publishing Co., 1979.

Zuk, G.H. "A Therapist's Perspective on Jewish Family Values," *Journal of Marriage and Family Counseling* 4:101–11, 1978.

SECTION II

Assessing Families with Life-Threatening Illness

5 Assessing families of infants with biliary atresia

Sheila M. Kodadek, RN, PhD
Associate Professor
Department of Family Nursing
School of Nursing
The Oregon Health Sciences University
Portland, Oregon

OVERVIEW

Families of infants with biliary atresia face a life-threatening illness requiring early diagnosis and surgical intervention if the child is to survive more than 3 years. Since the required long-term postsurgical care is characterized by medical crises, usually in the form of cholangitis, long-term survival is uncertain. The family must learn quickly both how to provide the complex care their child needs and how to cope with the child's disease. Nurses working with such families can have a significant impact by accurately assessing family needs and addressing them when planning care.

Less than 30 years ago, biliary atresia meant death within the first 3 years. Today, the families of affected children still face the knowledge that their child's disease remains little understood, with treatment a recent, and still experimental, option. These families and their children are pioneers, with the hopes and fears, uncertainties, and risks that accompany dramatic new therapies.

NURSING PROCESS

Assessment

The health problem: Biliary atresia. Five to 10 of every 100,000 live-born infants have biliary atresia. Biliary atresia was once believed to be a congenital malformation of the bile ducts, of unknown cause and with no known treatment; the average survival of diagnosed infants was 1.5 to 2.5 years (Behrman and Vaughan, 1983). The accepted medical advice to parents was to take their infant home and provide as much love as they could for as long as he survived.

Over the past 25 years medical research has demonstrated that biliary atresia is not only treatable, but, in some cases, curable (Altman, 1981; Kasai, 1974; Lilly, 1984). Among the most significant research findings was that biliary atresia is a liver disease, with related extrahepatic ductal involvement (Altman, 1981). The disease process causes the bile ducts to become fibrotic and, as a result, not patent. When the bile cannot move from the liver into the intestine, it builds up in the liver, leading to cirrhosis. Atresic infants cannot digest fats or absorb selected nutrients, including fat-soluble vitamins.

Infants with biliary atresia present at 2 to 3 weeks of age with severe jaundice, dark urine, acholic stools, hepatomegaly, early signs of failure to thrive, and irritability. Current diagnostic procedures include serial percutaneous needle biopsies of the liver, duodenal aspiration for the presence of bile, and nuclear scans (Altman, 1981). If biliary atresia has not been ruled out, surgical exploration is indicated.

The more common surgical intervention is biliary reconstruction by hepatoportoenterostomy. In this procedure, fibrous tissue at the porta hepatis is used to construct a biliary intestinal anastomosis. This tissue is used because microscopically patent biliary channels have been found in this tissue, making possible a functional biliary passage (Altman, 1981).

This surgery succeeds only when performed before the 12th week of life because, it is hypothesized, the patent biliary structures at the porta are destroyed sometime around 3 months. Why this is so is not known (Altman, 1981). If the surgery is to be attempted, early referral and diagnosis are imperative.

Bile drainage in infants who have undergone atresia surgery, usually present by the 10th to 12th week of life, does not mean that the infant is cured (Altman, 1981). Complications are common and include failure of the bile to drain, jaundice in spite of bile drainage, hepatic impairment, cirrhosis and portal hypertension, and gastrointestinal hemorrhage from esophageal varices. The most serious problem is ascending cholangitis, which causes most of the complications. Further surgery is sometimes needed after a severe case of cholangitis to reestablish bile drainage (Lilly, 1984). When the original or subsequent surgeries fail, or the condition is diagnosed after 12 weeks, a liver transplant offers the only hope of cure.

Approximately 40% to 50% percent of children who have atresia surgery have survived 5 or more years (Behrman and Vaughan, 1983). Most have had cholangitis, some with severe related complications. The oldest survivors, now in their late teens and early twenties, are in Japan (Kobayashi et al., 1984). The extended prognosis for children who do well postsurgically remains largely unknown. The biggest unanswered question is, what will the existing liver damage mean as survivors enter adulthood?

Impact of the diagnosis on the family. Families of infants with biliary atresia face a crisis for which they will have had little or no preparation. Typically, no signs of the disease are present at birth. Usually, at the first well-child visit at 2 to 4 weeks, the family learns that its infant may be seriously ill. Because prompt surgery is required for atresia, liver and biliary function tests should begin immediately. If the results are positive, surgery should be scheduled as soon as possible. The diagnostic workup and surgery are usually done in several days.

Because corrective surgery is usually done at the time of the laparotomy, most parents are urged to decide on treatment before the initial surgery. If they choose nontreatment, death before age 3 is almost assured. (For some families, a liver transplant is presented as an initial possibility. However, this is a rare first choice because of the scarcity of available organs.) These families do not have the time to consider and decide. If they wait, they will lose one of their options.

With surgery, the family must first wait for bile drainage and then contend with the fear of cholangitis. The first year is crucial and requires a full-time commitment to the infant's care, with vigilant monitoring of vital signs and frequent trips to the clinic or hospital. When a child's temperature can soar in a matter of hours, as it will with cholangitis, even an afternoon out can be hazardous.

Ample documentation suggests these families need support managing their child's illness (Drotar et al., 1981; Green and Solnit, 1964; Koocher and O'Malley, 1981; Lascari and Stehbens, 1973; McCollum and Gibson, 1970). The diagnostic period is a time of particular family crisis. When parents permit the necessary testing, they must consider that their child may be seriously ill. They must first learn how to obtain information from health professionals or through independent research, then learn enough about diagnoses and diagnostic tests to communicate with others. They must learn to care for their newly vulnerable infant in an unfamiliar setting. And they must learn to manage their other responsibilities—other children, jobs, commitments—around his demands.

Making decisions about treatment is often difficult for families of children with life-threatening illnesses (Burton, 1975). For families of children with suspected biliary atresia, this difficulty is intensified by the limited time in which decisions must be made. Families must obtain knowledge and develop trust in health care providers quickly enough to make decisions that will determine both their child's future and their own.

Once surgical or palliative treatment begins, the family must cope with the biliary atresia and meet the ill child's needs while enhancing the growth and development of the entire family.

Besides learning how to provide basic care for their child, parents must learn the signs and symptoms of cholangitis, dietary restrictions, vitamin supplementation, medication administration and monitoring, and, in many cases, stoma management. They must learn how to communicate with health care providers and with family, friends, and strangers about their child's care, appearance, and prognosis. They must also obtain the support they need as parents of a child with a life-threatening disease and provide support for each other and all members of their family. They must learn to "normalize" their situation by allowing all family members to capitalize on their strengths and abilities. In sum, they must learn to live with a chronic life-threatening illness.

A model of family stress. A growing body of research explaining how families cope with acute or chronic stress contributes to nursing study and practice. Clinicians who care for families facing life-threatening illness know that the diagnosis does not necessarily cause a family crisis. In 1949, Hill proposed the classic ABCX model of family stress, in which the characteristics of the stressor event (A), the family's crisis-meeting resources (B), and definition of the stressor (C) all contribute to the prevention or precipitation of a family crisis (X). The ABC factors—the stressor event, crisis-meeting resources, and definition of the event—affect the family's vulnerability to crisis.

McCubbin and Patterson (1983) have expanded Hill's original work with what they call the Double ABCX Model, adding such postcrisis variables as the pileup of other family stresses that makes adaptation more difficult (aA), the social and psychological resources and coping strategies with which the family manages crisis (bB), the meaning the family assigns to the event (cC), and the range of positive and negative outcomes possible in family adaptation. Awareness of these factors can help nurses explore the family process after the initial crisis, especially as the family's care responsibilities move from acute to chronic management.

Family assessment. McCubbin and Patterson's expansion of the ABCX model suggests that the nursing assessment of families dealing with a child's life-threatening illness is affected by the families' experiences. An initial assessment provides valuable baseline data, but it must be continually updated as the family's experience changes, in response either to the illness or to other situational or developmental changes.

Any family assessment strategy should include interviews with as many family members as possible. For infants with biliary atresia, this may include parents, siblings, and grandparents. Relying on only one family member for group perceptions may be misleading; it is better to interview all members individually and, if possible, as a group (Safilios-Rothschild, 1969). When family members have differing perceptions of their situation, it helps to bring them together for discussion so they can either work toward resolving differences or capitalize on their diversities.

Accurate family assessment often hinges on the nurse's approach. The Calgary Family Assessment Model (Wright and Leahey, 1984) offers a nursing approach to the family that yields structural, developmental, and functional information. In assessing structure, the nurse can prepare with the family a genogram and ecomap. These two tools can reveal much about how the family perceives available social support. This ecomap information is critical for the family whose infant has biliary atresia because of the need for long-term assistance in care management, as well as acute management of cholangitic crises and the stress of a chronic illness with an uncertain prognosis.

The ecomap can help the nurse assess the family's emotional, social, and economic resources. Besides asking questions about living arrangements, the nurse should probe for specific examples of support. For example, she might ask: "How are you managing at home? At work? Do you have family who live nearby? Who can you call on for help during this time? How are you managing financially?"

Understanding a family's developmental level helps the nurse identify the concerns that must be addressed if the family is to fulfill overall developmental expectations. Specific to families of infants with biliary atresia are problems related to the infant's sudden illness as he is just being integrated into the family. First-time parents are learning their roles as parents; the same may be true of grandparents. It is challenging enough to learn how to be a parent, but to learn how to be a parent of a child with a life-threatening disease about which little is known can be very difficult.

Finally, family functional assessment can provide invaluable information about how the family might cope more effectively. In biliary atresia, the nurse must have current knowledge not only of the disorder, but of diagnostic protocols, treatment, and prognosis. With this background knowledge, the nurse can assess what the diagnosis means to the family and their ability to manage the crisis. Specifically, the nurse should ask family members what they know about biliary atresia, listening not only for factual information but also for what that information means to the family. In some cases, she must ask directly, "What do you know about biliary atresia? What does the diagnosis mean to you? What does the diagnosis mean to your wife/husband/other children/

parents/in-laws?" For most families, the diagnosis will be new and strange, but its impact will depend on how well they understand the diagnosis, how much they trust health care providers, whether they have extended family support, and other factors that may not become evident until later.

As suggested above, the nurse needs to consider the family status relative to the diagnosis (Mailick, 1979). In the early stages, before and after diagnosis, she should focus on assessing immediate informational needs for managing the crisis at home and work and for making decisions. Although the nurse should think ahead to needs associated with long-term management, the family generally functions "one day at a time." The nurse must ask *repeatedly* if the family has questions about the diagnosis, tests, treatment, and/or prognosis. In addition, the nurse should be alert to nonverbal signs of confusion or doubt. Families generally need to hear explanations over and over to deal with the reality of the unthinkable; assessment of this need is critical, and its importance cannot be overstated.

Once the diagnosis is established and treatment decisions made, the family moves into the chronic stage of disease management (Mailick, 1979). In this stage, daily care management is transferred from health care professionals to the family. At this point, the nurse needs to assess the family's ability to provide direct care and long-term management, its perception of the situation, and its adaptation to date (Pless and Pinkerton, 1975). Questions the nurse might ask include: "How have your arrangements for managing home and work been holding up? What are your plans for going home? Who will provide daily care at home? Who will communicate with health care professionals? If your baby needs medical attention, who will you call? If you need a babysitter, who could help you? How has your understanding of biliary atresia changed since you first learned your child might have it? What does caring for a child with biliary atresia mean for you and your family now? How do you think you/your family are doing relative to the diagnosis and care?"

Besides assessing the family's skills at providing direct care, the nurse can assess demonstrations of care by all potential caregivers. While this can ensure that safe care will be provided at home, it can also help assess family members' comfort with the necessary procedures.

Periodic assessment should continue for as long as the family provides care for its child. Although models sometimes suggest that family stress is a linear process with adaptation at the endpoint, clinical practice and research suggest a much more complex process (Lawrence and Lawrence, 1979; Pless and Pinkerton, 1975). In chronic conditions, family coping strategies and resources often change in response to family members' growth and development as well as to fatigue, changing needs, and other factors. Clinic visits or periodic hospitalizations provide ideal opportunities to ask the family such questions as: "How are things going now? What has changed for the family since we met last? What events do you anticipate that may require new ways of managing care?"

Assessing the quality of adaptation is difficult. The family members' definition of the situation and their personal comfort provide good barometers. If open communication, sensitivity to others' needs, reasonable conflict-resolving ability, and shared goals are apparent, family members are probably adjusting well. But if individual members show signs of stress, if communication is troubled or there are signs of unresolved conflict, diagnosis- and management-related problems may exist. Questions that may give clues to adaptation and family functioning include: "How much does the family know about your child's diagnosis? Prognosis? How are decisions made in the family about your child's care? What do you do if there are disagreements about care? What changes have family members made to accommodate care?" Being alert to signs of potential problems also helps. For example, when a grandparent says to the nurse, "Well, I just don't understand this. There's never been anything like this on our side of the family," this belief should be explored with both the grandparent and the family.

Planning

Most infants with biliary atresia are cared for by their families, at home. Nurses in such cases must do numerous things. They must train relatives until they are experts in the infant's illness-related care. They must help them develop strategies for nurturing an infant with a chronic and potentially fatal disease. They should encourage family members to recognize their own and the family's growth and development needs. They must also prepare the family to interact with various professionals.

Many nursing strategies support achievement of these goals. For a start, the nurse can support parenting and caregiving activities during diagnosis and early treatment by allowing the parents to "room in" and by managing hospital routines around those of the family when possible. Parents should be encouraged from the start to perform as much of their infant's care as they can. Parents who are uncertain about their abilities should be allowed to decide what they can handle. Although the hospital staff may be experts in biliary atresia, the parents are experts regarding the infant and should be acknowledged as such. Through support and practice and a plan for help at home, parents can develop expertise and confidence in giving care.

The nurse can foster healthy family and child adjustment by approaching the infant as a normal one who happens to have biliary atresia. By focusing on an infant's normal growth and development and by emphasizing his strengths and achievements, a family can incorporate the infant's diagnosis into its definition of "normal."

With regard to both caregiving and communicating with professionals, family members should receive verbal and written information about their infant's diagnosis and management. They should be urged to ask questions; their questions should be treated with respect and answered fully. Parents can learn to keep their own medical records of the child's care and lists of questions they wish answered. Some parents benefit from role playing—that is, rehearsing asking their infant's physician questions or talking with an older child about his sibling's illness.

Families may also need assistance in thinking through the day-to-day management of the illness. They need to know how to ask for help and from whom. They need to think about how they will respond to questions about their child's diagnosis, how they will prepare others for the child's appearance and care, and what they will need in terms of respite. Individual family members may also benefit from identifying their personal needs.

CASE STUDY

Mary Anne and Robert Sawyer are the parents of Sarah, a 2½ year-old, and Jason, 3 weeks old at the time of his diagnosis of biliary atresia. The Sawyers have been married for 5 years and recently bought their first home. Robert has a new job and Mary Anne has taken a leave from her career as an elementary schoolteacher to become a full-time wife and mother.

Jason was 3 weeks old when a stranger stopped Mary Anne in a grocery store and told her that Jason was "awfully yellow." Mary Anne had noticed that Jason's color was unusual but thought he would outgrow it. She was upset by the encounter and called her pediatrician, who agreed to see Jason that afternoon.

The pediatrician found Jason to be markedly jaundiced and to have gained only 2 ounces over his birth weight. Mary Anne reported that Jason was eager to nurse every 2 to 3 hours but seemed hungry soon after feedings. She also reported that his urine was dark and his stools acholic. The pediatrician told Mary Anne that Jason should be evaluated immediately at the University Hospital. An appointment with a pediatric gastroenterologist was made for the next morning. The specialist's examination confirmed Jason's pediatrician's findings—Jason had the signs and symptoms of biliary atresia.

Jason was admitted to the hospital directly from the clinic. The admitting nurse, who would be the Sawyers' primary nurse, was experienced in working with infants and their families. Using the sketchy family information on Jason's clinic chart, she asked Mary Anne if she would like to call her husband before the admission interview. She did, and Robert arranged to come to the hospital immediately.

Next, the nurse asked about Jason's sister. Mary Anne called the family friend who was caring for Sarah and made arrangements for the friend to watch Sarah until evening.

The nurse then began admission procedures, taking care not to begin any teaching until Robert arrived. Upon his arrival, the nurse gave the couple time alone with Jason before she began interviewing them and preparing them for the next few days. She asked Robert and Mary Anne what they knew about biliary atresia, encouraging them to ask questions whenever they wished. She gave them paper and pencil to keep a log of questions. She asked how they would manage the sudden hospitalization and suggested ways they could support each other and Sarah during this time. The nurse emphasized the importance for Jason and for them of continuing the care routines they had established at home. In general, she concentrated on information that would help the Sawyers understand what would happen and how they might manage in the short term; a knowledge of crisis intervention told the nurse that this was the time for essentials.

The next two days were anxious ones for the Sawyers. Mary Anne stayed with Jason in the hospital, taking advantage of the rooming-in option. Robert juggled work and caring for Sarah with visits to the hospital. Sarah spent her days with the family friend and talked frequently on the telephone with her mother.

Because test results continued to suggest biliary atresia, an exploratory laparotomy was scheduled for the third day of hospitalization. Jason's parents consented to corrective surgery if the diagnosis was confirmed.

The nurse might have scheduled formal interviews during these three days to learn about the Sawyer family and to prepare them for the future, but she chose instead to concentrate on specific short-term needs. She helped the Sawyers stay in contact as a family and suggested how they might help Sarah understand what was happening. She recognized the long trial that was ahead for the family and provided information that would help them both now and in the future.

As suspected, Jason did have biliary atresia, and corrective surgery was needed. The next few days after surgery were a time of regrouping for this family. The strategies that had helped them during the first three days could not function indefinitely. The nurse set up a series of meetings with the Sawyers to help them think through their situation.

In advanced nursing practice, assessment can also be intervention, and the nurse used the assessment to provide information and to help the Sawyers reevaluate their situation. During the first meeting, a genogram and ecomap were completed to help both the Sawyers and the nurse understand who might help them. The Sawyers explored developmental issues during the second session, focusing on the needs of both their children and what caring for Jason would mean to them. During this session the nurse asked the Sawyers what they thought Sarah understood about her brother's illness and how she was responding to the family's disruption. The nurse also asked about Jason's needs and helped Robert and Mary Anne look at ways to balance their parenting. The next two sessions focused on what the diagnosis meant to them, what resources they could call on, how they would make decisions about care, and how they would manage any future hospitalization.

Because the nurse had observed this family during a time of crisis, she could point to their strengths as a family and help them recognize their resources. She gave them an opportunity to test solutions to future problems, thus helping them plan for Jason's long-term care.

Care planning included the expectation of routine clinic visits and the possibility of frequent hospitalizations. The hospital-based primary nurse would be available by telephone and by appointment during clinic visits to assist the Sawyers as they learned to cope with the chronic phase of Jason's illness.

CONCLUSIONS

Nurses working with families of infants with biliary atresia can make a significant impact by recognizing the importance of the family in assessing and planning care. A nurse who understands family responses to stress and has skills in family interviewing can provide care that supports the infant's primary caretakers, the family.

REFERENCES

Altman, R.P. "Biliary Atresia," *Pediatrics* 68:896–98, 1981.

Behrman, R.E., and Vaughan, V.C. *Textbook of Pediatrics.* Philadelphia: W.B. Saunders Co., 1983.

Burton, L. *The Family Life of Sick Children: A Study of Families Coping with Chronic Childhood Disease.* London: Routledge and Kegan Paul, 1975.

Drotar, D., et al. "A Family-Oriented Supportive Approach to Renal Transplantation in Children," in *Psychological Factors in Hemodialysis and Transplantation.* Edited by Levy, N. New York: Plenum Press, 1981.

Green, M., and Solnit, A., "Reactions to the Threatened Loss of a Child: A Vulnerable Child Syndrome," *Pediatrics* 34:58–66, 1964.

Hill, R. *Families Under Stress.* New York: Harper & Row Pubs., 1949.

Kasai, M. "Treatment of Biliary Atresia with Special Reference to Hepatic Portoenterostomy and Its Modifications," *Progress in Pediatric Surgery* 6:5–52, 1974.

Kobayashi, A., et al. "Long-Term Prognosis in Biliary Atresia after Hepatic Portoenterostomy: Analysis of 35 Patients Who Survived Beyond 5 Years of Age," *Journal of Pediatrics* 105:243–46, 1984.

Koocher, G.P., and O'Malley, J. *The Damocles Syndrome: Psychological Consequences of Surviving Childhood Cancer.* New York: McGraw-Hill Book Co., 1981.

Lascari, A., and Stehbens, J. "The Reactions of Families to Childhood Leukemia: An Evaluation of a Program of Emotional Management," *Clinical Pediatrics* 12:210–14, 1973.

Lawrence, S.A., and Lawrence, R.M. "A Model of Adaptation to the Stress of Chronic Illness," *Nursing Forum* 18:33–42, 1979.

Lilly, J.R. "Biliary Atresia and Liver Transplantation: The National Institutes of Health Point of View," *Pediatrics* 74:159–60, 1984.

Lilly, J.R. "Hepatic Portoenterostomy (the Kasai Operation) for Biliary Atresia," *Surgery* 78:76–86, 1975.

Mailick, M. "The Impact of Severe Illness on the Individual and Family: An Overview," *Social Work in Health Care* 5:117–28, 1979.

McCollum, A.T., and Gibson, L. "Family Adaptation to the Child with Cystic Fibrosis," *Journal of Pediatrics* 77:574–78, 1970.

McCubbin, H.I., and Patterson, J.M. "The Family Stress Process: The Double ABCX Model of Adjustment and Adaptation," in *Social Stress and Family: Advances and Developments in Family Stress Theory and Research.* Edited by McCubbin, H.I., et al. New York: The Haworth Press, 1983.

Pless, I.B., and Pinkerton, P. *Chronic Childhood Disorders: Promoting Patterns of Adjustment.* Chicago: Year Book Medical Pubs., 1975.

Safilios-Rothschild, C. "Family Sociology or Wives' Family Sociology? A Cross-Cultural Examination of Decision Making," *Journal of Marriage and the Family* 32:290–301, 1969.

Wright, L.M., and Leahey, M. *Nurses and Families: A Guide to Family Assessment and Intervention.* Philadelphia: F.A. Davis Co., 1984.

6 Assessing families of children with sudden injuries

E. Juanita Lee, RN, MN, EdD

Assistant Professor
Department of Nursing
University of Southern California
Los Angeles, California

OVERVIEW

Near drowning is a life-threatening crisis. It affects not only the physical and emotional health of the victim but the psychosocial functioning of the family as well. This chapter documents the need for family involvement in such a situation, and it suggests theories and techniques the nurse can use to assess how well the family is coping with the problem. The case study examines the role of the nurse in working with a family whose child has suffered injuries from a near-drowning incident.

NURSING PROCESS

Assessment

The health problem: Near drowning. In the United States, more than 6,000 deaths from drowning occur each year (U.S. Census, 1984). It is the fourth most common cause of accidental deaths in adults. More than half of the drowning victims are children under age 10, and nearly 40% of the victims are under age 4. According to Dietz and Baker (1974), drownings occur seven to eight times as frequently in males as in females, with the greatest incidence occurring between April and September. Goldfrank and Mayer (1979) report that 60% to 70% of all childhood drownings occur in fresh water in swimming pools, lakes, and bathtubs. Twenty percent of the toddler and preschool drownings occur in the bathtub. Accurate statistics are not available for near drownings.

According to Modell (1971), drowning is death from suffocation in fluid; near drowning refers to surviving the physiologic effects of hypoxemia and acidosis that result from suffocation due to submersion in fluid.

There are several differences between the effects of freshwater and saltwater aspiration (Bennett, 1976; Caudle, 1976). When the victim inhales fresh water, alveolar surfactants are displaced or removed, and the fresh water passes rapidly into the vascular system through the alveolar membrane. When large amounts of fresh water are aspirated, a mild, transient hemodilution and increase in blood volume can occur. Hoff (1979) states that hemolysis of red blood cells and platelets may damage the pulmonary vascular beds, which can lead to pulmonary edema.

Saltwater aspiration may also interfere with alveolar surfactants; however, its predominant effect is pulmonary edema, since the hypertonic salt water draws more fluid from the vascular space into the alveoli. With this fluid shift, hemoconcentration and severe hypovolemia can occur.

Regardless of the type of water, severe pulmonary infections such as pneumonia and atelectasis can occur if the victim has aspirated vomitus, sand, or algae during the near-drowning episode.

Near drowning can also damage the victim's neurological system. According to Siebke (1975), the severity of neurological effects depends on the duration of hypoxemia and on the temperature of the water. Cold water submersion produces hypothermia prior to the hypoxic insult. Hypothermia may reduce the body tissue's need for oxygen and help victims, particularly children, survive a respiratory arrest.

Need for family involvement. A life-threatening crisis such as near drowning creates anxiety in the family. Therefore, assessing the family's coping skills is an essential part of treatment.

Stichler and Showman (1981) state that both child and family are victims of a near-drowning incident. Curtis (1983) found the period immediately following an accident to be one of particular uncertainty for them. She suggests assessing family needs at this time in order to help them cope with the crisis.

Besides the fears generated by the unexpected injury, hospitalization itself places stress on families. Smitherman (1979) and Hymovich (1976) point out that the family does not always receive the assistance it needs to weather a child's hospitalization. Parents with fears of their own about the accident often have trouble helping their children. A study by Knox and Hayes (1983) revealed that parents could describe their anxieties and the causes and effects of those anxieties on their families. The findings of the study indicated that anxious parents often had difficulty dealing with their children.

Before planning care for the child, the nurse needs to understand the family. Crummette (1983) emphasizes the need for family involvement in caring for the acutely ill adolescent. She suggests seven categories for assessing the family: constellation, roles, interaction patterns, copying styles and strategies, values and goals, resources, and adaptation prior to illness.

In a classic study, Breu and Dracup (1978) identified the special needs of the spouse of a critically ill patient; these same needs apply to the families of children who are critically injured. These needs are to experience relief of initial anxiety, to be informed of the child's condition, to be with the child, to be helpful to the child, to be assured of the child's comfort, and to have an avenue for venting concerns and anxieties.

Using crisis intervention theory, Warmbrod (1983) advocates supporting families of acutely ill patients. The nurse, she says, should assess the family's knowledge of the crisis, its coping skills, the support systems available to the family, and alternative coping skills/support system options.

In another study, Griffin (1980) identified the family's three priorities in acute illness or injury: securing medical care, maintaining essential family services (food and shelter), and supporting the patient. These findings also indicate that nurses should become more involved in the care of families.

Finally, Gardner and Stewart (1978) report that staff-family interaction in acute care settings benefits all concerned. Close staff-family relations lead to decreased anxiety, increased reassurance, increased cooperation, improved rapport, and improved patient care.

Approaches to family assessment: Five theories. Several theories are available to help a nurse assess the family of a child with a sudden and life-threatening injury such as near drowning. However, no one model provides all the information necessary for comprehensive assessment. Five theoretical frameworks for family assessment will be briefly presented in this chapter.

In the **Systems Model,** the family is viewed as a social system composed of two or more people who share a strong emotional bond and who live in the same household. As a social system the family is "open" and comprised of different interdependent components—its family members. An event that affects one member of the family affects the others as well. Relationships within the family are described as "subgroups." Each of these subgroups (spouse-spouse, sibling-sibling, parent-child) greatly influences the functioning of the family. Furthermore, the family interacts with a "suprasystem," or larger system, of schools and work settings, the health care delivery system, etc. The systems theory views the family as a social system with a specific structure and function.

The **Structural-Functional Model** views the family as simply one component of a greater social system. The family interacts with and contributes to the greater system, called "society." At the same time, society's institutions, norms, and values affect the socialization of the family. For example, a father's unemployment places a strain on the family. The term "family" refers to family members and their relationships to one another, such as sister-brother, parent-child, husband-wife. According to Friedman (1981), the functions of the family benefit its individual members, the family as a unit, and society. She groups these functions into six categories: affective functions, socialization functions, physical care functions, reproductive functions, economic functions, and family coping functions.

Friedman offers a modified structural-functional model consisting of four areas that the nurse should assess: identification of data, environmental data, family structure, and family function. She also proposes a cultural assessment of the family as an essential area of data collection.

A **developmental framework** has been used for years by pediatric nurses for assessing the physical, psychological, and social well-being of both healthy and sick children. The work of Duvall (1977) offers a guide to understanding family development across the life cycle. This guide identifies the following eight stages of family development:
• married couple
• childbearing families
• families with preschool children
• families with school-age children
• families with teenagers
• families as launching centers
• middle-aged families
• aging families.

Duvall defines the stage of family development in relation to the age of the oldest child. For example, a family with a newborn and a 10-year-old child would be in the school-age stage of the life cycle. Family development theory, as described by Duvall, is based solely on the nuclear family (parents and children) and is not particularly useful for the single-parent family or a childless couple. The advantage of this approach is its focus on the whole family as well as its members.

Terkelson (1980) has expanded family development theory to include unpredictable life events, such as life-threatening injury, illness, divorce, and unexpected death, to which a family must adapt. They differ from normal events; they are unexpected and alter the normal sequence of the family cycle. When these events occur, each member of the family develops a new need. Indeed, the needs of one member often clash with the needs of others. But eventually, the family adapts by developing new methods of interrelating.

Interaction/role theory focuses on roles and role relationships among family members. Each member holds positions within the family (husband-father, wife-mother) in addition to positions in society, such as adult, teacher, nurse, etc. A "position" means a place in the system, and "role" is defined as the pattern of goals, attitudes, feelings, and actions that accompany that position (Robischon, 1969). Each member of the family has multiple roles. For example, the patient is not only a child but also a daughter, sister, granddaughter, and student. Therefore, relationships between parents and children and husbands and wives can be assessed for a range of interactions. Since this approach focuses on members' interactions with each other, it can be used with all types of families regardless of ethnicity, size, or social status.

Crisis theory offers the nurse a framework for assessing stressful family situations (Caplan, 1969; Aquilera and Messick, 1974; Leavitt, 1984). According to Caplan, a crisis occurs when a family cannot apply its usual problem-solving methods to a situation or event. He defines crisis as a "time-limited period of disequilibrium precipitated by an inescapable demand to which the family is temporarily unable to respond adequately." During this period the family approaches the problem by developing new resources and turning to others so that it can return to a normal state.

The crisis model is the nurse's best approach for assessing families of children with near-drowning injuries because it focuses on the immediate problem and sets aside the myriad other problems that may exist, such as marital discord or financial problems. A near drowning affects the entire family and, to some extent, alters family members' roles, routines, and expectations of one another. The emotional upheaval of sudden injury, the financial pressures of hospitalization, and sometimes the guilt and blame of its members place the entire family under stress.

For the nurse, assessment is the first step in crisis theory. It involves collecting data related to the crisis and its effect on the patient and the family. The three areas of assessment are:
• identifying the accident and the family's perception of the accident and the child's injuries
• identifying the family's strengths and coping skills
• identifying the nature and strength of the family's support system (Goldstein, 1978).

In identifying the accident and its meaning to the family, the nurse should ask the following questions: "What happened? When did it happen? How does this affect your family life *now*?" The nurse assesses how the family perceives the problem and the cultural and social factors that influence those perceptions. In near drowning, parents may become suicidal or feel haunted by their "sin" (Stichler and Showman, 1981). The subject of loss is often expressed. The death of a child by drowning is probably one of the most difficult situations for parents to face since most drownings occur because of varying degrees of neglect on their part. According to Hoff (1979), parental guilt reactions to the drowning of a child can be very severe and may require psychiatric care for resolution of the grief. Once the assessment is complete, the planning process starts.

In determining the family's strengths and coping patterns, the nurse should ask the following questions: "Has anything like this happened before? How have you handled other situations like this? How do you usually cope with anxiety and tension?" According to Caplan (1969), the answers to these questions indicate ways in which the family resolves its problems.

In identifying sources of family support, the following questions may be asked: "Is there someone with whom your family is particularly close? Are there friends available to assist you?" "Support system" refers to the family's relationship with other people who might help. Absence of friends and/or community involvement may indicate a need for support from others with similar problems.

Family assessment tools. The nurse may use a variety of standard tools to collect data for the family assessment. These tools help the nurse organize data, but they themselves do not constitute a complete assessment. Data collection must be combined with observations and discussions with family members. Instruments that help obtain this data include the Feetham Family Functioning Survey (FFFS) and Otto's Family Strengths Assessment.

The FFFS, developed by Feetham and Humenick (1982), is one way to assess family functioning under stress. The tool is comprised of questions that address six areas of functioning:
• household tasks
• child care
• sexual and marital relations
• interaction with family and friends
• community involvement
• sources of support.

The FFFS is a self-reporting instrument that takes the respondent approximately 10 minutes to complete and pinpoints specific areas of dysfunction in a family with a seriously ill or injured child. By identifying a specific stressor, the nurse can then identify ways to alleviate that stress.

Many indicators of family functioning are measured by this tool. These include assistance from relatives, friends, and spouse; problems with other children; emotional support from spouse, friends, and relatives; satisfaction with marriage and sexual relations; and the amount of time spent with spouse and children in household tasks and recreational activities. The respondent rates statements describing each area on a scale ranging from 1 (little) to 7 (much) relative to the present situation and ideal situation, and the importance of each area. When the "important" score is compared with the "discrepant" score (difference between present and ideal), the nurse can identify the respondent's degree of satisfaction or dissatisfaction with family functioning and can plan accordingly.

Otto (1973) developed a framework for assessing family strengths. It can be used as a tool to identify family assets, which can then be used to enhance the family's functioning. The nurse should assess how well the family is able:
- to provide for the family's physical, emotional, and spiritual needs
- to communicate with each other
- to assume responsibility for child-rearing practices and discipline
- to provide support, security, and encouragement to family members
- to use a crisis as a means of growth
- to initiate and maintain growth-producing relationships and experiences in and outside the family
- to be flexible in family functions and roles
- to provide self-help and to accept help from others when necessary
- to recognize, respect, and treat each other as individuals
- to grow with and through children
- to maintain family unity, loyalty, and intrafamily cooperation
- to assume and maintain responsible community relationships.

Johnson (1979) points out that marital relationships, family support systems, religious beliefs, and the family's ability to communicate feelings with others all affect how a family will adjust to a near drowning. The nurse must consider other stressors such as separation, divorce, and unemployment. These may have contributed to the unintentional injury.

Planning

Following a complete assessment of the family and the formulation of nursing diagnoses, the nurse works with the family to determine goals and interventions. Ideally, the goals should reflect the family's values and beliefs and be realistic and achievable. The entire family should be given the opportunity to ask questions and make suggestions related to the care plan. For example, if young children are involved, the nurse should explain situations using language appropriate to their level of understanding. The nurse organizing the care of the family should arrange to talk with teenage children separately. In many cases, teen-agers are more willing to discuss their concerns with an adult outside the family. However, talking with parents first may provide the nurse with insight into the family relationships.

When children survive drowning but suffer severe neurological dam-age, it can be agonizing for parents. The parents' initial joy and relief because the child survived are replaced with guilt, grief, and perhaps an inevitable desire for the child to die. Memories of their previously healthy child are replaced by the grim reality of a child with neurologi-cal damage. Also, previously supportive family members may be so affected by guilt and grief that they become hostile to each other and/ or to the nursing staff. Thus, the nurse must use all resources available to help the family cope with guilt and grief. These resources may include family, friends, neighbors, and various professional staff.

While planning interventions for families, the nurse must encourage the parents to continue normal parenting behaviors. The child's condition can cause parents to feel anger and frustration, and many parents repress such feelings because they are psychologically and socially "unacceptable." These repressed feelings, however, can alter normal parenting behavior. For example, parents who would normally set appropriate limits for the child's behavior might relax discipline and permit him to manipulate other family members. Parents who are over-burdened with the care of a disabled child sometimes become overpro-tective and encourage dependence rather than self-care. This behavior affects the disabled child and the parents' relationships with other children in the family. By helping parents identify appropriate and inap-propriate demands from the child and by teaching them to respond appropriately, the dependence cycle can be broken.

With the implementation of diagnostic-related groups (DRGs), in which hospitals receive a fixed amount of dollars from the government for a patient's particular illness, hospitals are offering more outpatient services and discharging patients more rapidly to reduce costs. For the child who survives drowning but suffers severe neurological dam-age, the cost of health care can be great. The survival places physical, financial, and emotional burdens on the family. Since nurses have 24-hour access to the patient, they can monitor the child's progress closely. They can ensure that hospital stays are shortened through early dis-charge planning and patient/family education. To make certain that the patient will be discharged to a safe environment, the nurse collaborates with the physician and the home health nurse. Depending on the type of assistance required (skilled nursing equipment, rehabilitation), the nurse teaches the family how to care for the patient prior to discharge. In the case of a near drowning, water safety, injury, and injury prevention instructions are given to the family by the nurse, and the family begins participating in the patient's care before leaving the hospital.

CASE STUDY

Pattie is a 3-year-old black female who has been admitted to the pediatric unit with a diagnosis of near drowning. She is accompanied by her mother. The data for this assessment were obtained through observation of and interviews with the family upon admission to the hospital.

Assessment

Family structure and function. This nuclear family consists of father Leroy, age 37, mother Dorothy, age 35, three sons ages 11, 10, and 1 year, and one daughter age 3 years. A grandmother lives approximately 10 miles away. Leroy is a physician and the primary source of financial support. Dorothy is a homemaker. Although she is a registered nurse, she does not work outside the home. The two school-age boys attend the neighborhood elementary school, and the 1-year-old son and the 3-year-old daughter are home with the mother during the day.

Household. The family lives in a five-bedroom home in an upper-middle-class neighborhood in the city. They also own a duplex located in a nearby city where Leroy's mother resides. The parents were born in Jamaica and immigrated to the United States 12 years ago. Both parents and the siblings of the patient are in good health. The family has relatives in New York and Jamaica; only the grandmother lives nearby.

Interaction with family and friends. The grandmother visits with the family at least once a week. Social engagements with friends occur rarely, but Dorothy is friendly with many of the women in her neighborhood.

Community involvement. Leroy is involved in the local medical association. Dorothy is active in the church and the parent-teacher association.

Other resources. The family has a private physician and is covered by private health insurance. There are no major economic concerns.

Problems Identified

Near drowning. Dorothy was home at the time of the incident. She says the child opened the sliding screen door to the outside and accidentally fell into the pool while the mother was talking on the telephone to a neighbor. The mother called the ambulance, provided the initial cardiopulmonary resuscitation, and accompanied the child to the hospital. A neighbor remained in the home with the mother's infant. Leroy and the other children were away at the time of the incident. At the hospital, emergency management included assisted ventilation and placement in the intensive care unit.

Marital difficulties. The parents explained that for the past few months they have argued with increasing frequency. Minor disagreements apparently end in a major argument. The father's demanding profession leaves very little time for him to be with the family. The couple states, with some reservations, that sexual relations have been satisfactory although the warmth of daily communication through touch is gone.

Planning

The nursing diagnosis for this family is potential parental distress related to the family crisis. The short-term goals for the family are:
• The family members will be able to communicate their feelings about the accident.
• The parents will be supported.

The long-term goal is to enable the family to cope with the crisis of the accidental injury. The interventions, rationales, and criteria for evaluation are presented in the accompanying care plan.

The Anderson Family Nursing Care Plan

Nursing Interventions	*Rationales*
• Encourage family members to express their feelings, such as guilt. The nurse may ask, "This must be a difficult time for you. What was it like for you when you found her?"	• Verbalizing feelings helps the family begin to adapt to the crisis situation.
• Empathize with the family's sense of loss and anxiety about the child's recovery. The nurse may say, "You took positive action in conducting CPR at the scene."	• Empathetic listening comforts members in their grief and uncertainty.
• Answer questions sensitively but realistically. The nurse may say, "We have a tube in Pattie's throat and it's connected to a machine which is breathing for her." Repeat information as necessary, and explain all procedures.	• Accurate information helps prevent misconceptions and fear.
• Encourage the family to participate in the child's care and to comfort the child. The nurse may say, "Feel free to touch Pattie or hold her hands."	• Interacting with the child and assisting in care reduce the parents' feelings of helplessness and reaffirm the parent-child relationship.
• Refer the family to a counselor, as necessary. The nurse may say, "We have several chaplains available. Would you like me to call one for you?"	• Encourage the use of additional resources for coping or being assisted by others.

Evaluation: The family demonstrates adaptive coping behaviors.

CONCLUSIONS

Sudden, life-threatening injuries can occur at any time. They affect the lives of family members by altering their roles, routines, and expectations of each other. The emotional upheaval of sudden injury places the entire family under stress. Crucial to decreasing the stress and resolving the crisis is the quality of the nursing service and the compassion of the nurses. The case study offers a means of exploring the role of the nurse in working with families of children with grave injuries. In the case presented, the family did not view the care of the child as a burden. Instead, the care was seen as a family responsibility, and the family preferred rehabilitation of its disabled child at home rather than in an extended care facility.

REFERENCES

Aquilera, D., and Messick, J. *Crisis Intervention: Theory and Methodology.* St. Louis: C.V. Mosby Co., 1974.

Bennett, R. "Drowning and Near-Drowning: Etiology and Pathophysiology," *American Journal of Nursing* 76:919–21, 1976.

Breu, C., and Dracup, K. "Helping the Spouses of Critically Ill Patients," *American Journal of Nursing* 78:50–53, 1978.

Caplan, G. *Principles of Preventive Psychiatry.* New York: Basic Books, 1969.

Caudle, J. "Emergency Nursing of Near-Drowning Victims," *American Journal of Nursing* 76:922–23, 1976.

Crummette, B. "Assessing the Impact of Illness upon an Adolescent and Family," *Maternal-Child Nursing Journal* 12:155–67, 1983.

Curtis, N. "Caring for Families During the Unknown Period," *Dimensions of Critical Care Nursing* 2:248–54, 1983.

Dietz, P., and Baker, S. "Drowning: Epidemiology and Prevention," *American Journal of Public Health* 64:303–11, 1974.

Duvall, E. *Family Development.* Philadelphia: J.B. Lippincott Co., 1977.

Feetham, S., and Humenick, S. "The Feetham Family Functioning Survey," in *Analysis of Current Assessment Strategies in the Health Care of Young Children and Childbearing Families.* Edited by Humenick, S. East Norwalk, Conn.: Appleton-Century-Crofts, 1982.

Friedman, M. *Family Nursing—Theory and Assessment.* East Norwalk, Conn.: Appleton-Century-Crofts, 1981.

Gardner, D., and Stewart, N. "Staff Involvement with Families of Patients in Critical Care Units," *Heart & Lung* 7:1–3, 1978.

Goldfrank, L., and Mayer, G. "Salt and Fresh Water Drowning," *Hospital Physician* 15:32–39, 49, 1979.

Goldstein, D. "Crisis Intervention: A Brief Therapy Model," *Nursing Clinics of North America* 13:657–63, 1978.

Griffin, J. "Physical Illness in the Family," in *Family-Focused Care.* Edited by Miller, J., and Janosick, E. New York: McGraw-Hill Book Co., 1980.

Hoff, B. "Multisystem Failure: A Review with Special Reference to Drowning," *Critical Care Medicine* 7:310–20, 1979.

Hymovich, D. "Parents of Sick Children: Their Needs and Tasks," *Pediatric Nursing* 5:9, 1976.

Johnson, S. *High Risk Parenting: Nursing Assessment and Strategies for the Family at Risk.* Philadelphia: J.B. Lippincott Co., 1979.

Knox, J., and Hayes, V. "Hospitalization of a Chronically Ill Child: A Stressful Time for Parents," *Issues in Comprehensive Pediatric Nursing* 6:217–26, 1983.

Kruger, S., et al. "Reactions of Families to the Child with Cystic Fibrosis," *Image* 12:67–72, 1984.

Leavitt, M. *Families at Risk: Primary Prevention in Nursing Practice.* Boston: Little, Brown & Co., 1982.

Leavitt, M. "Nursing and Family-Focused Care," *Nursing Clinics of North America* 19:83–87, 1984.

Miller, J., and Janosik, E. "Evaluation of Family Progress," in *Family-Focused Care*. Edited by Miller, J., and Janosik, E. New York: McGraw-Hill Book Co., 1979.

Modell, J. *The Pathophysiology and Treatment of Drowning and Near-Drowning*. Springfield, Ill.: C.C. Thomas, 1971.

Otto, H. "A Framework for Assessing Family Strengths," in *Family-Centered Community Nursing: A Sociocultural Framework*. Edited by Reinhardt, A. St. Louis: C.V. Mosby Co., 1973.

Robischon, P. "Role Theory and Its Application in Family Nursing," *Nursing Outlook* 17:52–57, 1969.

Satir, V. *Conjoint Family Therapy*. Palo Alto, Calif.: Science and Behavior Books, 1967.

Siebke, H. "Survival after 40 Minutes' Submersion Without Cerebral Sequelae," *Lancet* 1:1275–77, 1975.

Smilkstein, G. "The Family APGAR: A Proposal for a Family Function Test and Its Use by Physicians," *Journal of Family Practice* 6:1231–39, 1978.

Smitherman, C. "Parents of Hospitalized Children Have Needs Too," *American Journal of Nursing* 79:1423, 1979.

Stichler, J., and Showman, T. "A Child Drowns: A Nursing Perspective," *Maternal-Child Nursing* 6:324–28, 1981.

Terkelson, K. "Toward a Theory of the Family Life Cycle," in *The Family Life Cycle: A Framework for Family Therapy*. Edited by Carter, E., and McGoldrick, M. New York: The Gardner Press, 1980.

U.S. Bureau of Census. *Statistical Abstract of the United States*. Washington, D.C.: Department of Commerce, 1984.

Von Bertalanffy, L. *Robots, Men and Minds*. New York: Braziller, 1967.

Warmbrod, L. "Supporting Families of Critically Ill Patients," *Critical Care Nurse* 3:49–52, 1983.

<table>
<tr><td rowspan="1">7</td><td>

Assessing families of school-aged children with cancer

</td></tr>
</table>

Debra B. Rose, RN, MS, PNP
Clinical Research Associate
Triton Biosciences Inc.
Alameda, California

OVERVIEW

This chapter describes the nursing process used to assess and plan care for the family of the school-age child with cancer. Current information concerning this health problem is included.

The need for a family approach when assessing the management of a cancer-afflicted child is also explored. References to current theories, research findings, and available tools are presented. The author describes her own conceptual method for the spiral of family health, coping, and development as a basis for understanding and developing the nurse's role.

The process for planning nursing care examines the nurse's role as well as health care delivery trends. The chapter concludes with a case study that illustrates the concepts and theories described.

NURSING PROCESS

Assessment

The health problem: Childhood cancer. Childhood cancer, once regarded as an acute, invariably fatal disease, is now viewed as a life-threatening chronic illness (Koocher and O'Malley, 1981; Ruccione and Ferguson, 1984).

In children under age 15, the 5-year survival rate for all forms of cancer has been estimated to be greater than 84% (Krulik, 1982). In 1983, American Cancer Society estimates revealed 6,100 cases of cancer in such children with mortality of 2,300 (Sutow, 1984). Leukemia remains the most lethal chronic childhood disease (Harkey, 1983).

Despite advances in diagnosis and treatment, cancer accounted for 13% to 15% of all deaths of children aged 5 to 14 in 1984 (Sutow,

1984). It is the leading cause of death in this age population, exceeding accidents. Children are particularly prone to developing second or third tumors, and to late relapses (Van Eys, 1977). Also prevalent are such difficult-to-treat cancers as brain tumors, or those which require such intensive care interventions as bone marrow transplants.

Common childhood cancers. Leukemias, brain tumors, and lymphomas account for 63% of all childhood malignancies (Sutow, 1984). Symptoms of acute lymphoblastic leukemia include fatigue, bone pain, weight loss, unexplained fever, and bleeding. Physical examination often reveals hepatosplenomegaly accompanied by lymphadenopathy. Bone marrow aspiration is a key diagnostic procedure, allowing differentiation of affected cell types. If the child's white blood cell count exceeds 50,000 (initially), the prognosis is guarded.

Advanced treatments, including use of monoclonal antibodies, bone marrow transplants, and granulocyte transfusions in conjunction with chemotherapy, have produced longer remissions with fewer complications, however. The overall 5-year childhood cancer survival rate approaches 90% (Pegelow, 1983).

In the case of osteosarcomas, the addition of high-dose chemotherapies to childhood treatment regimens has led to a 90% disease-free survival ratio (Wilbur, 1983). Other types of malignant neoplasms often seen in children include Ewing's sarcoma, retinoblastoma, Wilms' tumor, neuroblastoma, and rhabdomyosarcoma. Ruccione and Ferguson (1984) estimate that, "by the late 1980s, 1 in 1,000 individuals reaching the age of 20 will be a survivor of childhood cancer."

Physiological sequelae of treatment. Physiological changes in many organ systems can occur as late sequelae of treatment protocols (see Table 7.1). Nurses must be aware of these changes in order to assess the full impact of the illness on the child and family.

Need for a family approach. If a family's purpose is to help individuals meet changing needs (Kaplan et al., 1973), children cannot be treated in isolation from their families; therefore, effective nursing assessments take the family approach. Reciprocal relationships must be recognized (Doherty, 1985); indeed, reciprocity is central to an assessment model presented later in this chapter. As Doherty has observed, "a corresponding opportunity emerging from the modern development of a better-trained and more confident nursing profession is the greater leadership nurses are taking in family-centered health care." Therefore, nursing assessments must consider a range of family variables.

Prior research (Krulik, 1982; Kupst et al., 1984; Sabbeth, 1984; Barbarin et al., 1985; Koch, 1985) has focused on a number of these variables: developmental status (physical and emotional) in relation

Table 7.1 Summary of Organ System Disruption Associated with Childhood Cancer Treatments

System	Physiological Changes
Musculoskeletal	Shortness Scoliosis and/or kyphosis Increased susceptibility to fractures Bone pain Osteoporosis
Endocrine	Selective growth hormone deficiency Pituitary ablation Hypo- or hyperthyroidism Thyroid nodules Infertility Gonadal hormone abnormalities
Neurological	Leukoencephalopathy Neuropathy: central (affecting gray matter) or peripheral (affecting extremities) Neuropsychologic dysfunction
Respiratory	Pneumonitis Pulmonary fibrosis
Gastrointestinal	Nausea/vomiting, weight loss Strictures Obstruction Enteritis, ulceration Malabsorption Hepatic fibrosis Cirrhosis Portal hypertension
Urinary	Nephritis Chronic cystitis Renal dysfunction
Skin	Radiation burns Rashes
Miscellaneous	Sensory deficits (vision, hearing, speech) Dental abnormalities Immunosuppression (anemias) Surgical deformity (for example, amputation) Alopecia

to the illness, communication, family strengths and roles, and stress associated with chronic illness.

Coping is a predominant issue (Spinetta et al., 1981), since numerous and often conflicting demands, coupled with restrictions imposed by the disease itself, influence development. A delicate balance exists between family needs, developmental tasks, and chronic illness (Robinson, 1985), making forced change particularly disruptive.

Spinetta et al. (1981) examined 23 sets of parents coping effectively with the death from cancer of a child. In these cases, communication consistent with the child's age and developmental level allowed continuing expression of both positive and negative feelings during the illness. A support system, or simply a single significant other, as well as a consistent theology or philosophy of life, also appeared important in effective coping. Neither the child's age nor sex seemed significant.

A recent study (Kupst et al., 1984) of families with a child 5 years post–cancer diagnosis revealed ineffective coping in the presence of multiple problems, such as poor marital or family relationships, weak support systems, and closed or distorted communication. These family variables significantly affected fulfillment of the child's psychosocial and physiological needs.

Other authors have described sibling reactions as an important determinant of the impact of cancer on the child-patient and family. One consequence of directing available resources to the ill child is the aggravation of ambivalence in a sibling (Siemon, 1984).

Beardslee and Neff (1982) emphasized the need to evaluate the personal meanings of disease for children in terms of their strengths and concerns rather than their vulnerabilities. Perception of the illness by both children and families involves assigning specific meanings to the conditions, several researchers have noted (Van Eys, 1977; Anderson, 1981; Kupst et al., 1982; Zurlinden, 1985). Although the medical prognosis in childhood cancer has changed over the past two decades, "the initial emotional meaning of the diagnosis, for many parents, remains much the same" (Koocher and O'Malley, 1981). However, a different approach views the child, according to Wilbur (1983), as one who is "going to do well, unless proven otherwise."

Studies of illness perception have also described such issues as preparing the child for hospitalization. Various authors, including Rutter (1981), have stated that children are affected as much by parental attitudes toward hospitalization as by hospital procedures or routines. Therefore, nursing assessments need to include information about parental as well as children's outlooks.

Successful family assessment takes into account the feelings and needs of *all* members. This author has encountered a range of needs and attitudes among parents, siblings, and children facing hospitalization during the terminal stages of leukemia and solid tumors. Although families provide comfort and reassurance for the young patient, the school-age child with a life-threatening illness sometimes finds more relief from his fears in the knowledge that familiar physicians and nurses, as well as emergency equipment, are nearby. The increased availability of hospice care allows many children in the terminal phase of cancer to remain at home.

Whether at home or in the hospital, a child's coping abilities are influenced by developmental issues and illness severity. Early research by Spinetta (1977) validated Waechter's observations of higher anxiety levels in children with life-threatening illnesses. Twenty-five 6- to 10-year-old leukemia patients were compared to 25 children of the same ages with diabetes, asthma, and renal and heart defects. The cancer patients were more preoccupied with threats to bodily integrity and function than were the controls. However, since family function has been shown to influence a child's coping capacity as much as the disease itself does (Whitt, 1984), a complete nursing assessment of such cases incorporates the family's effect.

Family assessment models and tools. Many approaches to family assessment have developed in conjunction with theories regarding stress and the crises, roles, development, systems, communications, and conflicts of family life. Interaction and social learning theories have also been applied to nursing practice.

Other approaches to assessment use tools based on specific strengths (Welch et al., 1982) and, more recently, on coping strategies (Miles and Carter, 1985). Such tools may have been developed for use in one setting, such as the pediatric intensive care unit, or with one group of chronically ill children, and may or may not be useful for oncology patients.

Another important question is the reliability/validity of the assessment model: is the instrument sensitive to family health problems in childhood cancer? Tools developed by the Pediatric Ambulatory Care Treatment Service (Stein and Jessop, 1982) were designed for families of children with a variety of chronic illnesses, including cancer. For example, the *Clinician's Overall Burden Index* incorporated the medical and nursing tasks that parents face, the disruption in family routines, the fixed deficits in the child necessitating changed parental behavior and activities, and the psychological burden of the prognosis. The child's sleeping, eating, and elimination habits are assessed in the *Functional*

Status Measure. Both of these tools have been used in the school-age cancer population.

McCubbin and associates (1982) used healthy families to develop assessment tools of potential relevance to families of children with cancer. Stress, vulnerability, resources, support systems, esteem, communication, mastery, health, and (parental) coping are among the assessed concepts.

Reliable assessment tools address physiological, psychological, or cognitive issues at different times. The selection of any tool is based upon prior knowledge as well as current information about the family.

Table 7.2 Family Assessment Tools

Instrument	Type	Purpose
Family Impact	Structured interview	Evaluates impact of childhood illness on family
Family Environment Scale	Structured interview	Assesses social environment (to differentiate disturbed and normal families in terms of interpersonal relationships, growth, and organization)
McMaster Family Assessment Device	Structured interview	Screens for family health; measures problem solving, communication, roles, affective responsiveness involvement, behavior, and overall function
Chronicity Impact and Coping Instrument: Parent Questionnaire	Parent questionnaire	Assesses parents' experience coping and caring for a chronically ill child
Family Apgar	Closed-end questionnaire	Screens for overview of adaptability; partnership, growth, differentiation, and resolve
Family Function Index	Semistructured interview	Evaluates psychological adjustment of healthy and chronically ill children
Family Adaptability and Cohesion Evaluation Scale II	Self-report	Measures cohesiveness, adaptability, and social desirability

Adapted from Speer & Sachs, 1985.

Nurses must try to assess such factors as language skill and cognitive development (Hodges et al., 1982), as well as family structure, roles, and individual perceptions of family function (Barnard, 1984). Appropriate tools exist for decoding most of these variables, but such concepts as family function have so many meanings that they are beyond measure.

For a more detailed analysis of how to choose an assessment tool, the reader is referred to relevant chapters in nursing research texts (Polit and Hungler, 1978; Skodol-Wilson, 1985). Several pertinent tools are summarized in Table 7.2.

Reliability	Ages	Author(s)
Internal consistency data, alpha coefficients of .60 to .88 reliability and validity; studies in progress	Mixed	Stein and Reissman
Test/retest .68 to .86; internal consistency of .64 to .70	Mixed	Moos and Moos
.72 to .92 internal consistency	Mixed	Epstein, Baldwin, and Bishop
Field testing; item/total of test/retest, internal consistency of .83; split half of .93	Mixed	Hymovich
Test/retest of .83, split half of .93	Mixed	Smilkstein
.72 interspouse reliability still being evaluated	School	Pless and Satterwhite
Test/retest .84, split half .78 to .90	Mixed	Olson, Russell, and Sprenkle

The Spiral of Family Health, Coping, and Development: A Conceptual Framework

Several assumptions form the basis of this model, among them:
- The client family is within the childbearing, child-rearing years.
- Ongoing changes in family dynamics affect certain family developmental processes over time.
- Actual concepts are dynamic, fluid, interrelated, and vary according to stages in the family's life cycle (Otto, 1973).
- Changes occur according to four principles (Rogers, 1970):

    Reciprocity. Interactions between people and their environment cause repatterning of both.

    Synchrony. Changes depend on the respective states of people and their environment (at any given moment).

    Helicy. Life processes are rhythmic probabilities—sequential, innovative, and diverse, but organized.

    Resonance. Patterns of change are wavelike.

Processes. At the core of the spiral framework depicted in Figure 7.1 is an assessment of all family physical and emotional needs. In this instance, the family meets Hymovich's (1974) definition: "a group of two or more individuals living together and interacting with one another through mutually defined roles." Interactions within such units provide individual support and encouragement through communication and modeling processes.

Communication has been defined in part as a "behavioral process based on shared symbols whereby meanings are conveyed and interpreted among social interactants" (Meleis, 1975). To be more explicit, "positive communication skills (for example, empathy, reflective listening, supportive comments) enable couples and families to share with each other their changing needs and preferences as related to cohesion and adaptability." (Olson et al., 1983).

Modeling is defined as an observational type of vicarious learning. Individuals have a tendency to reproduce actions, attitudes, or emotional responses seen in real life or in symbolic models.

Strengths. Family strengths develop from the previously described family processes. Strengths have been defined as "factors or forces that contribute to family unity, solidarity, and that foster the development of the potentials inherent within the family" (Otto, 1973). Family strength has several dimensions, including competence in problem solving (to be discussed later) and group pride. The latter manifestation requires mutual respect, trust, and loyalty and provides a basis for shared values and attitudes, such as optimism (Olson et al., 1983) and cooperation (in relationship to decision making, particularly regarding child rearing).

Figure 7.1 The Spiral of Family Health, Coping, and Development

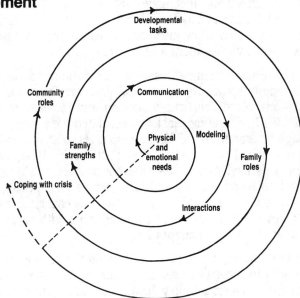

Roles. Over time, roles are clarified by expectations, rituals, and shared meanings. Primarily, however, roles depend on prior experience. The interactionalist view of role theory interprets a role as something learned from others and as a function of position or status. A role is not "merely a set of behaviors or expected behaviors but a sentiment or goal which provides unity to a set of potential actions" (Meleis, 1975). Behavioral expectations or roles may also be defined in terms of developmental tasks (Rowe, 1966). In that context, family roles provide a mechanism for balancing interpersonal interactions against intrapersonal needs (Janosik and Miller, 1979), and thus are reciprocal.

Conflict and coping. Any conflict contains the potential for developmental crisis—that is, an interruption of necessary tasks. When and if the crisis is averted, growth continues.

Crisis situations produce, and often arise from, stress, which in itself may unravel the spiral of development. In fact, vulnerability occurs when there is a "variation in the family's ability to prevent a stress or event of changes in a family system from creating some crisis" (Holaday, 1984).

Problem-solving strategies—in other words, coping styles—allow families to overcome crises and further their development. But families must implement these strategies as a unit. If parents take opposing positions at an early stage in the coping process, the entire unit's coping ability is jeopardized (Aguilera and Messick, 1974).

One of the keys to successful adaptation/conflict resolution is the mastery of problem-solving techniques (Spinetta, 1977) derived from family roles and interactions both at home and in the community (Hill, 1965). These techniques allow members to reason out the answers to questions on their own (Aguilera and Messick, 1974).

Nursing implications. Nursing assessment and planning occur at every phase of the family spiral. Recognition of prior family coping strategies is essential. Unresolved conflicts compound and increase tensions (Pless et al., 1972), including tensions associated with illness. For a more thorough interpretation of family responses to stress and coping, the reader is referred to McCubbin and Patterson's (1983) double ABCX model. This model describes an event or stressor (A) interacting with the family's resources (B) and the family's perception of the event (C) to produce a crisis (X). The double component allows for the addition of preexisting A's, B's, and C's interacting with coping methods to produce adaptation or maladaptation.

Although the nursing assessment focuses on the coping process, nurses also need to recognize existing strengths and become aware of how family members negotiate key developmental transitions (Drotar, 1981).

Assessing knowledge of planned procedures. Nurses need to determine whether or not the child-patient wants to know more about his illness and when it would be most valuable to inform him. Children's views on cancer are best understood from a developmental perspective. Children, like adults, attempt to integrate changes in their personal reality with their newly developing values and beliefs. It is important to assess their capacities and expectations.

"Cognitive coping strategies" are one aspect of the "response range" (Ross and Ross, 1984) that must be assessed in children with leukemia. An accurate, helpful nursing history in such cases should include information relevant to the child's overall level of functioning and address physiological, psychological, and cognitive issues (see Table 7.3).

Anderson (1981) reports that one parent compared the procedures and treatments necessary for her child's cancer to necessary, daily hygiene practices. This helped the child to appreciate the continuing need for interventions.

Questions to ask the child. Most nurses find it helpful to ask questions regarding the child's knowledge of planned procedures. Even very general questions can be useful; for example, Dorn (1984) suggested asking siblings as well as cancer victims, "What do you think is making _____ sick?" Other examples are, "How is your day different from days before diagnosis or treatment?" (Ahmann, 1984) or "What do you

Table 7.3 Assessing a School-Aged Child with Cancer

Illness/Treatment-Related Stressors (Inpatient/Outpatient)	Issues		
	Physiological	*Psychological*	*Cognitive*
Separation from family/peers	Alteration in daily activity patterns, gross and fine motor coordination, balance, and strength, as well as sleep habits	Changes in communication and interaction patterns, possibility of isolation	Changing awareness of time (past and future)
Disrupted school attendance	Interference with basic learning skills (perceptual, motor, language, and memory); possibility of delays	Changes in problem-solving abilities and attention span (confusion regarding classroom explanations, impaired capacity to enjoy school and tasks); changed self/body image related to need for prosthetic devices (wigs for hair loss, crutches or artificial limbs)	Changes in cause/effect relationships, logic and abstract reasoning, concept formation and organization (categorizing, serializing, conserving, reversing); increasing familiarity with bodily and organ functions/processes
Increased contact with health care providers	Changes in living space/distance between self and others	Fear of losing control, increased dependence on others	Increasing familiarity with authority figures (members of treatment team)

usually do when you are in a new place with different kinds of things?" (Zurlinden, 1985). The last question aims at assessing the child's or sibling's reaction to numerous clinic visits or hospitalization.

Other questions for nurses to ask children and siblings may pertain to their understanding of health, bodily functions, and illness. For instance, what is their understanding of cancer and its progress? Exploring issues of fairness and responsibility can also be useful (Siemon, 1984).

Assessing prior coping strategies. A 5-year study of families of children with leukemia and meningitis (Schulman, 1983) raised the issue of variations in reactions *over time.* One of the findings was that "approximately 85% of the families coped very well." The definition of coping, however, required a history of prior good coping, which apparently excluded families with poorly developed skills.

Questions to ask the family. The nurse assessing family members dealing with childhood cancer might ask what has helped them cope with the disease and its treatment, which problem has been most difficult and how they have resolved it, and whether their approach has been effective or ineffective.

One assessment of prior successful coping strategies was described to the author by the father of a 6-year-old receiving intravenous chemotherapy for relapsed leukemia. When this patient was initially diagnosed and treated at age 3, he overcame his fear of the painful blood transfusions associated with chemotherapy by playing a game of chasing the "red worm" back into his cave. Additional approaches suitable for a child of the patient's age were also provided. Chemotherapy became a positive rather than a frightening experience, and the treatment provider could administer further therapy.

Role strains and stresses. Role flexibility is often mentioned as a significant variable in coping with cancer diagnosis (Koch, 1985). Another useful aspect of role theory is the concept of role insufficiency, which is defined as the inability to meet one's own perceived obligations and expectations or those of significant others (Meleis, 1975). Assessing changes in the child's school performance, peer relations, and home situation broadens the nurse's perspective of the burdens posed by the illness on the family.

Parents sometimes question the need for continued academic achievement or the importance of limit setting for a terminally ill child. Nursing assessment of child/family issues must address these concerns and explore feelings and plans affecting the child's developmental progress. If the parents indicate that they feel further school achievement is unnecessary or discipline unimportant, the child is likely to interpret their signals as portents of death. Withdrawal, accompanied by disappointment, anger, or depression, may result.

Working directly with the teachers of children with cancer throughout the diagnostic and treatment processes improves the educational experience (Perin and Manchester, 1984). The significance of continuing school achievement should be emphasized to the parents; many institutions demonstrate their commitment to that ideal by employing inpatient teachers on pediatric units. Such situations also create unique opportunities for nursing assessment and planning.

Further areas to assess. The nurse assessing the family of a child with cancer must consider a broad range of individual, social, and interpersonal issues. General questions might include: What is the family's primary stress? Is it the illness itself or the painful treatment procedures? Are the parents dominated by fear of relapse? What about the child's concerns regarding changes in daily routines? Is the child worried about impairment of future abilities and roles? Do the parents reinforce their child's existing stresses, particularly those associated with developmental issues? Does the child passively accept his disease or actively attempt mastery? How do the parents' concerns mesh with those of the child? Is communication open or limited? Do the children participate in family decisions? Finally, the nurse might consider how the parents have approached the school, particularly the child's classroom teachers, regarding their child's disease.

Encouraging the child to participate in family decisions, particularly those concerning treatments, is a common parental "normalizing" tactic (Krulik, 1980) and should be considered in nursing assessment. The nurse must recognize that the parents' strategies for managing the school-age child's chronic illness should include strengthening the child's coping abilities and resources as well as changing the environment (Krulik, 1980).

Assessing family and marital functioning. Current research also focuses on marital functioning in families of children with cancer (Barbarin et al., 1985). Thirty-two families of children with cancer (40% of whom were between the ages of 6 and 11 years) were interviewed using a semistructured questionnaire. During the 60- to 90-minute sessions, family cohesion, marital quality, spousal support, medical stress, and involvement in medical care were all measured. The range of identified coping strategies included information seeking, problem solving, help seeking, maintenance of emotional balance, religion, optimism, denial, and acceptance. Fifty-four percent of the families displayed improved marriage and family life quality. Interestingly, wives' and husbands' ratings of their situations agreed closely. However, as the child's number of hospitalizations increased, perceived marital quality and spousal support decreased.

A significant issue raised by this study was the timing of the interview. The degree of marital discord may depend upon *when* (in terms of the child's illness) the assessment is performed. Families at diagnosis are different from those 6 months, 2 years, or 5 years postdiagnosis. A further complication is the fact that stress increases developmental differences.

Assessment questions. When evaluating marital and family functioning in childhood cancer, the nurse should ask several basic questions: Are there problems in marital or family relationships? To whom do family members turn for support? What problem-solving abilities do family members display? How is information obtained and by whom? What is the family's overall outlook on life?

Planning

The nurse's role. A nurse's planning for family intervention begins with the examination of her own feelings and role. As Sabbeth (1984) has stated, "Each time I sit with a parent, I am faced with the difficult decision of how involved do I want to get?... Are my questions intrusive?... If the parent gets very upset, what will I do?" It is important to consider who else on the treatment team might be addressing similar issues. What information can be obtained from prior assessments? How will nurses interact with other providers?

Effective planning for complications arising from cancer and its treatment requires a multidisciplinary, team health care approach. Nurses have encouraged this strategy by developing case-oriented educational programs for a variety of health professionals. One way to promote awareness of patient needs is nursing grand rounds (Mazonson et al., 1981). By sharing literature, standardizing care plans, and providing outreach, nurses expand their expertise and upgrade their planning techniques.

A related development is the increasing participation of nurses on various hospital and community committees. The advocacy role for patient care needs, particularly the needs of clients in the middle years of childhood, extends beyond the immediate pressures and constraints familiar to many nurses. This requires sharing information with parents, children, and other health professionals. Reintegrating the child with cancer into the classroom, for instance, is a significant planning activity. Providing written information for teachers and speaking at continuing education conferences are other methods of outreach.

As nursing roles have changed, so have those of parents. Increasing consumer participation in health care means that parents of children with serious illnesses are becoming involved in surgical recovery (Kuhn, 1985), acting with parent consultants (Pitel et al., 1985), performing more tasks in the hospital (Algren, 1985), and becoming increasingly active in self-help groups (Yoak et al., 1985). Involving parents as members of the health care team requires greater nursing sensitivity; finding time to help parents define their roles involves careful planning.

Awareness of health care delivery trends. Major economic, technological, and educational changes currently affect nursing service delivery. One specific economic change is the development and use of diagnostic related groups (DRGs). Another related trend, necessitated by earlier discharge, is the increased use of complex care devices in the home.

The most recent economic development, however, has been the consolidation of hospitals with insurance companies. The joint venture between Voluntary Hospitals of America and Aetna Life and Casualty Company is one example of this *(San Francisco Chronicle,* August 7,

1985). One explanation for this trend is that, since 1970, losses to commercial health insurers have exceeded $6 billion (Mitchell, 1984). Cost-effectiveness is an issue for all health care providers in the eighties, and it has a significant impact on families of children with cancer.

Patient acuity systems directed toward budgetary management have altered delivery of inpatient nursing services (Walker, 1983). For example, more primary nurses are now being used on pediatric units. Other options include offering patients the opportunity to purchase extra services. These changes will hopefully have a positive effect on nursing services.

Furthermore, benefits are being revised, both contractually and legislatively, with lower premiums available for those who practice wellness. Premiums are also being withdrawn or limited for specified treatments, such as the Hickman catheter. Instead of reimbursement for unlimited supplies on discharge, insurance companies limit the amount of reimbursable supplies for discharge planning. The result is that nurses and families must try harder to purchase these supplies in clinics or pharmacies. Complications arise for those living in rural areas whose pharmacies have limited access to the most recent products.

As inpatient benefits have decreased, ambulatory care payments have increased (Mitchell, 1984). In general, ambulatory and home care services have intensified, with the development of "hospitals without walls" (Stein, 1978).

Technological advances also necessitate an increased sensitivity to ethical dilemmas. Unresolved questions for nurses and families planning care include: How aggressive should treatments be in relation to quality of life and expectations for cure? When should active therapy be discontinued in the hospital? At home? How can parents ensure adequate care of the child at home? (Allen and Klunder, 1985).

Meeting the complex needs of children with cancer also involves selecting vendors and maintaining needed equipment. Nurses must be aware of any written material families may need to maintain and operate equipment. Close collaboration is imperative if continuity in patient education and appropriate use of devices is to be maintained (Hartsell and Ward, 1985).

CASE STUDY

Lily Layton was an 8-year-old Caucasian female with recurrent Wilms' tumor. Despite removal of her involved kidney 2 years ago, she required chemotherapy for metastatic disease.

Her family consisted of her parents and a 4-year-old sibling. They lived more than 50 miles from the treatment center, a factor which, combined with her father's changes in employment, limited his involvement in her frequent clinic visits and hospitalizations.

Initially, Mrs. Layton expressed concern about caring for Lily's Hickman catheter. Lily's lack of cooperation and, indeed, active resistance, resulted in frustration and discipline problems. As her disease progressed, so did Lily's acting-out behavior, which included throwing temper tantrums in the computerized tomography scanning department, locking herself in the clinic's bathroom, and refusing nursing care on the inpatient pediatrics unit. She even refused such simple procedures as taking oral medications or having her temperature taken. Since communication with Lily's father was limited, Mrs. Layton assumed increasing responsibility for Lily's care.

What were this family's physical and emotional needs? Were food, clothing, and shelter adequate? What was the health status of Lily's family members? Were they aware of their strengths and resources? Did they use resources outside the system? Did they encourage and support each other? Did they have sufficient rest, activity, time alone, and time together? How did the family respond to the ill child? The assessing nurse realized that ascertaining the family's responses to the illness and to changes associated with the disease's progress was as significant as obtaining the history of the somatic illness itself (Mutter and Schleifer, 1966).

Other questions pertained to family communication. Was active listening used? Did the family communicate with the school? Further, what type of modeling occurred and what was the outcome? What roles were developed and what expectations evolved? Specifically, who provided support during procedures, scans, and treatments? How did Lily's sibling respond?

What difficulties arose, if any, in relation to child-rearing practices? Were there problems with trust, optimism, and cooperation?

For this family, it was crucial to assess problem-solving abilities. How were prior, similar conflicts resolved? How did the family handle stress?

Answering questions like these involved more than one clinic or hospital encounter. It became obvious that Lily's frequent hospitalizations had altered her family's communication and support processes. Changes in family roles were evidenced by altered levels of cooperation. Lily's development seemed to cease and compliance with treatment regimens deteriorated. Her problems involved an increasing dependence on her mother and on health care providers. She had an ongoing struggle to understand her disease and its effects upon her. One example of this struggle occurred during a waiting period in the clinic's examination room, when she role played with dolls a cardiac procedure she had experienced several months earlier. Encouraging expressions of her feelings about this and other procedures was helpful.

Planning care

A conference involving physicians, staff and head nurses, Lily's mother, a social services case worker, the hospital-based teacher, and a clinical specialist was held to review the family's problems and develop a cooperative plan. Refocusing Mrs. Layton on her parental, rather than nursing role, supporting her use of discipline (specifically, limit setting), clarifying behavioral expectations, and continuing (in the hospital) specific care routines developed at home all served to strengthen both family and hospital staff members.

Lily's father was included in a second conference held a few months before her death. Her medical treatments, including future chemotherapy for widespread metastases, were discussed at that time. Lily's own preferences were considered, although she did not attend the meetings. She had explained to her parents, "I don't want to die fast...I want to die slow."

Following the conference, the nurse planned strategies for reinforcing the family's own strengths. Open communication, particularly regarding death and dying, helped Lily and her family maintain a sense of equilibrium and reorganize their lives. Active participation in decision-making by both child and family also reinforced coping strategies.

CONCLUSIONS

The family-centered nursing process delineated in this chapter will help promote nursing competence and coping ability, while offering comfort and supporting family growth along the developmental spiral. "Cooperative caring" (Robinson, 1985), as well as "empathy, interest, objectivity, and involvement" (Leininger, 1970) were underlying themes.

REFERENCES

Aguilera, D.C., and Messick, J.M. *Crisis Intervention: Theory and Methodology.* St. Louis: C.V. Mosby Co., 1974.

Ahmann, E. "The Child at Home with Chronic Pain," *Maternal-Child Nursing* 9:264–66, 1984.

Algren, C.L. "Role Perception of Mothers Who Have Hospitalized Children," *Children's Health Care* 14(1):6–9, 1985.

Allen, M., and Klunder, V. "Human Responses to High Technology," *Maternal-Child Nursing* 10:247, 1985.

Anderson, J.M. "The Social Construction of Illness Experience: Families with a Chronically Ill Child," *Journal of Advanced Nursing* 6:427–34, 1981.

Barbarin, O.A., et al. "Stress, Coping and Marital Functioning among Parents of Children with Cancer," *Journal of Marriage and the Family* 47:473–80, 1985.

Barnard, K.E. "The Family as a Unit of Measurement," *Maternal-Child Nursing* 9:21, 1984.

Beardslee, C., and Neff, E.J. "Body Related Concerns of Children with Cancer as Compared with the Concerns of Other Children," *Maternal-Child Nursing* 11:121–24, 1982.

Doherty, W.J. "Family Intervention in Health Care," *Family Relations* 34:129–37, 1985.

Dorn, L.D. "Children's Concepts of Illness: Clinical Applications," *Pediatric Nursing* 11:325–27, 1984.

Drotar, D. "Psychological Perspectives in Chronic Childhood Illness," *Journal of Pediatric Psychology* 6:211–28, 1981.

Epstein, N., et al. "The McMaster Family Assessment Device," *Journal of Marital and Family Therapy* 9:171–80, 1983.

Harkey, J. "The Epidemiology of Selected Chronic Childhood Health Conditions," *Children's Health Care* 12:62–71, 1983.

Hartsell, M.B., and Ward, J.H. "Selecting Equipment Vendors for Children on Home Care," *Maternal-Child Nursing* 10:26–28, 1985.

Hill, R. "Generic Features of Families Under Stress," in *Crisis Intervention: Selected Readings.* Edited by Parad, J. New York: Family Services Association of America, 1965.

Hodges, K., et al. "The Development of a Child Assessment Interview for Research and Clinical Use," *Journal of Abnormal Child Psychology* 10:173–89, 1982.

Holaday, B. "Challenges of Rearing a Chronically Ill Child, Caring and Coping. *Nursing Clinics of North America* 19:361–69, 1984.

Hymovich, D.P. "Incorporating the Family into Care," *Journal of the New York State Nurses' Association* 5:9–14, 1974.

Janosik, R.H., and Miller, J.R. "Theories of Family Development," in *Family Health Care,* vol. 1. Edited by Hymovich, D.P., and Barnard, M.U. New York: McGraw-Hill Book Co., 1979.

Kaplan, D.M., et al. "Family Mediation of Stress," *Social Work* 18:60–69, 1973.

Koch, A. "'If Only It Could Be Me': The Families of Pediatric Cancer Patients," *Family Relations* 34:63–70, 1985.

Koocher, G.P., and O'Malley, J. *The Damocles Syndrome: Psychological Consequences of Surviving Childhood Cancer.* New York: McGraw-Hill Book Co., 1981.

Krulik, T. "Helping Parents of Children with Cancer During the Midstage of Illness," *Cancer Nursing* 5:441-45, 1982.

Krulik, T. "Successful 'Normalizing' Tactics of Parents of Chronically Ill Children," *Journal of Advanced Nursing* 5:573–78, 1980.

Kuhn, P. "In My Opinion... Benjamin's Surgery—Mommy Was There," *Children's Health Care* 14:10-11, 1985.

Kupst, M.J., et al. "Coping with Pediatric Leukemia: A Two-Year Followup," *Journal of Pediatric Psychology* 9:149–63, 1984.

Kupst, M.J., et al. "Family Coping with Childhood Leukemia: One Year after Diagnosis," *Journal of Pediatric Psychology* 7:157–76, 1982.

Leininger, M. *Nursing Anthropology: Two Worlds to Blend.* New York: John Wiley & Sons, 1970.

Mazonson, P.D., et al. "Oncology Grand Rounds for Nurses: The Need for Case-Oriented Continuing Education Programs in Cancer Nursing," *Cancer Nursing* 4:107–13, 1981.

McCubbin, H.I., and Patterson, J.M. "The Family Stress Process: The Double ABCX Model of Adjustment and Adaptation," in *Social Stress and Family: Advances and Developments in Family Stress Theory and Research.* Edited by McCubbin, H.I., et al. New York: The Haworth Press, 1983.

McCubbin, H.I., et al. *Family Stress, Coping and Social Support.* Springfield, Ill.: Charles C. Thomas, 1982.

Meleis, A.F. "Role Insufficiency and Role Supplementation: A Conceptual Framework," *Nursing Research* 24:264–71, 1975.

Miles, M.S., and Carter, M.C. "Coping Strategies Used by Parents During Their Child's Hospitalizations in an Intensive Care Unit," *Children's Health Care* 14:14–21, 1985.

Mitchell, K. "Possible Trends in Commercial Insurance," *Pediatric Nursing* 10:249, 1984.

Moos, R.H., and Moos, B.S. "A Typology of Family Social Environments," *Family Process* 15:357–71, 1976.

Mutter, A.Z., and Schleifer, M.J. "The Role of Psychological and Social Factors in the Onset of Somatic Illness in Children, Part 1," *Psychosomatic Medicine* 28:333–43, 1966.

Olson, D.H., et al. "Circumplex Model of Marital and Family Systems II: Empirical Studies and Clinical Intervention," in *Advances in Family Information, Assessment and Theory.* Edited by Vincent, J.P. Greenwich, Conn.: JAI Press, 1980.

Olson, D.H., et al. *Families: What Makes Them Work.* Beverly Hills, Calif.: Sage Pubns., 1983.

Otto, H.A. "A Framework for Assessing Family Strengths," in *Family Centered Community Nursing.* Edited by Reinhardt, A., and Quinn, M. St. Louis: C.V. Mosby Co., 1973.

Pegelow, C. *Acute Lymphocytic Leukemia in Childhood.* Lecture, Feb. 14, 1983.

Perin, G., and Manchester, P.B. "Pediatric Oncology Nursing," in *Clinical Pediatric Oncology.* Edited by Sutow, W.W., et al. St. Louis: C.V. Mosby Co., 1984.

Pitel, A.U., et al. "Parent Consultants in Pediatric Oncology," *Children's Health Care* 14:46–51, 1985.

Pless, J.B., and Satterwhite, B. "A Measure of Family Functioning and Its Application," *Social Science and Medicine* 7:613–21, 1973.

Pless, J.B., et al. "Chronic Illness, Family Functioning, and Psychological Adjustments: A Model for the Allocation of Preventive Mental Health Services," *International Journal of Epidemiology* 1:271–77, 1972.

Polit, D.F., and Hungler, B.P. *Nursing Research: Principles and Methods.* Philadelphia: J.B. Lippincott Co., 1978.

Robinson, C.A. "Double Bind: A Dilemma for Parents of Chronically Ill Children," *Pediatric Nursing* 11:112–15, 1985.

Rogers, M.E. *The Theoretical Basis of Nursing.* Philadelphia: F.A. Davis Co., 1970.

Ross, D.M., and Ross, S.A. "Stress Reduction Procedures for the School-Age Hospitalized Leukemic Child," *Pediatric Nursing* 10:393–95, 1984.

Rowe, G.P. "The Developmental Conceptual Framework Applied to the Study of the Family," in *Emerging Conceptual Frameworks in Family Analysis.* Edited by Nye, F.I., and Benardo, F.M. New York: Macmillan Publishing Co., 1966.

Ruccione, K., and Ferguson, J. "Late Effect of Childhood Cancer and Its Treatment," *Oncology Nursing Forum* 11:54–65, 1984.

Rutter, M. "Stress, Coping and Development: Some Issues and Some Questions," *Journal of Child Psychology and Psychiatry* 22:323–56, 1981.

Sabbeth, B. "Understanding the Impact of Chronic Childhood Illness on Families," *Pediatric Clinics of North America* 31:47–57, 1984.

Schulman, J.L. "Coping with Major Disease: Child Family Pediatrician," *Journal of Pediatrics* 102:988–91, 1983.

Siemon, M. "Siblings of the Chronically Ill or Disabled Child," *Pediatric Clinics of North America* 19:295–307, 1984.

Skodol-Wilson, H. *Research in Nursing.* Menlo Park, Calif.: Addison-Wesley Publishing Co., 1985.

Smilkstein, G. "The Family Apgar: A Proposal for a Family Function Test and Its Use by Physicians," *The Journal of Family Practice* 6:1321–29, 1978.

Speer, J.J., and Sachs, B. "Selecting the Appropriate Family Assessment Tool," *Pediatric Nursing* 11:349–55, 1985.

Spinetta, J.J. "Adjustment in Children with Cancer," *Journal of Pediatric Psychology* 2:49–51, 1977.

Spinetta, J.J., et al. "Effective Parental Coping Following the Death of a Child from Cancer," *Journal of Pediatric Psychology* 6:251–63, 1981.

Stein, R.E.K. "Pediatric Home Care: An Ambulatory 'Special Care Unit,'" *Journal of Pediatrics* 92:495–99, 1978.

Stein, R.E.K., and Jessop, D.J. "A Noncategorical Approach to Chronic Childhood Illness," *Public Health Reports* 97:354–62, 1982.

Stein, R.E.K., and Reissman, C.K. "The Development of an Impact on Family Scales: Preliminary Findings," *Medical Care* 18:465–72, 1982.

Sutow, W.W. "General Aspects of Childhood Cancer," in *Clinical Pediatric Oncology.* Edited by Sutow, W.W., et al. St. Louis: C.V. Mosby Co., 1984.

Van Eys, J. "The Outlook for the Child with Cancer," *Journal of School Health* 47(3):165–69, 1977.

Walker, D.D. "The Cost of Nursing Care in Hospitals," *Journal of Nursing Administration* 3:13–18, 1983.

Welch, D., et al. "The Development of a Specialized Nursing Assessment Tool for Cancer Patients," *Oncology Nursing Forum* 9:37–44, 1982.

Whitt, J.K. "Children's Adaptation to Chronic Illness and Handicapping Conditions," in *Chronic Illness and Disability Throughout the Lifespan.* Edited by Eisenberg, M.G., et al. New York: Springer Publishing Co., 1984.

Wilbur, J.R. *Osteosarcoma.* Lecture, February 18, 1983.

Yoak, M., et al. "Active Roles in Self-Help Groups for Parents of Children with Cancer," *Children's Health Care* 14:38–45, 1985.

Zurlinden, J.K. "Minimizing the Impact of Hospitalization for Children and Their Families," *Maternal-Child Nursing* 10:178–82, 1985.

8 Assessing families of adolescents with central nervous system trauma

Karin M. Buchanan, RSW
Social Worker and Clinical Instructor
Department of Clinical Neurological Sciences
University Hospital
University of Saskatchewan
Saskatoon, Saskatchewan, Canada

OVERVIEW

The time is 2 a.m. Sunday. The plaintive siren of an approaching ambulance grows louder. As they hear it, nurses in the emergency room, the intensive care unit, and the neurosurgical ward all shudder with the same thoughts: "Another accident...another teenager?...another family..."

This chapter focuses on the nurse's assessment of the family with an adolescent who has suffered serious head or spinal cord injury. The emphasis will be on the critical, initial phase, which starts in the emergency room and ends when the patient dies or stabilizes (usually in 1 to 3 weeks). The Calgary Family Assessment Model (Wright and Leahey, 1984) forms the framework for pertinent assessment issues; suggested assessment strategies are based on the author's 12 years of clinical experience as a medical social worker (in neurosurgery) working primarily with families of injured adolescents.

NURSING PROCESS

Assessment

The health problem: Head/spinal cord trauma.
What injuries are most common? In the author's experience, many adolescents break bones. While most of these heal, a few orthopedic injuries lead to amputation of a limb. Severe burns are relatively rare, but they can be profoundly disfiguring and disabling. Grave multiple internal injuries are sometimes seen in this age group, although it is rare for an adolescent to be left with a colostomy or permanent tracheostomy, or

with kidney damage requiring dialysis. Most teenagers survive multiple internal injuries and recover well.

The most common serious injury in adolescents is central nervous system (CNS) trauma—head and spinal cord injuries. Head injury, for instance, causes approximately 70% of the accidental deaths in this age group (Rimel and Jane, 1983). (In all age groups, 25 to 30 million cases of spinal cord injury are reported annually.) The adolescents who survive serious injury—and their families—pay a heavy toll in medical costs and, more significantly, in lost human potential (Charles et al., 1974).

Who suffers head and spinal cord injuries? Rimel and Jane (1983) found that approximately 35% of all head-injured patients are age 10 to 19, with 62% being between ages 10 and 29. Although most studies report that such injuries are two or three times more common in males, they find the greatest sex-related differences between ages 15 and 24. In the author's catchment area (Saskatchewan, Canada), approximately 85% of all head-injured patients who survive after a week or more of hospitalization are male (Saskatchewan Coordinating Council on Social Planning, 1984). During the year ending in March 1985, 90% of all spinal cord–injured patients were male (Canadian Paraplegic Association, Saskatchewan Division, 1985).

How do these injuries occur? Head and spinal cord injuries in rural communities often result from farm accidents, especially at harvest time when a fatigued and inexperienced teenager may be asked to operate heavy equipment. Shooting accidents—suffered while hunting, cleaning guns, or playing—are also common, as are diving and contact sports injuries. Most significant, however, are the dirt bike, motorcycle, snowmobile, bicycle, and automobile accidents. Automobile accidents account for approximately 50% of all head and spinal cord injuries (Bond, 1975).

Why do these accidents happen? There is no simple answer to this question. Whereas serious injuries in small children generally occur when adults are nearby (for example, a child darts out between parked cars with parents or other adults not far away), increasing numbers of adolescent CNS traumas occur during expeditions away from the family (farm accidents are the main exception to this trend). Excessive risk taking and/or showing off often result in serious injury; alcohol consumption is a significant contributing factor.

Theoretical framework for family assessment. Few, if any, theoretical models of family assessment exist that are entirely practical for the nurse in the initial critical phase after a serious injury. It is even more difficult to find a model that encompasses the unique features of family response to CNS trauma, particularly when an adolescent is affected.

The existing literature (familiar enough to the nurse not to warrant review here) concentrates on the common emotional responses of *individual* family members—on artificially "staging" these individual emotional responses with the very naive assumption that the nurse will be rewarded by the patient's, as well as the entire family's, arrival in some static state known as "acceptance." The family itself, as an interacting dynamic unit with its own history and form, has been largely ignored. These models do not reflect reality, and their standards become major sources of frustration, helplessness, and feelings of failure for nurses. Nurses soon realize that not only has the patient not fully recovered physically, but the family is not "all better," emotionally or functionally. To protect both nurse and patient, a broader view is necessary.

Family assessment in critical adolescent injury is intricately interwoven with intervention. Therefore this chapter focuses on the assessment issues that the nurse faces in such a situation. The Calgary Family Assessment Model (CFAM) (Wright and Leahey, 1984) provides an excellent framework for general family assessment and gives the nurse the "mind set" necessary to organize and interpret her observations.

The exigencies of time, place, and potential family cooperation make it difficult to apply the CFAM without modification. Readers are referred to Wright and Leahey's own volume for a complete explanation of this model; this chapter discusses only those assessment issues specific to families of injured adolescents.

Family structural assessment (Calgary model).
Internal structure. In adolescent CNS trauma, it is important to understand the *family composition*—for instance, who lives at home and who lives away? How many "families" support this adolescent? Given today's high incidence of divorce and the proliferation of single-parent families, understanding family composition becomes a complex task. Indeed, the nurse in such cases must often assess family superstructure as well as structure. Say, for instance, that the nurse encounters a 36-year-old single mother and the patient's 14-year-old sister. The father, along with his wife of 5 years, may also be present. He may or may not have been close to his son since the divorce 6 years previously; he may or may not have had contact with his ex-wife; she and his present wife may or may not be willing to speak to one another; he may or may not want to assume the role of father and try to usurp his ex-wife's role as prime decision maker regarding treatment.

Such things do happen. The author has seen the father of an 18-year-old quadriplegic, who had had no contact with his son or ex-wife for 12 years, arrive at the hospital the day after the boy's accident and expect to make decisions. In fact, he openly accused his former wife of irresponsible and inadequate parenting and held her responsible for the accident. But, long before the son's discharge from hospital 3 months later, when the mother assumed full responsibility for the disabled teen's care, he was gone.

A nurse must also ascertain whether or not the family has endured past losses or crises as a result of death or serious illness. In many cases the nurse does not even have to ask this question, since the information will have been volunteered. Life-threatening circumstances cause many people, including patients and their families, to relive previous similar situations, especially if they never adequately acknowledged and worked through their painful feelings about the incident. The author has found that more than half of her clients had to talk at length about previous grief before they could sort out their feelings about the present situation.

In addition to assessing past losses, it is important for the nurse to recognize family "gains." Has the mother, for instance, just remarried, or the grandmother/father just moved in? Has the 15-year-old daughter just brought home her 5-day-old son? Whatever the losses or gains, has the basic family unit reestablished equilibrium?

Although not strictly considered part of the family "structure," each family member's *health status* is another appropriate area of inquiry. Mother may be hypertensive, or father a severe diabetic. A sibling may have juvenile arthritis. Any of these existing conditions might be exacerbated by the natural tendency of individuals to ignore their own health during a relative's time of crisis. Eating and sleeping patterns may be disturbed, prescription drug compliance may be poor, and drug and alcohol abuse may increase, in addition to the general physiological effects of excessive distress. At this time, a gentle question about "nerve problems" can reveal existing or potential psychiatric illness. On the other hand, it may not be appropriate to ask about alcohol-related illnesses at this early stage, especially if there is a suspicion that alcohol contributed to the traumatic event (unless, of course, the family volunteers this information). If the accident *is* alcohol-related and there is alcohol abuse within the family, members may perceive this questioning as blaming—especially if questions are asked before a trusting relationship has been established with the nurse.

Rank order within the family. This has major implications for all members, including the injured adolescent's parents. Fathers may have a particularly difficult time when their eldest son is injured. That child may have represented the father's dream of having the son follow in his footsteps or go on to something better (Toman, 1976). Fathers identify particularly strongly with their eldest sons, the ones who "carry on the family name." Such statements as, "If only I could take his place," or "I've lived my life, he has his whole future ahead" are common in such cases. With an older, sexually active adolescent, the father might have derived vicarious (although unacknowledged) pleasure at the thought of his son growing up in a more sexually liberal time than he did. Middle-aged fathers engaged in long-established relationships may especially appreciate this identification/proximity to their sons' sexual prowess, since they may be concerned about the waning of their own sexual powers. Such fathers are particularly devastated when a spinal cord injury impairs a son's sexual function. The father may just keep repeating, "He is not even a man anymore, not even a man..."

Mothers have more difficulty facing head or spinal cord injury in the youngest son or daughter, particularly if the child's life is threatened. This may reflect a maternal willingness to see the potential disability as a way to restore them to the familiar role of caretaker or prime nurturer. Mothers may plead for "life at all costs," particularly for the youngest in the family. When her 13-year-old daughter sustained a severe head injury, one mother said, "I'll look after her no matter what it takes. I'll do it forever. I won't let death empty my nest." Obviously, this woman had little sense of her own identity beyond that of mother and would have had difficulty even when her daughter left home under normal circumstances. But a sudden death at age 13 would have brought an abrupt and devastating end to the mother role.

An injured adolescent who is much younger than his siblings (the so-called "afterthought child") prompts particular concerns in *both* parents. The couple may describe how their maturity, parenting experience, and financial security at the time of this belated offspring's arrival afforded them an unusually relaxed but very close relationship with the child. They may make statements such as, "He was our best, all we were capable of. We learned from our past mistakes, but now we may have nothing to show for it."

Family *subsystems* are probably best observed, rather than asked about, at this early assessment stage. When everyone is feeling the effects, good or bad, of his individual relationship with the patient, it is difficult to probe into the subsystems without creating more guilt and anxiety. Both nurse and family are better served by simply noting obvious references to subsystems. If such references seem to reflect anxiety and/or guilt, the nurse can explore them further and explain that such subsystems are virtually universal.

Serious illness also plays havoc, in both the short and the long term, with family *boundaries*. A 17-year-old girl, for example, might have to "parent" her three younger siblings while her mother and father remain at the bedside of her head-injured twin. A 19-year-old male who has just left home may parent his mother, a single parent, when his 15-year-old sister suffers a spinal cord injury. As his mother's anxiety abates, however, he may not willingly give up the power that accompanies his new role. (Many of the "boundary" issues, are, of course, also functional-expressive-role issues.)

External structure. Culture and religion both influence a family's ability to speak with physicians, touch the seriously injured patient, or show emotion in front of strangers comfortably. These factors help determine how and where they ask for help, how much help they think is available, and even how much help/information they believe is necessary and appropriate (McGoldrick et al., 1982). Religion may also determine a family's values and coping style or even dictate the limits of health care, as in the case of Jehovah's Witnesses' refusal of blood transfusions. Even more complex is the impact of religion on family coping patterns and overall functioning. When religion provides the family members with the confidence that they can cope, when it tells them that they have reserves of strength beyond their own and that good may eventually come from the present tragedy, then it will facilitate stress resolution and healthy adjustment. Such family members may pray for the strength to cope with whatever lies ahead, while still acknowledging and expressing their own hopes. They show little reality distortion and certainly appear strengthened by their faith.

On the other hand, if religious beliefs magnify the family's need to find a reason or meaning for every accident, such beliefs can easily lead to the feeling that this "unnatural" phenomenon has been visited on the family as a form of punishment. This can lead to guilt and conjecture over the cause of the accident, as well as to prayer for solutions contradicting all laws of nature. This is illustrated by the case of an 18-year-old who suffers a severe head injury and arrives at the hospital with brain tissue oozing from skull and nasal fractures. He remains deeply comatose for many weeks, maintained only by sophisticated life support systems. Yet, the family, despite thorough medical explanations, continues to pray that he will instantly sit up in bed, look around, and ask, "Where am I? What happened?" Although it is possible that this teenager may survive, he cannot have an immediate and complete recovery. When their totally unrealistic petitions are not granted, the family may attempt to distort reality in order to maintain their faith, or instead blame themselves for being "weak" believers.

Social status, particularly as evidenced by occupation, educational attainment, and income, will affect the family's general comfort within the typically middle-class health care milieu (Warner, 1962). The severity of the financial burden of prolonged hospitalization and permanent severe disability is obviously proportionate to family income, assets, and insurance coverage. The treatment *environment,* both in the short and long term, is another important factor. The family that stays close to the referral center, possibly far from home, faces issues of cost, comfort, and convenience. Even more important is the long-term environment for the permanently disabled adolescent. This, of course, has tremendous implications for the monumental instrumental tasks facing the family, all of which are similar to those confronting the nurse.

Both *extended family* and close friends can be important sources of support for the family faced with instrumental and expressive tasks associated with head or spinal trauma. Serious injury either tightens family networks or pushes them apart, but it never leaves family dynamics unaltered. There are several ways in which severe trauma pushes a family apart. It is common, for instance, for people to judge the coping strategies of others, thinking that their own methods are right. When parents receive an accurate assessment of their teen's prognosis after a severe head injury, they may decide that death would be preferable. However, the grandparents may feel that even discussing the possibility that death may be preferable in some way complies with death or disability. They may feel that the parents should instead insist that the child will recover fully. (This reflects the superstition that talking about a possibility can make it happen.)

The crisis associated with severe trauma can also bring unresolved past developmental conflicts within the family network to the surface. For example, the patient's grandparents may attempt to use the divorced mother's present distress to prove that they were right in advising her not to leave home and get married when she became pregnant at age 16. Nurses should be careful in such situations; extended family members will often try to draw the nurse into their conflict to "score points" for their side of the dispute.

Although a good structural assessment of the family helps the nurse in such cases, it is doubtful whether, outside of her personal records, there is a need for genograms or ecomaps, at least in the initial phase. Although a patient's family will in time reveal its internal structure, members first need to believe that the nurse's focus is on the patient.

Family developmental assessment. Very few families of injured adolescents fit perfectly in the CFAM Stage V—Families with Teenagers (Wright and Leahey, 1984). Divorce, remarriage, an age spread of more than 7 years between the parents or between the oldest and youngest offspring, or cultural factors can result in a family facing concomitantly the tasks of several stages (Aldous, 1978). The more tasks they face, the more likely they are to have fallen into disequilibrium even before the adolescent's injury, and the less likely they are to restabilize after the injury, particularly if the patient survives but remains severely disabled. Nevertheless, families of injured adolescents do have to accomplish the CFAM Stage V tasks in addition to the other tasks they face. For that reason, these tasks will be addressed here.

The issue of the patient's developing *autonomy* is crucial to thorough assessment in head or spinal cord trauma. The actual accident may represent to the family, realistically or symbolically, the child's "failed autonomy." One illustrative incident involves a 16-year-old who was injured the first time he was allowed to take his peers to the family cabin without adult supervision. He persistently argued with his parents for this privilege, continuously countering their concerns with the claim that he was an adult and that they should stop treating him like a baby. The boy's father eventually relented and, although his mother disagreed, let the boy make the trip. Three hours after arriving at the lake, by which time he was inebriated, the boy dove off the bank into 2 feet of water, suffering a fracture dislocation of C4-C5 and immediate quadriplegia.

Regardless of the circumstances of the accident, the paralyzed or comatose adolescent's complete helplessness will conjure up in parents images of the same dependence on them that their child displayed as an infant. They balance this against the sight of a body that may be 6 feet long and weigh 180 pounds. This disparity almost always elicits ambivalence, if not overt guilt, over how the family had dealt with the adolescent's increasing need for autonomy. They may also feel repressed anger about how the adolescent mishandled his end of the autonomy bargain, but parents can seldom admit this, at least not without additional guilt.

If the adolescent survives the initial injury, the family's future or long-term tasks relating to his autonomy are even more complex and are often dealt with poorly. In the author's experience, families have great difficulty treating a spinal cord–injured member like a young adult. The patient's obvious and overwhelming physical disability almost always leads to family overprotectiveness, despite the fact that he may have matured significantly in even the first few months after the injury. On the other hand, some families of head-injured adolescents err in the opposite direction. The patient may go home with little or no obvious physical impairment and, consequently, may be given age-appropriate (or beyond) independence as a reward for surviving the traumatic ordeal, to cheer him up, and/or to challenge him to further improve. This can be dangerous. Head-injured patients who have problems with abstraction, concentration, attention, judgment, problem solving, impulse control, and frustration tolerance do not fare well with too much "challenge." Instead, their minds perceive it as excessively stressful; regressed behavior is the almost inevitable result.

Parents of CNS-injured adolescents may find their situation further complicated by their own developmentally normal *refocusing on midlife marital and career issues.* Parents who have, by the time of the accident, successfully reinvested in their marital relationship tend to handle the injury best, probably because they have been strengthened by mutual comfort and intimacy. Partners who are "out of practice" in attending to each other's emotional needs may have difficulty "relearning" these skills quickly enough. On the other hand, a woman who has just reinvested in a career may be so overwhelmed by a teenager's severe disability that she will leave the work force, at least temporarily, to provide rehabilitation and/or long-term home care. (This is by far the most common scenario: the woman, not the man, modifies work responsibilities.) When an adolescent dies, a woman who has reestablished a career may cope better over the long term than would a full-time housewife and mother; a career is one way in which men and women establish identities for themselves beyond their roles of partner and parent.

The family of a CNS-injured adolescent may have already begun a *shift toward concern for the older generation,* which is usually put "on hold" after the traumatic event. Especially when the youngest in the family is injured, parents worry about who will look after him when they no longer can.

Individual and family *attachments* are difficult to assess immediately after injury, when everyone is feeling (or making it seem that they are) deeply attached to the patient. Only after more extensive contact will the nurse be able to distinguish clearly between adaptive and maladaptive attachments and/or guilt-ridden attempts to create new bonds. From the start of the nurse/client relationship, however, the nurse will be able to observe family interactions and ascertain relationships within the family network. The nurse might also be alert to the difficulty that parents have, when facing their child's distraught friends, acknowledging for the first time the strengths of his attachments outside the family. They may have to juggle this with the blame and resentment they feel toward friends present at and/or involved in the accident.

Functional assessment.
Instrumental functioning. Every nurse is well aware of the short- and long-term instrumental issues surrounding an adolescent's head or spinal cord injury and can usually assess the family's instrumental needs in this area quickly. However, the same nurse, if unaware of the far-reaching influence of instrumental issues, may denigrate the role of intervention. Failure to solve, or at least ease, practical problems can have devastating emotional consequences: self-esteem may be lowered, anxiety heightened, frustration created, relationships stressed, depres-

sion complicated and intensified, and, most significantly, feelings of helplessness created, magnified, and reinforced. Consequently, the nurse who can assess instrumental needs and initiate effective strategies for meeting those needs is an invaluable ongoing asset for families of CNS-injured adolescents. Success in this area eventually produces more confidence and a greater sense of control, which first reduces anxiety and then has a positive effect on other areas.

Expressive functioning. Expressive functioning is the keystone of family functioning and equilibrium. CFAM's parameters are excellent. Although the nurse may have only limited chances in the initial phase to question the family in this area, she will have ample opportunity to assess by observation. Since, in the author's experience, these issues are not unique to adolescent injury, only a few comments need to be made here.

A family crisis of the magnitude of a head or spinal cord injury in an adolescent can reveal the full range of emotional and nonverbal communication of which the family is capable. Understandably, sadness, anger, anxiety, as well as happiness at any "good news" might each be expressed at any time. The time immediately after the injury is one for tenderness, concern, touching, holding, hugging, and stroking. For many families, such a range of emotions may never have been demonstrated before, and the sheer unfamiliarity of the situation may be overwhelming for some.

The quality of family members' emotional and nonverbal communication with extended family and close friends must also be assessed at this time. As her 17-year-old daughter lay comatose, one mother, a single parent, walked through the halls of the hospital tightly embracing a friend. The mother wanted to walk from the intensive care unit to the maternity ward in the same hospital, "back to where it all began, 17 years ago." Her friend understood. Because of this kind of emotional intensity, many people flounder for words, but offer comfort eloquently.

Verbal communications often include statements of great protectiveness or concern for other family members, but in reality only reflect the speaker's need for control, power, or a sense of importance. The patient's aunt may volunteer to be the spokesperson with the medical profession, claiming that her sister and brother-in-law are "just too upset to talk to doctors right now." She may be heard boasting to other patients' families in the intensive care waiting room that she has not left the hospital in 3 days, and that "the others left several times because they just couldn't take it anymore." This woman thrives on life-and-death drama that meets her own power needs.

The nurse must notice when the family's need for control deteriorates into a power struggle with the health care system or the physicians.

Unfortunately, when the family focus shifts from the patient to "who is right" and "who can score points," physicians sometimes join in the game. One father and physician disagreed over the prognosis of a severely head-injured teen, with the father insisting that his son's "will to live" would "bring him around" and that "you doctors don't know anything but your bank balance." When the son improved faster than expected, the father showed as much pleasure at having "outsmarted" the physician as at his son's improvement.

The interrelated *roles* of siblings within the family network are also important. Death or severe disability constitutes a devastating end to sibling rivalry. In one case, two brothers had always competed fiercely for grades, for tennis honors, for part-time jobs, for dates, and for their parents' affection. When a motorcycle accident killed one brother, it meant that the other had "won" the competition, but at high personal cost. If the disabled or deceased sibling was brighter, more talented, more successful, or significantly more likely to realize parental hopes and aspirations, the "survivor" sibling is left painfully aware of what he perceives to be the parents' preference. He may feel that he should have been injured instead. Siblings suffering this kind of "survivor guilt" are very high suicide risks. Their depression, guilt, and perceptions of parental disappointment may be coupled with the romantic notion that their death would expiate the disappointment. At a rational level, they realize that their death will not "resurrect" the sibling, but on an emotional and superstitious level, it may seem the only recourse.

Family *beliefs* and values influence whether or not members believe that death is preferable to severe disability and to what extent disability is acceptable. For a family that has stressed hard physical labor and contact sports for recreation, paraplegia is a devastating blow. On the other hand, for a family of professionals, even a mild head injury may be far more frightening than a spinal cord injury.

Planning

Whether in the emergency department, intensive care unit, or neuro-surgical ward, the hospital-based nurse does not have the luxury of long, uninterrupted sessions with the family. Instead, she must gather information at the bedside, in the hallway, and hopefully, in a quiet private family or waiting room nearby. Seldom does she have access to the entire nuclear family at one time. Family members may be visiting the hospital and sleeping in shifts, young children may be at home in another community when the adolescent is in a tertiary care facility, and/or the family may not feel any need to be seen as a unit. Indeed, given the high level of emotional intensity, the nurse will often find it simpler to request to see the parents alone first, before embarking on contact with the patient's siblings, grandparents, and remaining extended family, even if they are available and willing to be seen.

The nurse must remember that the family members' focus at this time is on the adolescent patient. They may not have requested family nursing or family therapy. Therefore, they are apt to interpret poorly timed and/or numerous questions about family structure, development, and function as irrelevant, intrusive, or a nuisance, or, even worse, to conclude that the nurse is shirking her patient care responsibilities. To avoid this, always begin the contact by answering the family's questions about the patient. Reducing initial anxiety is essential, and the most effective way to do this is through brief, accurate, informative explanations. Fear of the unknown is a major component of anxiety, and even the simplest explanation can help. Although many forms of "teaching" cannot be absorbed while anxiety is high, small amounts of understandable information can help families plan how to cope with traumatic events, making them feel less dependent and more in control. *Realistic* reassurance about the medical staff's competence and experience, coupled with information about the treatment facility, is usually appreciated.

After an accident, people may become "locked into" the event and may require release through *recreating the scene*. Whether the relative(s) actually saw the incident, found their loved one after the fact, or, as is most common, were engaged elsewhere when they received the news, mentally revisiting the scene can be cathartic. A mother may recreate in vivid detail what she was wearing and what she was doing when a police officer arrived at the door to inform her that her teenaged son had just been in an accident. To the nurse these details may seem boring, superfluous, and time consuming. They are *never* superfluous, however. People in shock freeze a time frame, and the sooner they are given the time and audience to recreate that frozen moment, the sooner they will be able to return to the present. With gentle prodding, this usually leads to an explanation of how the accident happened and who else was involved. A certain number of patients will have been involved in accidents where other people were killed, perhaps through their own or someone else's negligence, as in drunken driving.

In addition, accidents are much more common at times of high individual and/or family distress. Family members may feel responsible for the accident; these feelings have profound implications that need to be addressed by the nurse planning intervention. Even when no one is directly or indirectly responsible, family members almost always experience guilt after an accident. Such feelings are typified by statements beginning, "If only..." or "If I had not..." Why do families add to their suffering in this way? Like the patient, they are looking for an answer to the question, "Why?" Death, even death by "natural" causes in anyone except the very old, is seen less and less as natural in our society. When there is an accident, families search for concrete explanations and recall previous safety lessons. Everyone has heard that *accidents are preventable.* Family members, desperate to justify what has happened, can always find a reason to feel responsible and to blame themselves. For our purposes here, it is enough to say that the nurse should never prevent family members from expressing feelings of guilt, even when such expressions are painful for the family or seem inappropriate or irrational to others. The cathartic act of "pointing the finger" at oneself, while being exonerated by another, has a tremendous calming effect. It allows the nurse to gently suggest that she would like to know a little more about the entire family. By answering questions, reducing anxiety, hearing about the accident, and listening to the expression of feelings of guilt, the nurse is not ignoring "assessment"; she is merely developing trust, initiating crisis intervention, engaging the family, and already filing in her mind a great deal of information about this family. Depending on mutual time constraints and the family's level of cooperation, the nurse may now have an opportunity to fill in any information gaps. The CFAM can give form and meaning to what is already known and offer direction for future questioning.

CASE STUDY

Jason Henderson, a 17-year-old male, is admitted to the intensive care unit, deeply comatose and decerebrating, having suffered a closed head injury in a single-vehicle accident. He is a star athlete, the youngest of four, with married sisters aged 26, 28, and 29. He lives with his mother and father, aged 55 and 60, respectively, in a small town where the parents own and operate the local garage and convenience store. A good student, he has just been honored as "athlete of the year" at a community dance. Happy and inebriated, he was driving his 16-year-old girlfriend, Lori, home from the dance when he lost control of the vehicle on a gravel road. The car flipped through the air twice and landed upside down in the ditch. Lori was killed on impact.

The charge nurse in the intensive care unit the night of admission makes a point of meeting with Mr. and Mrs. Henderson in a nearby "quiet room." They are distraught, overwhelmed by shock and anxiety. They describe in detail their pride during the dance, juxtaposing it with their shock when, as they were preparing for bed, the police arrived to tell them about the accident. They keep repeating unfinished sentences: "If only we'd driven Lori home ourselves...," "If only we hadn't let him drink to celebrate...," "If only the dance hadn't..."

The nurse allows the parents to recreate the scene, express their perceived guilt, and share their disbelief. Gently, she says, "It must seem so unreal, like a nightmare. In one evening you've gone from being the proudest of parents to the most scared." She lets the family respond to this and then slowly and simply informs them of Jason's condition, the treatment plan, and their involvement. She also introduces them to the treatment facility (explaining, for example, the location of coffee, washrooms, and telephones). Mr. and Mrs. Henderson are calmer; more importantly, a relationship has been established.

Already, by sensitive listening and careful observation, the nurse has started both structural and functional assessment. By allowing the parents to talk first, she has established a relationship that will allow her to probe for more information about the Henderson family and the impact of Jason's injury.

CONCLUSIONS

When the ambulance arrives at the hospital carrying an adolescent with a head or spinal cord injury, the nurse faces a complex array of assessment and intervention tasks on behalf of both patient and family. Despite severe limitations of time, place, and cooperation, she will have the opportunity, even during active patient treatment in the initial phase, to assess family structure, development, and function.

This chapter has focused on the unique characteristics of nursing assessment in families facing the possibility of death or profound disability in an adolescent member. The family relies on the nurse to care for the patient. The nurse, however, knows that this injury will have devastating effects on the whole family. Therefore, family assessment and effective intervention go hand in hand.

REFERENCES

Aldous, J. *Family Careers: Developmental Change in Families.* New York: John Wiley & Sons, 1978.

Bond, M.R. "Assessment of Outcome after Severe Brain Damage," *Lancet* 1:489, 1975.

Buchanan, K.M. *Coping When Life Is Threatened.* Regina, Canada: Weigl, 1984.

Canadian Paraplegic Association, Saskatchewan Division. *Annual Report.* Canadian Paraplegic Association, 1985.

Charles, E.D., et al. "Spinal Cord Injury—a Cost Benefit Analysis of Alternative Treatment Models," *Paraplegia* 12:225, 1974.

McGoldrick, M., et al. *Ethnicity and Family Therapy.* New York: Guilford Press, 1982.

Rimel, R.W., and Jane, J.A. "Characteristics of the Head-Injured Patient," in *Rehabilitation of the Head-Injured Adult.* Edited by Rosenthal, M., et al. Philadelphia: F.A. Davis Co., 1983.

Saskatchewan Coordinating Council on Social Planning. *A Study of the Rehabilitation Needs and Services in Saskatchewan for Persons Who Have Suffered a Brain Injury.* Saskatchewan, Canada: Saskatchewan Coordinating Council, 1984.

Toman, W. *Family Constellation—Its Effects on Personality and Social Behavior,* 3rd ed. New York: Springer Publishing Co., 1976.

Warner, W.L. *American Life: Dream and Reality.* Chicago: University of Chicago Press, 1962.

Wright, L., and Leahey, M. *Nurses and Families: A Guide to Family Assessment and Intervention.* Philadelphia: F.A. Davis Co., 1984.

9 Assessing marital responses to the threat of breast cancer

Janice M. Bell, RN, MS, PhD
Assistant Professor
Faculty of Nursing
University of Calgary
Calgary, Alberta, Canada

OVERVIEW

The discovery of a breast lump or other abnormality has implications for the individual that ripple through the marital and family systems. Evidence suggests that this is a stressful time, with the fear of breast cancer a major concern. This chapter proposes that early assessment of the woman and her partner during the prediagnosis phase may have a prophylactic effect, reducing both individual distress and family disruption. An interview guide based on the Calgary Family Assessment Model (CFAM) suggests specific questions to ask the couple. The importance of creating an opportunity for partners to express emotional concerns and receive accurate information is emphasized.

> I have not been sleeping well. In the middle of the night I keep thinking "What if...?" and I just go crazy. In the daytime I can just say I am not going to think about it and I don't. But at night it is harder not to think about it because you are just lying there. (woman, age 48)

A woman's discovery of a lump or other abnormality in her breast often triggers thoughts of breast cancer and raises a multitude of fears about dying, disfigurement, and abandonment by her partner. This intensely emotional response is well documented in the popular and scientific literature. The most stressful stage of the breast cancer experience seems to come immediately after discovery of the lump (Jamison et al., 1978), yet health professionals have given relatively little attention to this prediagnosis period.

This chapter reviews what is known about the impact of the breast cancer threat and identifies a nursing assessment framework for working with the marital subsystem before biopsy. While breast cancer is known to occur in males, female breast cancer is the focus here.

NURSING PROCESS

Assessment

The health problem: Breast cancer. Breast cancer, the most common female malignancy, strikes approximately 1 in every 11 women. It is the leading cause of death of women aged 35 to 54. The American Cancer Society predicted that, in 1985, 119,000 women would be newly diagnosed as having breast cancer and 38,400 of all women with breast cancer would die from it (Silverberg, 1985). Although concern about the alarming increase in the incidence of this disease continues to grow, 80% of abnormal breast conditions, including tumors, are benign (National Institutes of Health [NIH], 1982). Surgical removal of breast tissue for biopsy is commonly used to make an accurate diagnosis.

Among the factors associated with increased breast cancer risk are aging, family history of breast cancer, a high-fat diet, and high socioeconomic status (Helmrich et al., 1983; NIH, 1982).

Family implications. Empirical studies and clinical observations of female breast cancer reported in the literature have focused almost exclusively on individual patients in the postdiagnosis treatment phase. Women's psychological adjustment following breast cancer diagnosis and surgical breast removal (mastectomy) has received wide attention in the literature (Ervin, 1973; Lewis and Bloom, 1978–79; Morris, 1983; Morris et al., 1977; Scott, 1983b). However, little is known about individual experience during the critical prediagnosis period when the *possibility* of breast cancer is the primary concern.

Scott (1983a) interviewed 85 women with benign tumors at the prebiopsy phase and at 6 to 8 weeks postbiopsy to determine their anxiety levels and critical thinking ability. Patient anxiety levels prior to knowledge of diagnostic results were extremely high; 6 weeks later, anxiety was significantly reduced. Scott made no attempt to involve family members.

Maguire (1976) included prebiopsy measures in his study of 95 mastectomy and 65 benign breast disease patients. On admission to the hospital for the biopsy procedure, 40% of the women rated themselves as very anxious or depressed. Again, data were not collected from any other subsystems.

How does the psychological distress related to the threat of breast cancer affect the marital system? No empirical evidence could be found describing marital or family subsystem experience during the prediagnosis period; this is not surprising because in most settings where women receive breast care, the partner is involved only peripherally, if at all. Furthermore, there is usually little provision for partner involvement in patient education or in the selection of treatment. A comprehensive listing of breast cancer services identified only one program that offered women *and their families* prebiopsy education sessions with a nurse (NIH, 1982).

The impact of a confirmed breast cancer diagnosis and mastectomy on the marital and whole family systems has also received limited attention. One of the few relevant studies found that husbands involved in presurgical decision making reported greater postsurgical sexual satisfaction than those who were less involved. A significant number of men in the sample also reported psychosomatic and psychological reactions, including sleep disorders, appetite loss, and work disruption, during their partner's diagnosis and surgery (Wellisch et al., 1978).

Further justification for including the partner in breast cancer assessment is provided by Cooper (1984), who found that lung cancer diagnosis affected the openness of a married couple's communication. Most spouses reported not sharing their fears and concerns with the patients, and more spouses than patients reported signs of stress and isolation.

Obviously, the male partner appears affected by a woman's breast cancer experience. Yet he is largely neglected in present health care delivery and research efforts.

Taylor et al. (1985) reported that the more disfiguring the breast cancer surgery, the more likely it is that the patient will report a decline in marital affection and sexual behavior. Spiegel et al. (1983) found better patient adjustment to breast cancer in families that encouraged open discussion of feelings and problems. These observations further strengthen the importance of including the partner in prediagnosis assessment.

Theoretical bases. Traditional disease models have centered on the dualism of mind vs. body and individual vs. context, recognizing no relationship between the parts. The systems perspective clearly demonstrates the fallacy of such a dichotomy. This chapter offers an assessment tool based on systems theory; it postulates that the world comprises complementary, hierarchical components (von Bertalanffy, 1950). Living systems contain levels ranging from the biological to the societal, with each level being organizationally distinct but communicating with others. Therefore, change at one hierarchical level effects change at other levels.

This theory modifies conventional views of illness in several ways. First, it suggests that illness affects the patient's psychological *and* organic subsystems. Moreover, it suggests that illness has an impact on several subsystem levels, as well as on interactions between levels

(Beavers, 1983). This challenges nurse clinicians and researchers to examine illnesses in context and to look beyond the individual when planning nursing assessment and intervention.

Nurses in any setting who wish to include the partner or significant other in the critical prediagnosis assessment can use this framework. The assessment provides a unique opportunity for marital partners to share their concerns through the presence of a third party. Questions invite expression of feelings and concerns and allow the couple to broach sensitive issues that they might otherwise have been reluctant to explore. In this way open marital communication can be enhanced and future adjustment difficulties prevented.

Herz (1980) suggests that, in addition to open emotional communication, another factor affects family responses to illness: the nature of the illness itself. This finding is especially significant for those facing the threat of breast cancer because of the breast's association with nurturing, femininity, and sexuality (Goin, 1982). Added to this is cancer's widespread image as a cause of pain, suffering, and death. These associations may vary with individual or cultural values, but they speak eloquently to the sensitive nature of the illness and the importance of including the marital/sexual partner in assessment.

Why perform a prediagnostic nursing assessment? As suggested by the literature, this phase is critical (Scott, 1983b); although four out of five breast biopsies are benign, the patient and family will feel in limbo until the results are known. As one woman remarked, "I felt I could not plan for next month or next year until I knew." Often the prediagnosis phase consists of waiting—for an appointment with a surgical oncologist, for mammogram results, and for biopsy scheduling. This phase can take anywhere from a few days to several weeks, creating what Welch (1981) calls the "worry and waiting syndrome."

Lambert and Lambert (1985, p. 71), although concentrating on implications, support nursing involvement during the prediagnosis phase. They define the nurse's role in prediagnosis as

> ...assisting the individual in obtaining appropriate medical evaluation; dealing with the impact that the detection of a lump has upon one's life; being cognizant of the possible ramifications of a mastectomy, and utilizing appropriate support systems.

The assessment process. A prediagnostic assessment provides information and support as it encourages anticipatory coping. As such, it may also reduce distress and family disruption.

The assessment tool contains several questions that may be used as a guide during a joint interview with the woman and her partner. By using Wright and Leahey's CFAM (1984), questions can be developed to assess specific areas of family structure, development, and function. A home interview allows the nurse to see the couple in their physical and social environment, thus enriching the data collected; however, the session can be conducted in any quiet and private setting.

Family structure. Involving the couple in preparing a genogram or diagram of the family constellation (Wright and Leahey, 1984) helps begin the interview and engage their interest. To enhance engagement efforts, it is best to begin with the male partner, and then ask parallel genogram questions of the woman. These questions are usually willingly and enthusiastically answered, and it is amazing to watch the degree of rapport that develops when the nurse interviewer conveys genuine interest in family information. After the genogram has been constructed, the couple can be shown their "family map" as evidence that important and valued information has been shared.

Besides eliciting information about the family's structure, the questions used to generate the genogram can illuminate such other important issues as previous experience with illness, family history of breast cancer, the quality and quantity of supportive relationships, and even self-fulfilling health prophesies.

Research comparing various methods of obtaining family information found that the semistructured genogram interview was useful and efficient, yielding four times as much information as the informal health interview. Ninety-six percent of all patients respond favorably to its use (Rogers and Durkin, 1984).

Family development. The timing of the illness in the family life cycle also needs to be assessed. Because breast cancer tends to be a "middle-aged" illness, such developmental tasks as relinquishing parental control and reinvesting energies in the marital relationship and individual pursuits (McCullough, 1980) may influence and be influenced by the illness. The genogram provides the information needed to determine the family's developmental stage and identify related tasks. Additional questions, such as "How does what you're doing to face this illness now compare with what you would have done 10 years ago (or 10 years from now)?" may also elicit useful information about the illness's impact on family development.

Family functioning. Assessment of family functioning must encompass the following topics (see also Table 9.1):

Beliefs. This area explores the couple's knowledge of breast lump diagnosis and treatment. Lazarus and Folkman's (1984) theoretical work emphasized that some situations have the potential to create threat, harm, and challenge, depending on a dynamic interaction between several personal and situational factors. Individual interpretations of an illness or the possibility of illness might be related to previous experience with the illness itself; exposure to media or personal reports about the condition; uncertainty about how the illness will develop or respond to treatment, or the mental confusion that comes from having to consider several possible outcomes; the length of the anticipation time; and timing of the illness in relation to other life events. All of these factors may contribute to or diminish the perceived threat.

An exploration of family beliefs (see Table 9.1) not only assesses the couple's perceived threat but also identifies information deficits. Seeking information about the illness, its treatment, and the probable outcomes is an important skill in coping with acute health crisis (Moos, 1982). However, anxiety, uncertain diagnosis, and lack of partner involvement in discussions of treatment alternatives can hinder information processing and result in an incomplete and unclear understanding of the health crisis. Nurses can provide necessary patient education in such specific areas as diagnostic testing procedures (for example, the mammogram); expectations and sensations associated with various types of biopsies (including when results are expected); and general health care, such as management of postoperative pain, swelling, bruising, and fatigue.

Table 9.1 Assessing Family Function in Potential Breast Cancer

Area Assessed	Appropriate Questions
Beliefs (Perception of threat)	• What do you understand will be done about the breast lump? • What previous experience do you have with major illness/surgery? • What does the word "cancer" mean to you? • Do you know someone who has or has had cancer? What happened to that person? • What other major events are happening in your life right now?
(Information deficit)	• What do you want to know about your illness, diagnosis, and/or treatment?
Emotional communication	• What concerns you most about the possibility of breast cancer? • What changes have you noticed in your partner since you were told about the need for a biopsy? • Who seems to be most affected by this situation?
Problem solving	• What have you as a couple found to be most helpful in dealing with your current situation? What else would help you cope? • What do you need most from your partner at this time?

It is crucial that the nurse allow the couple to guide the education process by asking what *they* want to know. Research suggests that a need *not to know* may serve a protective function (Bean et al., 1980; McIntosh, 1974). Learner readiness is an important aspect of any health teaching and one that nurses are frequently least sensitive to in their eager attempts to help clients.

The client couple may also ask the nurse, "What if they find cancer?" Recent media attention and an abundance of conflicting information about breast cancer treatment make this a question that must be dealt with carefully and accurately. Several publications might be recommended to interested couples (Kushner, 1984; Morra and Potts, 1980; NIH, 1982).

Emotional communication. Even in well-functioning families, the ability to express thoughts and feelings may be threatened by the intensity and duration of the illness (Herz, 1980). The nurse must encourage the couple to communicate openly, even about emotional concerns that are difficult to discuss.

In most cases, the woman facing a possible breast cancer diagnosis is concerned primarily with the biopsy and the likelihood of a positive diagnosis. Knowing this allows the nurse to probe empathetically for more specific fears about pain, breast loss, and death. The partner is generally most concerned about his wife's health and the possibility of her death; he may feel that the potential breast loss is less important or not important at all. Sharing his feelings with the patient may allay her concerns about sexual attractiveness and abandonment. In this way, assessment of emotional communication may, in a sense, become intervention by initiating ventilation and verbal intimacy.

Another useful strategy is to ask each partner for information about the other, thereby acknowledging and normalizing behavior changes that, while normal in the context of coping with the breast cancer threat, may be causing anxiety for one or both partners.

Wright and Leahey (1984, p. 107) suggest that "clarification of differences between individuals is a significant source of information about family functioning." By allowing partners to share their concerns and behaviors in relation to the threat of illness, the nurse can facilitate a clearer understanding of their present experience and encourage mutual support.

Problem solving. The nurse should encourage the couple to consider what problem-solving approaches they will use to deal with the threat of breast cancer. Focusing specifically on marital subsystem solution patterns will at least demystify current patterns and may encourage consideration of new coping techniques.

Planning

Should breast cancer be diagnosed, several interventions, based on the prebiopsy assessment, will require planning. Information deficits noted in the prediagnosis phase may direct the nurse to explore what the couple wants to know about cancer treatment alternatives, so she can plan appropriate education. The nurse might also encourage more specific emotional communication about the cancer diagnosis and examine problem-solving methods used to compensate for differing communication styles.

CASE STUDY

The following are excerpts from an interview with Susan and Dave Rennie. After the surgeon suggested a biopsy of Susan's breast lump, a nurse called and arranged to see the couple in their home a few days before the test. When constructing the genogram (Figure 9.1), the nurse learned that the Rennie family consisted of the father, Dave (43), an accountant, and the mother, Susan (41), a part-time sales clerk. Their children were Michelle, 14, and Todd, 11— students in grades 8 and 5, respectively. The couple has been married 19 years. Dave is the older of two adopted children. Heart disease tends to run in his family of origin, but he is in good health. His family lives in the area and Dave sees them once a month. Susan is the oldest of three children. Her mother had a mastectomy 20 years ago and her father died of liver cancer in 1983. She sees her family several times a year.

Nurse:
What do you two understand about the breast lump? How was it found and what will be done with it?

Dave:
Well, my wife found it. It has scared the hell out of both of us. We have been told it needs to be looked at. Unless in the odd chance it turns out to be something worse, it's just a matter of having it removed.

Susan:
I think I have known about it for a while. I never thought anything of it and then all of a sudden it seemed to feel different. I decided to go to the doctor. By the time I had my mammogram it was another week to wait. I gave my resignation at work and gave them a week's notice. I thought since I have to start going to the doctor's I might as well just finish right now. Then I saw my doctor again and he referred me to the surgeon. I wish they could find a faster system. It would certainly help. I've been waiting a month and a half. It is a long time to be held in limbo. Do you go on with your life or what? I'm still waiting to hear when the biopsy will be. I'm just waiting for the hospital to call.

Nurse:
What have you been told about the biopsy?

Susan:
I haven't been told anything, basically. I think they just take it for granted. The doctor said if it was serious, we would talk later about what would be done. My husband was waiting for me in the doctor's office but I really never thought

Figure 9.1   Genogram—The Rennie Family

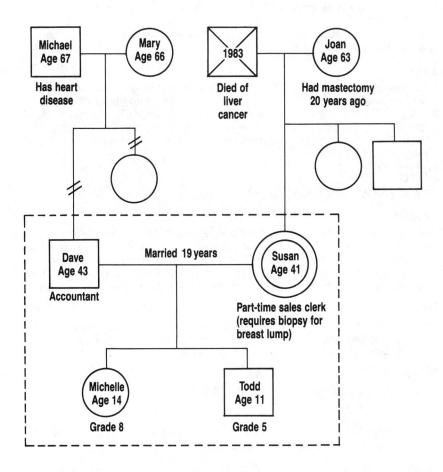

he should be in there with me. It wasn't really that big of a deal to me but maybe I should have had him in there with me. We haven't really talked about it that much.

Nurse:
Do you have any questions that I might help you with?

Dave:
Yes, I have millions of questions. (Discussion about these ensues.)

Nurse:
What previous experience have you had with major illness or surgery?

Susan:

My mother had a mastectomy 20 years ago, so I started to think back to that time. I wondered if I should connect the two. For the first time in my life I may have the possibility of really having a disease other than taking an aspirin and staying in bed for a day.

Dave:

You have to look at the odds. With the history in the family, it's like flipping a coin: heads or tails. But I think you have to get away from being afraid of the big "C." When you hear the word "cancer," automatically you switch to dying. I'm not saying it's always curable, but there are controllable types of cancer. (Discussion ensues regarding the husband's experience of his father having a heart attack.)

Nurse:

What is your greatest concern now?

Susan:

Oh, my biggest concern is that it not be malignant. That is my only main concern. I'm not looking forward to the biopsy procedure but I'm not...that is not terrifying me...Sometimes I think "What if...?" and I have to tell myself to stop it. I wouldn't say all the time. But I think, "Oh my goodness, I have two kids. What would happen?" I'll wait until the results are in and go from there.

Dave:

Both of us are quite capable of handling any news, but just not knowing is the worst of it. To say, okay, half the breast is gone or the whole breast is gone, so what, that's all. I just want her to come out healthy.

Nurse:

Dave, what changes have you noticed in Susan?

Dave:

She has changed a bit. This is difficult to describe. She has been spending more time with the kids. She's also been grouchier!

Susan:

My emotions are high. I'm on edge. I have the odd cry, but I'm okay.

Dave:

I think I would be a bit that way too.

Nurse:

Susan, what changes have you noticed in Dave?

Susan:

The uncertainty is very hard on us. He's not a big talker about such things anyway. I think we have become more affectionate. Like, he phones me every day a couple of times, more than he did before. We both started smoking again. We had both quit smoking before this happened. I know I shouldn't be smoking right now but I can't seem to stop.

Nurse:

Who do you think is most affected by this situation?

Dave:
Oh, Susan, definitely. Sure, it bothers me, but I'm sure it bothers her more. My role is to be the support person. You have to be supportive, and yet you are a little scared too.

Susan:
Yes, but you don't show your inner feelings. He tries to be strong for me all the time no matter what.

Nurse:
Is that helpful to you?

Susan:
Yes, but I wish he would let his guard down once in a while! (Laughter)...I share emotions for both of us...You don't like me to talk about things like this so you say "Oh, Susie!" I tend to be very abrupt when I say things. He doesn't like it when I say things like, "What if I die?"

Nurse:
What do you need most from your husband at this time?

Susan:
Just the support, and being able to talk about it. They say sometimes this makes or breaks a couple. It either drives you closer together or farther apart. Like, will he still love me if I'm lopsided?

Dave:
I like to take things one step at a time. It is fine to try and plan ahead but you can only go so far and then you start tripping yourself up. She tends to look at the grim side of things.

Nurse:
Yes, but what do you need most from Susan at this time?

Dave:
Nothing really. I just want her to know that I am worried too and I'll stick with her through thick or thin.

Nurse:
What has been helpful for you as a couple in dealing with this experience?

Susan:
Each other. Knowing that you have each other for support. I think work helps too. Keeping very busy.

Dave:
I think having information is helpful. That's why this interview is a good idea. A person needs clear explanations of what is going to happen and why. Also, this interview has given me a chance to understand Susie's concerns better.

It is clear from the interview that Susan's family cancer history plays a significant role in this couple's belief system about breast cancer. Susan reflects on her mother's experience and realizes that, while her mother survived the illness, she may not be so fortunate. Themes of death and dying emerged several times in the interview. The threat is so large that Susan has chosen to quit her part-time job in order to free more time for family relationships. By asking the assessment questions, the nurse provided an opportunity for increased emotional communication and identification of what the couple needed most from each other. Susan requested more communication from Dave and he responded by sharing feelings of fear, concern, and support. At this point, no further intervention appears necessary.

CONCLUSIONS

Nurses wishing to provide family-focused care (Wright and Bell, 1981) should initiate assessment soon after a lump is detected and before final diagnosis. The questions in this framework are specifically designed for the prediagnosis period, and are based on the assumption that the breast cancer threat will have a ripple effect on the family—specifically, on the marital subsystem. The interview facilitates change within the marital subsystem: increased understanding about what to expect during the operative procedure, more realistic perceptions of the illness, enhanced emotional communication, and overt rather than covert expression of each partner's needs from the other. These changes may result in less individual distress and family disruption. In this way, assessment becomes intervention.

REFERENCES

Bean, G., et al. "Coping Mechanisms of Cancer Patients: A Study of 33 Patients Receiving Chemotherapy," *CA—Cancer Clinician* 30(5):256-60, 1980.

Beavers, W.R. "Hierarchical Issues in a Systems Approach to Illness and Health," *Family Systems Medicine* 1(1):47–55, 1983.

"Cancer Statistics," *Cancer* 34:7–23, 1984.

Cooper, E.T. "A Pilot Study on the Effects of the Diagnosis of Lung Cancer on Family Relationships," *Cancer Nursing* 7(4):301–08, 1984.

Ervin, C.V. "Psychologic Adjustment to Mastectomy," *Medical Aspects of Human Sexuality* 7:42–65, 1973.

Goin, M.K. "Psychological Reactions to Surgery of the Breast," *Clinics in Plastic Surgery* 9(3):347–54, 1982.

Helmrich, S.P., et al. "Risk Factors for Breast Cancer," *American Journal of Epidemiology* 117(1):35–45, 1983.

Herz, F. "The Impact of Death and Serious Illness on the Family Life Cycle," in *The Family Life Cycle: A Framework for Family Therapy.* Edited by Carter, E.A., and McGoldrick, M. New York: Gardner Press, 1980.

Jamison, K.R., et al. "Psychological Aspects of Mastectomy: I. The Woman's Perspective," *American Journal of Psychiatry* 135:432–36, 1978.

Kushner, R. *Alternatives.* Cambridge, Mass.: Kensington Press, 1984.

Lambert, V.A., and Lambert, C.E. *Psychosocial Care of the Physically Ill,* 2nd ed. Englewood Cliffs, N.J.: Prentice-Hall, 1985.

Lazarus, R.S., and Folkman, S. *Stress, Appraisal, and Coping.* New York: Springer Publishing Co., 1984.

Lewis, F.M., and Bloom, J.R. "Psychosocial Adjustment of Breast Cancer: A Review of Selected Literature," *International Journal of Psychiatry in Medicine* 9(1):1–17, 1978–79.

Maguire, P. "The Psychological and Social Sequelae of Mastectomy," in *Modern Perspectives in Psychiatric Aspects of Surgery.* Edited by Howells, J.G. New York: Brunner-Mazel, 1976.

McCullough, P. "Launching Children and Moving On," in *The Family Life Cycle: A Framework for Family Therapy.* Edited by Carter, E.A., and McGoldrick, M. New York: Gardner Press, 1980.

McIntosh, J. "Processes of Communication, Information Seeking and Control Associated with Cancer: A Review of the Literature," *Social Science and Medicine* 8:167–87, 1974.

Moos, R.H. "Coping with Acute Health Crisis," in *Handbook of Clinical Health Psychology.* Edited by Millon, T., et al. New York: Plenum Pubs., 1982.

Morra, M., and Potts, E. *Choices: Realistic Alternatives in Cancer Treatment.* New York: Avon Books, 1980.

Morris, T. "Psychosocial Aspects of Breast Cancer: A Review," *European Journal of Cancer and Clinical Oncology* 19:1725–33, 1983.

Morris, T., et al. "Psychological and Social Adjustment to Mastectomy," *Cancer* 40:2381–87, 1977.

National Institutes of Health. *The Breast Cancer Digest. A Guide to Medical Care, Emotional Support, Educational Programs, and Resources,* no. 82–1691. Bethesda, Md.: National Cancer Institute, 1982.

Rogers, J., and Durkin, M. "The Semi-Structured Genogram Interview: I. Protocol, II. Evaluation," *Family Systems Medicine* 2(2):176–87, 1984.

Scott, D.W. "Anxiety, Critical Thinking and Information Processing During and After Breast Biopsy," *Nursing Research* 32(1):24–28, 1983.

Scott, D.W. "Individual Response to Breast Cancer," *Topics in Clinical Nursing* 4(4):20–37, 1983.

Silverberg, E. "Cancer Statistics, 1985," *CA—A Cancer Journal for Clinicians* 35(1):19–35, 1985.

Spiegel, D., et al. "Family Environment as a Predictor of Adjustment to Metastatic Breast Carcinoma," *Journal of Psychosocial Oncology* 1(1):33–44, 1983.

Taylor, S.E., et al. "Illness-Related and Treatment-Related Factors in Psychological Adjustment to Breast Cancer," *Cancer* 55:2506–13, 1985.

von Bertalanffy, L. "An Outline of General Systems Theory," *British Journal of the Philosophy of Science* 1:134–65, 1950.

Welch, D. "Waiting, Worry and the Cancer Experience," *Oncology Nursing Forum* 8:14–18, 1981.

Wellisch, D.K., et al. "Psychological Aspects of Mastectomy: II. The Man's Perspective," *American Journal of Psychiatry* 135:543–46, 1978.

Worden, J.W., and Weisman, A.D. "Psychosocial Components of Lagtime in Cancer Diagnosis," *Journal of Psychosomatic Research* 19(2):69–79, 1975.

Wright, L.M., and Bell, J.M. "Nurses, Families and Illness: A New Combination," in *Treating Families with Special Needs.* Edited by Freeman, D., and Trute, B. Ottawa: The Canadian Association of Social Workers, 1981.

Wright, L.M., and Leahey, M. *Nurses and Families. A Guide to Family Assessment and Intervention.* Philadelphia: F.A. Davis Co., 1984.

10 Assessing families and open heart surgery patients

Kathleen M. Gaglione, RN, MS
Phase III Coordinator
Maywood Cardiology Associates
Cardiac Treatment Center
Westchester, Illinois

OVERVIEW

Because patients are members of families, holistic care of the cardiac surgical patient demands assessment of and intervention for the needs of the family as well as the patient. Surgical treatment of cardiac disease is both radical and life-threatening and affects each member of the family. A growing body of literature describes the importance of addressing family needs to enhance the system of support for healthy and ill members alike. The patient can only benefit from the support offered by a family that is less anxious and better able to contribute to the recovery process.

This chapter helps the nurse anticipate and assess the needs of cardiac surgical families. Specific assessment and planning recommendations are made for the admission, hospitalization, discharge, and rehabilitative periods. The author intends to convey readily applicable guidelines for working with the cardiac surgical family.

NURSING PROCESS

Assessment

The health problem: Cardiac surgery. Roughly 20% of all Americans, it is estimated, suffer from one or more forms of cardiovascular disease. Of these, an estimated 40% annually require coronary artery bypass grafting (CABG) (American Heart Association, 1985). CABG has come under increasing scrutiny in recent years but remains one of the most viable interventions for symptomatic coronary artery disease.

The advent of such procedures as percutaneous transluminal coronary angioplasty clearly reflects cardiac researchers' dedication to developing less traumatic interventions for coronary artery disease. This procedure involves introduction of a balloon-tipped catheter into a partially occluded coronary artery. Once inflated, the balloon compresses the atheromatous plaque into the vessel wall, thus reducing the obstruction. Research and clinical trials also continue to perfect the use of the laser to open occluded or narrowed vessels.

CABG has become fairly standardized. Following preoperative preparation, the patient is anesthetized and respiratory support provided. The chest is opened and the heart exposed while acceptable vein grafts are harvested from the leg. The patient is then prepared for placement on the heart/lung bypass machine, which redirects the patient's blood from the right atrium or the superior and inferior venae cavae through the machine; carbon dioxide and oxygen exchange replace normal lung function. Metabolic byproducts and electrolytes are also kept in balance through the machine. A second cannula pumps freshly oxygenated blood through the ascending aorta and on to the rest of the body.

The heart is stopped by induction of a cardioplegic solution, customarily a chilled, high-potassium saline fluid. Surgeons then attach one end of the vein graft at a point past the coronary artery occlusion and sew the other end of the graft onto an opening created in the aorta. When the required number of grafts are completed, blood flow is restored to check for graft patency. Tubes are placed in the chest to prevent fluid build-up around the heart. The body is gradually warmed and the heart defibrillated to restore electrical activity. The leg graft sites and chest are sewn and dressed. The patient then returns to the cardiac surgical intensive care unit.

Need for family involvement. The term "family" has been defined as "a group of two or more individuals living together and interacting with one another through mutually defined roles. Because of its dynamic state, any change in one results in changes in all other family members" (Hymovich, 1978, p. 19). Williams notes that "when one person leaves a system each member of the system is affected. Part of the way in which each person maintains his view of himself is undermined. Therefore, when one family member is hospitalized, each family member experiences stress" (1974, p. 38). Illness disrupts not only the afflicted member's life, but the whole family's life as well. Of the family's particular stress, Roberts observed that "while remaining on the periphery, the family quietly experiences its own special stress, the sources of which have to do with the illness itself and the threats it implies" (1976, p. 356).

Cardiac disease has a tremendous impact on both patients and their families. Heart damage, actual or potential, threatens not only physical functioning but also self-image. "In our culture, the heart is a symbol which is used to represent emotion, character, and psychological traits far beyond its physical function" (Carnes, 1971, p. 1187).

For the cardiac surgical patient and his family, the threat to life may be twofold. Preexisting cardiac disease, whether symptomatic or asymptomatic, requires significant life-style changes for most persons—changes that, along with symptoms, constantly remind them and their families of the health problem. The cardiac patient requiring CABG faces threats far beyond the normal risks of surgery. Despite the technical improvements made in recent years, a great likelihood of intra- and postoperative complications remains, and the psychological impact of such a grossly invasive procedure cannot be overlooked.

As CABG has been increasingly commonplace, nurses have assumed more direct interventional responsibility for both patient and family care. The importance of family support in effective recovery from critical illness is well documented (Gaglione, 1984; Molter, 1979; Rasie, 1980; Rogers, 1983). Like any illness, a cardiac event is experienced collectively; family needs must be assessed and incorporated into the nursing care plan. In turn, the patient benefits from the support offered by a healthy, relaxed family (Gaglione, 1984, p. 432).

A theoretical model of family assessment. Viewing the CABG patient and the family as a system provides an efficient means of assessing the needs of both. Family assessment must consider the cardiac patient as part of the whole and vice versa; an important interplay exists between assessing and meeting the needs of both segments of the family. A systems approach to assessment also affords the nurse a succinct approach to planning effective and comprehensive care.

Due to the life-threatening nature of cardiac disease, the nurse should approach needs assessment from three perspectives: patient needs, family needs exclusive of the patient, and family needs including the patient. This framework allows the nurse to anticipate need variance and tailor care to specific groups or subgroups.

Given the collective impact of change in any single family member, the family's systemic equilibrium can best be maintained or restored by recognizing and working with the crucial members of the family. Viewing the cardiac patient and his family from this perspective is essential for effective recovery.

Family assessment and intervention. Just as the surgical patient's needs change throughout hospitalization, so do the needs of the family. Nursing awareness of this aspect of assessment and planning represents an important step toward total patient care for the open-heart surgery candidate. Table 10.1 summarizes the basic family needs, as well as assessment and intervention strategies, common to cardiac surgical care.

Table 10.1 Family Assessment and Intervention in Cardiac Surgical Care

Need	Assessment Questions	Intervention
Preoperative Period		
Information about the procedure	• What are your specific questions about the surgery? • What do you already know about the procedure? • What have the physicians told you about the procedure?	• Include the family in patient instruction about the surgical procedure, preoperative routine, and immediate postoperative period. • Arrange consultation with appropriate health professionals.
Reassurance that the best care is being provided	• What would you like to know about the staff who will be caring for your (relative)?	• Provide open, direct information within an appropriate scope. • Offer direct reassurance and examples of quality care provision.
Postsurgical information	• Have the surgeons told you when they will tell you how the operation went?	
Familiarity with the hospital setting and postoperative routine	• Have you seen an intensive care unit before? • Would you like to tour the unit here? • Do you know where to find something to eat or drink or make a phone call while you are waiting?	• Tell family members where to find the surgical waiting area, chapel, cafeteria, etc. • Advise the family of other available services, for example, overnight accommodations, special parking permits, social services.
A predictable schedule	• Do you know what time surgery is scheduled and how long it should last?	
Stress management		• Help family members identify effective coping mechanisms. • Meet with family members regularly, away from the patient's room; encourage questions and ventilation of thoughts and concerns.

Need	Assessment Questions	Intervention
Intraoperative Period		
Information about the patient's status during surgery	• Do you have any questions at this time?	• Meet intermittently with family members to convey information; offer emotional support. • Use auxiliary personnel to help keep the family informed.
Privacy		• Allow family members some time alone.
Additional information about the surgery and its aftermath (for example, duration of the procedure, what to expect in the ICU)		• Help family members understand the time frame for surgery.
Spiritual/emotional support	• Has the chaplain been by to see how you are doing? • Do you know where the chapel is located?	• Use touch to convey support and comfort.
Individual needs	• Are you hungry? • Is there anyone you would like to call? • Would you like to freshen up?	
Postsurgical contact with the surgeon/radiologist	• Have you thought about what you would like to ask the surgeons when they are finished?	• Arrange for the operating physician to meet with the family after surgery.
Immediate Postoperative Period		
Reassurance that the best care is being provided	• What would you like to know about your (relative's) care?	• Schedule regular (daily) meetings with the family.

(continued)

Table 10.1 Family Assessment and Intervention in Cardiac Surgical Care *(continued)*

Need	Assessment Questions	Intervention
Immediate Postoperative Period (continued)		
Ability to help the patient directly	• Would you like to help me make your (relative) more comfortable?	• Involve the family in care (giving back rubs, assisting with personal care). • Encourage physical contact (for example, hand holding). • Include the family in any formal or informal patient teaching.
Confidence that the family will be informed of any change in the patient's condition		• Reassure relatives.
Regular contact with the patient	• Do you know what visiting hours are?	• Make the visitation schedule as flexible as possible. • Reorient relatives to the ICU environment so they can comfortably visit and help the patient.
Prompt, clear, direct answers to questions		• Answer questions honestly and openly.
Ability to contact health care personnel whenever necessary	• Do you know how to contact us from outside the hospital?	• Provide the unit phone number.
Postoperative Step-Down/Predischarge Period		
Concise, shared, individualized home care instructions	• What questions do you have about bringing your (relative) home?	• Prepare the family for all aspects of home care: patient activity/exercise, personal/incision care, resumption of sexual activity, return to work, follow-up appointments. • Arrange formal and informal instruction.

Need	Assessment Questions	Intervention
Postoperative Step-Down/Predischarge Period (continued)		
A primary contact person	• Would you like to be able to call someone about questions or problems that arise after you return home?	• Stress the importance of follow-up. Ensure that patient and family have a workable understanding of and adequate supply of postoperative medications. • Be sure all necessary follow-up appointments have been made. • Determine whether or not a rehabilitation program has been arranged and educate the family accordingly.
Ventilation of fears and concerns		• Educate patient about cardiac recovery. • Anticipate questions about post-surgical/chest pain, the likelihood of another attack, incision drainage. • Use ancillary personnel to provide education and emotional support. • Orient the family to step-down routines and the rationales for care procedures. • Arrange a private meeting with the family to answer questions and provide direction. • Use a spouse—or family—support format to encourage expression and resolution of concerns and questions.
Rehabilitation Period		
Emotional/educational support		• Invite relatives to participate in teaching sessions, observe cardiac exercise groups, and/or join support groups.
Coping assistance		• Suggest cardiopulmonary resuscitation instruction for all family members.

Recognizing family members' responses to their relative's surgery is an integral part of family assessment and planning, since needs and responses to illness are interrelated. Reactions to illness may vary depending on the coping techniques available. However, anxiety has been cited as the primary response to illness for both patient and family members (Gaglione, 1984, p. 428).

Nursing assessment of family needs requires several important skills, but none more critical than observation and communication. In addition, the professional nurse with clinical experience and/or familiarity with current family nursing literature should be able to anticipate family needs. Family members will exhibit and experience common responses to the cardiac surgical event. This does not preclude family assessment, but should enhance it.

The preoperative period. Family needs assessment should begin with the patient's preoperative admission. A staff nurse who worked with the patient and family previously could be reassigned to the case. This is possible where step-down units accommodate both medical and surgical cardiac patients. Many patients are also readmitted to the floors where they received cardiac catheterization. From the nurse's standpoint, familiarity with the patient, family, and history will facilitate needs assessment.

Routine nursing admission responsibilities such as taking a history and obtaining vital signs offer an excellent opportunity to assess family interaction and initial responses to the pending procedure. Note facial expressions, voice tone, and physical appearance for clues to family coping. Including family members in the nursing history interview may prompt questions that illuminate educational needs; separate meetings with patient and family members will often prompt more specific questions and expressions of concern. Finally, the nurse can use the patient history to help relate past experiences with a critical event and identify effective coping mechanisms.

Many nursing interventions can be planned for and anticipated during the open-heart hospitalization period, but attention to changing individual needs must be maintained. Based on the anticipated preoperative needs of family members, specific interventions can be developed in the nursing care plan.

The intraoperative period. One frequently overlooked area of nursing assessment and intervention is the status of the family while the patient is in surgery. Family members are often left alone at this time, and their need for privacy and isolated meditation should be respected. However, this is also a time when relatives need information. The situation is out of their hands, leaving many of them with feelings of powerlessness.

Institutions accommodate open-heart patients' families in different ways. Many provide a private waiting room; others ask family members to remain in the intensive care unit (ICU) waiting area. Some facilities do not provide for these families, who must spend the time in cafeterias or lobbies.

The professional nurse, often in concert with social support personnel, can use this time to assess and plan to meet family needs. All resources should be used, including the social workers and clergy who are often involved with routine open-heart follow-up for the patient and family.

Nursing assessment of family needs during surgery can be made through observation and discussion with family members. Other intraoperative needs may be anticipated based on past reactions to critical illness.

Nursing interventions, when feasible, can extend into the intraoperative period as well. Indeed, this should be encouraged, especially in settings where primary nursing is implemented. Intraoperative interventions can be incorporated into the nursing care plan before surgery on the basis of anticipated needs.

The immediate postoperative period. Families need new and diverse information after surgery, when the patient has been transferred to the ICU. The nurse's role at this time becomes crucial. Because different nurses may have divided care responsibilities, the preoperative floor nurse should inform the intensive care staff of identified family needs. In some institutions the patient and family may have been able to meet the intensive care nurse preoperatively. When they cannot, it becomes even more important that information regarding the family members be transmitted.

A verbal report and the nursing history and care plan provide the basis for continued assessment of family needs in the ICU. Meeting with the family members outside the unit and observing them at the bedside can offer the nurse clues to their specific needs.

Family needs change dramatically once the patient is transferred from surgery to intensive care; the need for information becomes critical. This requires planning several new interventions.

The postoperative step-down/predischarge. Following an uncomplicated 24 to 48 hours in surgical intensive care, most coronary bypass patients are transferred to a cardiac step-down unit. Specialized nursing care remains available, along with facilities for monitoring and meeting the specific needs of the cardiac surgical patient in a less critical setting. Families of patients in this setting might have divergent needs. The patient is now past the most critical phase of the process, and new family concerns may surface. Mixed emotions are common—excitement that the patient no longer requires intensive care may be offset by fear that the patient's needs will not be readily or adequately met outside the ICU.

Other family concerns can create challenging opportunities for the professional nurse. Members often harbor a variety of fears, including fear that the staff cannot meet the patient's needs well enough, which is often rooted in individual family members' fears that they cannot help the recovering patient. In the ICU, the family's chief concern was to have the ill relative "pull through"; now reality has set in and family members begin to face the fact that the patient will be coming home. They are likely to be surprised to find (even if instructed preoperatively) that, assuming there are no complications, cardiac patients are commonly discharged within 5 days of transfer to the step-down floor. This sometimes leaves family members feeling unprepared for the patient's homecoming.

At this stage, families need information about the impending discharge and appropriate home care techniques. They may sublimate fears and concerns by displaying anger or indifference. The attentive nurse recognizes this and incorporates family anxieties into care planning and delivery.

Assessment of family needs at this stage can begin at the time of transfer from the ICU staff. Observed interactions between patient and family often offer clues to the needs of both; the patient can also help identify family needs. Finally, one-to-one discussions with family members can reveal specific needs and concerns.

After the patient's transfer to the step-down unit, care plans should be updated to reflect the patient's and family's changing needs. Planning to meet family needs at this stage can begin with information reported by the intensive care nurse.

The rehabilitation period: Role of the cardiac rehabilitation nurse. In many facilities a cardiac rehabilitation nurse addresses the needs and concerns of open-heart surgery patients and their family members. In such a setting, the collaboration of nurses, the surgical team, the cardiac rehabilitation staff, nutritionists, cardiologists, and social service personnel is vital. Each team member contributes to patient treatment and recovery and to meeting family members' needs.

Preoperatively, the cardiac rehabilitation nurse may become acquainted with the patient and family and review the nursing goals and purposes of the immediate postoperative rehabilitation program. These goals usually include assisting with progressive ambulation, meeting educational/instructional needs, and providing emotional support.

Postoperatively, the cardiac rehabilitation nurse can pursue these goals through daily interaction on the step-down unit. Individualized or group sessions with patients and families can provide needed information as well as support through interaction. The cardiac rehabilitation nurse can define specific home care instructions and can serve as a postdischarge resource and liaison.

Planning

Planning nursing intervention for CABG patients and their families demands accurate need identification, followed by careful determination of appropriate nursing diagnoses. Family interventions need to address the family as a whole as well as individual members. The nurse must always plan to meet a variety of changing client needs.

The professional nurse uses two tools when planning for family members' needs—the nursing history and the nursing care plan. The nursing history forms the basis for identifying patient and family needs amenable to intervention. In many institutions it contains an abbreviated care plan for initial identification of nursing diagnoses and cursory intervention.

The nursing care plan is the worksheet for intervention planning. Based on the nursing diagnoses noted therein, specific individualized nursing interventions may be planned and documented.

For CABG patients and their families, the care plan maps out specific, individualized interventions. As noted previously, accurate nursing assessment and familiarity with potential anticipated needs facilitate effective planning.

CASE STUDY

Dr. Ravin, a 48-year-old white male and a cardiologist with a busy Midwestern practice, was admitted to the emergency department following cardiac arrest at home. He collapsed after 48 hours of vague, flulike symptoms and indigestion. Risk factors were significant: a very positive family history, a stressful occupation, and inconsistent exercise habits. Following admission, an inferior-posterior myocardial infarction and cardiogenic shock were diagnosed and the patient immediately taken for cardiac catheterization. Disease was diagnosed in three vessels; Dr. Ravin underwent an emergency triple bypass and was transferred to intensive care in stable condition.

The sudden nature of Dr. Ravin's illness did not allow family preparation. However, family assessment and intervention began when the family arrived in the emergency department. The patient's wife, daughters, and son were encouraged to ask questions and received direct, open answers. Mrs. Ravin was allowed to be with her husband before he was taken for cardiac catheterization. Such support persons as the patient's minister and colleagues were identified and summoned. The catheterization procedure was briefly explained to the family; since Mrs. Ravin was a nurse, the explanations were more comprehensive than in some other cases. The surgery itself was explained by the patient's peers.

Following the CABG, family members were given the most liberal visiting privileges allowable in the intensive care unit. Mrs. Ravin was allowed to call the unit from home and her husband's peers provided frequent updates and explanations. Nursing staff provided emotional support and encouraged hand holding between family members and the patient as they met immediate educational needs regarding recovery.

Following Dr. Ravin's transfer to the cardiac step-down unit, a more comprehensive patient-spouse education program was initiated. By mutual agreement, they received the same information, care, and rehabilitation as any other cardiac patient and family. Special attention was given to visitor restriction to allow rest and privacy.

Family members received both formal and informal education and were included in daily ambulation/exercise sessions with the cardiac rehabilitation staff. Family life-style changes and risk factor modification were discussed; members agreed to undertake a more structured exercise regimen, eliminate fast-food meals, investigate stress management classes, and reevaluate job work loads. A registered dietician reviewed advice on a prudent diet.

Discharge instructions were reviewed with the patient and his spouse. The importance of intrafamily communication was stressed. Explicit guidelines for activity resumption and exercise were discussed and arrangements made to have the patient and his wife participate in Phase II and Phase III cardiac rehabilitation programs. The patient's return to work was also discussed at length in a session that included his spouse and partners in practice.

The nursing and cardiac rehabilitation staffs met separately with Mrs. Ravin several times before and after discharge to discuss her fears and concerns. She was allowed to cry and to ventilate the feelings she did not wish to share with her husband.

Mrs. Ravin was encouraged to follow her husband's course through a Phase II cardiac exercise program. She observed exercise sessions, participated in educational offerings, and was invited to spouse support groups. Over the long term, they planned to participate in a Phase III maintenance exercise program together.

CONCLUSIONS

Family involvement is critical to comprehensive care provision. Due to the nature of the physiological insult involved in cardiac surgery, it becomes paramount in such cases. Preparation, involvement, and effective family coping will benefit the patient as well as the family and can contribute significantly to recovery.

REFERENCES

American Heart Association. *Heart Facts, 1985.* Washington, D.C.: American Heart Association, 1985.

Carnes, G.D. "Understanding the Cardiac Patient's Behavior," *American Journal of Nursing* 6:1187–88, 1971.

Gaglione, K.M. "Assessing and Intervening with Families of CCU Patients," *Nursing Clinics of North America* 19:427–32, 1984.

Hymovich, D. "Incorporating the Family into Care," *Journal of the New York State Nurses' Association* 5:9–14, 1978.

Molter, N.C. "Needs of Relatives of Critically Ill Patients: A Descriptive Study," *Heart and Lung* 8:332–39, 1979.

Rasie, S.M. "Meeting Families' Needs Helps You Meet ICU Patients' Needs," *Nursing80* 10:32–35, 1980.

Roberts, S.L. *Behavioral Concepts and the Critically Ill Patient.* Englewood Cliffs, N.J.: Prentice-Hall, 1976.

Rogers, C.D. "Needs of Relatives of Cardiac Surgery Patients During the Critical Care Phase," *Focus on Critical Care* 10:50–55, 1983.

Williams, F. "The Crisis of Hospitalization," *Nursing Clinics of North America* 9:37–45, 1974.

11 Assessing families and burns

Betsy C. Blades, MSW, PhD Candidate
School of Social Work and Social Research
Bryn Mawr College
Bryn Mawr, Pennsylvania

OVERVIEW

Since most burn victims do survive, the primary goals for improved outcome are qualitative. A literature review indicates that the family, while having needs of its own, plays a major role in ensuring the quality of patient recovery. During even the earliest assessment procedures, the nurse can provide the family with valuable support, build trust between family and health team members, and begin planning the multiple interventions necessary to optimize the outcome for all. An example of family systems assessment based on a burn case illustrates this potential and demonstrates an improvement in family care through a multidisciplinary, integrated team effort.

NURSING PROCESS

Assessment

The health problem: Burns. Improvements in medical and surgical technology, wound care, and rehabilitation have all contributed to improved survival, shorter initial hospitalization, and fewer cases of readmission among burn patients. However, burn care remains both a painful and lengthy process for the patient, his family, and the treatment staff. Scarring and skin contracture, as well as vocational and psychosocial adjustment problems, continue well beyond the period of acute hospitalization.

Each year in the United States, 70,000 persons are burned seriously enough to require hospitalization. The 21,000 who require the highest care level are admitted to one of 178 specialized regional burn services (American Burn Association, 1985). Such individuals have burns involving more than 10% (in young children and older adults) or 20% (in the middle age range) of total body surface. Burns of the hands, face, feet, or perineum, electrical injuries, circumferential burns, and burns accompanied by respiratory damage or other complications also require burn unit admission.

Analyses of large-scale data sets from hospital burn units indicate that 70% of admitted patients are male (Feller and Flanders, 1979). The most frequent place of injury is the home, where 70% to 85% of all serious burns occur. The work site is the second most frequently reported site (Feck et al., 1981; Feller, 1970). Burn injuries are highly preventable. An estimated 70% occur as a direct result of the injured party's actions, and only 20% of such patients are innocent bystanders. Assault or abuse, unusual medical risk, and rescue efforts are responsible for the remaining 10% (Feller, 1970). Significant numbers of burn patients are considered predisposed to such injury by virtue of behavioral, mental, or physical characteristics (MacArthur and Moore, 1975).

A burn victim's chances of survival depend largely on the total burn size, the extent of third-degree injury, sex, and age. A majority of the patients are between 5 and 34 years old, and this group has the highest survival rate for all burn sizes. Within all age groups, male survival rates are higher than female. Survival for all of those who are seriously injured now exceeds 87%, and only the very old have death rates above 50% (Feller et al., 1979). Organ failure and infection, which may occur several weeks or even months after admission, are the major causes of death. However, because the health care commitment is to quality as well as sustainment of life, an integrated team approach to burn injury treatment demands that rehabilitation efforts begin before survival is ensured.

Finally, burn care is expensive. Burn patients have been identified as having the highest average cost of all diagnostic groups, with an average of $55,000 per patient (Fleming et al., 1985). Indirect costs are more difficult to calculate, but the loss of income for this predominantly male working-age population is a major consideration. The social and psychological costs to patients and families are often incalculable.

Need for family involvement. Although studies of the long-term effects of burn injury date from the 1940s, most of the literature on psychosocial recovery was developed in the early 1970s, with the rise of regionally organized burn care centers. The importance of the relationship between the burn patient and his family was first studied in children; specific family needs in adult cases were identified later, and a family adjustment process was described. To date, however, the role of the family in the recovery process has rested more on a theoretical than empirical basis; only recently has it begun to be explicated by research.

The family-related literature has four foci:
• preinjury family characteristics
• long-term psychosocial sequelae
• identification and exploration of the major issue areas or family

reactions (for example, guilt, anger, and helplessness)
• delineation of stages of family adaptation.

While these studies and discussions are burn specific, there are many similarities between burns and other catastrophic health events, and the general critical care literature may be drawn on as well.

Preinjury characteristics. Studies of preinjury family characteristics have come primarily from child-patient populations and have been characterized by higher than expected representation from the lower socioeconomic groups, a higher number of single-parent families, larger than expected family sizes, and high degrees of family stress, as well as by preexisting behavior problems in the injured child (Gladston, 1972; Libber and Stayton, 1984; Martin, 1970; Wilkins and Campbell, 1980). Gladston and Martin have suggested a relationship between the parents' emotional resources and lapses in preventive behavior.

Research into preinjury characteristics of adult patients has rarely considered family resources, although one study did identify a high degree of family disturbance (Andreasen et al., 1972). Studies of predisposing factors have focused on the patient's physical and psychiatric states, although many significant stress factors, such as alcoholism and financial worry, are family problems (Noyes et al., 1979).

No study has yet identified the characteristics or strengths of families who are not living in deprived or depleted circumstances. Nevertheless, the existing work is important because it highlights some of the problems that burn patient families bring with them and that might continue or recur during and after hospitalization. Findings support the need for assessment of family resources to identify potential areas of nursing intervention.

Long-term sequelae. The literature relating to the long-term sequelae of burn injury is, again, heavily weighted toward families of affected children. Parents seem to have problems related to guilt and shame (Bernstein, 1976). They often see the child's visible scars as reminders of their failure to provide adequate protection. Bernstein also describes injury-related changes in family dynamics: some parents become overprotective, affording the injured child special treatment or attempting to overcompensate for changed appearance. Whatever coping strategies a family may develop, the sequelae are often enduring. Some researchers, for instance, have reported long-lasting emotional disturbance in mothers. However, none have related these to preinjury functioning, so it cannot be determined if these were new, ongoing, or exacerbated conditions.

Early research into long-term adjustment among burned adults yielded inconsistent findings. While one study reported a high incidence of postinjury divorce (Chang and Herzog, 1976), others indicated improved family relationships (Andreasen et al., 1977; Blades et al., 1979). Two recent studies, both involving large sample populations, identified both time and social support as significant in good long-term adjustment (Davidson et al., 1981; Knudson-Cooper, 1981). The patient's perception of a supportive social system was especially important in mitigating the effects of large injuries or disfigurement. How intervention or lack thereof affects the support system is unknown, but these studies strongly encourage the need for family involvement and for planned intervention to bolster the patient's support mechanism at all stages.

Family issues. There is wide agreement in the literature that the major family issues during burn hospitalization are guilt, the assigning of blame for the injury, helplessness, and anger. These conclusions are based largely upon family interviews and reports from family support groups (Abramson, 1973; Bowden and Feller, 1973).

Some degree of guilt and/or associated attempts to blame burn injuries on others seems universal, as families seek to fit the experience into an understandable framework. Knudson-Cooper (1981) has found guilt in all parents studied whether or not they had any direct role in their child's injury. Likewise, individuals with no direct role in the incident can find themselves blamed by the patient's family. For instance, a parent, absent through divorce or separation, may be blamed for not having stayed with the family to protect them.

Families of burn patients also feel helpless. They are suddenly thrust into a situation so threatening to their sense of equilibrium that usual coping defenses fail. The shock associated with the traumatic event, the unfamiliarity of the treatment setting, lost feelings of invulnerability, fear of death, and the patient's changed appearance have all been cited as contributing to feelings of helplessness.

Anger may help families counteract feelings of helplessness. Relatives sometimes direct the anger toward each other, in intensification of previous conflicts. More often they vent it on the treatment staff, whom they perceive to be purposely causing patient discomfort by, for instance, failing to relieve pain. Much of the literature mentions families suppressing anger for fear that staff members will retaliate through the patient. Unresolved anger thus contributes to family mistrust of care personnel and reduced energy for supporting the patient.

Ultimately, however, many family needs are family specific. Bernstein (1976), for instance, notes family-to-family variations not only in needs, but in ability to assist in patient care. The special problems of divorced families have also been recognized (Ahrons and Arnn, 1981). Families that have experienced deaths in a fire as well as critical injury are coping with multiple family changes simultaneously. All of these factors support the need for individualized family assessment and planning.

Family adjustment process. Several researchers have attempted to divide burn families' major problems and needs into distinct stages, either by interviewing families throughout hospitalization (Brodland and Andreasen, 1974) or by other means (Steiner and Clark, 1977).

Most researchers have found that, in the initial postinjury stage, the family's main concerns are quantitative. Patient survival is most important, and few concerns about appearance and function are expressed. As in any crisis, the incident's suddenness and unpredictability produce family disequilibrium; relatives first attempt to reestablish a base for effective coping. Family needs in this stage (identified through work in a nonburn critical care setting) are related to anxiety reduction and include knowing what to expect, what treatments are being provided, and what, if any, changes occur (Daley, 1984). Lower-ranked but also important needs are staying with or near the patient, receiving emotional support, and having the opportunity for ventilation.

The second stage has been labeled "psychological emergency" because it occurs primarily during acute hospitalization. The patient, family, and staff interactions are best understood in this stage. Once patient survival seems ensured, relief and the resurgence of the family's psychological defenses can be tremendously buoying. This optimism, however, may not reflect the patient's actual physical condition, and relatives' denial may need to be tempered with doses of realism. At this stage, families believe that old problems will never recur and the future will be wonderful. They feel very positive about the staff and the work they are doing; similar optimism often serves the patients as they attempt to sort out what has happened to them.

In time, however, the stress of pain, discomfort, and forced dependence wears down patient defenses; family defenses falter beneath the demands of balancing home life and hospital visitation, supporting the patient, and comprehending the patient's appearance and behavior. Patients experience periodic depression and regression which, while normal under the circumstances, lead them to focus almost exclusively on pain and treatment. Any thoughts of the future center on the day of discharge, when things promise to be better. Families often insulate the patient from what is happening at home, and the patient may try to protect the family from his concerns as well. Attempts to maintain comfort by avoiding painful issues can produce feelings of isolation on both sides, however. Staff-patient-family conflicts are most likely to arise in this period. The patient feels staff expectations are unreasonable, and the family, trying to be helpful, agrees or experiences internal conflict over not "protecting" the patient. Additionally, the family can see farther ahead than the patient and may become concerned about cosmetic changes and how the injured relative will manage in the future.

The third stage is that of social emergency—what life will really be like when the patient returns to his original social milieu. Discharge, long viewed as the end of the ordeal, becomes an anxiety-producing concept. Families and patients begin to doubt their readiness for the move but rarely share their concerns; indirect delaying tactics are common.

Some authors have divided the social emergency stage to form a fourth stage, home emergency. However, Goodstein (1985) combines family intervention for this stage with the previous one, acknowledging that little is known about home emergency as a separate entity. At home, the need for exercise, splinting, and care of fragile skin continues. Nightmares about the trauma may recur, and sleep disturbances affect the whole family. The patient also needs encouragement to resume former social contacts, and family routines developed during the patient's absence must be altered to accommodate both the patient's presence and changed state.

Although the long-term effects on the family system have not been well documented, the complexity of the entire burn recovery process and the potential for complications at multiple points emphasize the need for family-based assessment for both short- and long-term planning.

Theoretical models. Since most of the burn literature reviewed specified no assessment model, our task is to work backward, looking at areas of functioning considered in burn assessment, and to identify a model.

The conception of the family as a system is consistent with nursing theory (Wahl, 1981). A family system is a unique whole that, while composed of the interacting subsystems of its members, has a character different from the sum of its parts. The system is in simultaneous and mutual interaction with its environment. The unique characteristics of the family include interaction and communication patterns, role relationships, and characteristic stability and attachment patterns.

The individual family unit has its own psychological, social, and physical subsystems, each with permeable boundaries; an attack on the physical system, for example, affects both the social and psychological components. Every individual's unique characteristics evolve over time. Daily behavior and the development of dreams and goals are influenced by the past, the present, and the future.

In response to stress, all systems seek to maintain equilibrium or reduce distress; this is true whether the stress is general or confined to one or more subsystems. Adaptation—that is, the incorporation of stressful change into the individual system—is one means of accomplishing this. Patterns of adaptation, both functional and dysfunctional, develop over time. For example, the psychological defense of denial can be adaptive shortly after injury because it slows down the potentially overwhelming amount of information entering the system. Likewise, regression is adaptive when the patient is suddenly forced to be more dependent than usual. However, if these coping patterns persist, they become dysfunctional, blocking the person's ability to adjust to change and to participate in rehabilitation. The nurse who enhances effective coping will most successfully intervene at the time of crisis.

A family's sense of past, present, and future also bears on its ability to cope with change. Both present and future are changed by crisis, and ingrained patterns determine response. Individual members and the family system as a whole have different levels of stability or adaptive capacity, and each family system has both strengths and weaknesses, all of which bear an adaptive capacity. Examples of these situations abound in nursing practice. A family might try to protect a weaker member or to slow the introduction rate of unpleasant information; a more articulate relative may serve as family spokesperson; someone else may be adept at solving problems.

Still, many families have difficulty reaching a natural equilibrium. Overprotection can leave a perceived weak member with little opportunity to adapt. Several members may compete to be the spokesperson or leader, thus intensifying old conflicts. Such disruptions can only divert family attention from the task at hand—the need to recognize what has happened, how it changed the family, and what must be done to adapt to and incorporate the change.

The family systems model used in much nursing assessment is simply a conceptualization of the family and does not necessarily require assessment of every facet of the system. When death is expected within a short time, for instance, contact with the family is expected to be brief. Therefore, although family assessment is not omitted, it focuses only on the immediate issues. When the involvement will be of considerable duration, as in the case of most burns, more than superficial information is desirable to plan the multiple interventions necessary for recovery.

In general, the literature on families of burn victims has focused on three areas: the individual subsystems of the injured and other key members; such interactional patterns as role relationships and communication; and patient and family relationships to the environment, including the hospital (Bernstein, 1976; Bowden et al., 1979; Goodstein, 1985). The unique characteristics of the whole system, however, have been largely neglected. Thus, the family has been viewed as a system not including the patient, and the patient has been viewed as separate from but interacting with the family.

The literature also reflects a second, usually unstated, model, which is also related to general systems theory. This model places family, hospital, treatment staff, and community within an environment centered around the patient. The individual patient becomes a system of overlapping components in complex interaction with that environment. Bowden (1979) organized an extensive review of the psychosocial burn literature according to this person-environment (P-E) fit model, theorizing that adaptation or behavior at any particular time results from synchrony between person and environment. A supportive environment that satisfies a patient's needs facilitates adaptation to the changed situation. In this model, changes in the patient affect the family, and changes in the family affect the patient, but here the family including the patient does not form the unique whole that it does in the family systems model.

The family assessment literature on burn patients remains insufficient for productive debate on the fine points of competing models. Several points, however, can be made. Family systems theory was developed with family units in mind. Individual subsystems need not have a biological or legal relationship to fit this model, but they must have a common history. Crises, however, often bring together disparate and sometimes competing assemblages of individuals who share nothing but their membership in the patient's social system. While some of these groups work well together to support the patient, competition between them can threaten to overwhelm patient and staff, forcing them to choose sides and delaying assessment.

Both the family assessment and P-E fit models recognize the treatment team's potential impact on families and patients. In some family systems models, staff members are considered part of the family energy field, affecting and affected by that relationship (Wahl, 1981); in the P-E fit model, staffers are part of the patient's environment. In any case, long-term social support by staff members has been recognized as potentially important to outcome, especially when the patient or family has a depleted support system (Bernstein, 1976; Bowden et al., 1979).

The placement of the patient within an environment can have a marked effect on nursing care. Treatment goals differ, however subtly, when the patient moves from one environment to another rather than staying in one place. The dynamic symbolism of the latter seems to weigh heavier in family-centered care. Additionally, not viewing the family as a unique whole may make the P-E model inconsistent with nursing theory (Wahl, 1981).

Ultimately, the appropriate model for burn care probably depends upon professional perspective. A social worker or another health team member not providing direct critical care might find it easier to view the system as a whole. The critical care nurse or the therapist conducting painful rehabilitation procedures is more likely to focus on the patient and regard everything else as environment. A family assessment model may need to be modified to take these factors into consideration. If a team approach is the goal, then theory should be, at the least, consistent with the theory of the professional disciplines involved.

Family assessment instruments. Few assessment instruments or tools have been described in the burn literature. One exception is Talabere and Graves' (1976) multidisciplinary assessment tool for use with families in pediatric burn settings (see Table 11.1). It provides the interviewing nurse or social worker with a format for organizing information according to observations, problem identification, plans, and action taken. Family systems theory serves as the base.

Table 11.1   Talabere and Graves' Model of Pediatric Burn Assessment

Elements
• History of the burn crisis —Family response —Expressed concerns
• Identification of family members —Individual roles —Family support system
• Patient's developmental history and history during other health crises and at equilibrium —Response to separation —Fears —Responses to pain, discipline

Source: Talabere and Graves, 1976.

The literature emphasizes that a guide is preferable to a set of questions (Talabere and Graves, 1976; Wahl, 1981). Observed verbal and nonverbal cues are often as important as responses, and reliance upon a formal set of questions may interfere with such observation and discourage verbalization. Talabere has also emphasized the supportive aspects of open-ended questions. By encouraging family members to discuss crises and express feelings, the nurse can help them begin grief work. Assessment also provides an opportunity to establish a trusting relationship with the family.

Wahl's (1981) assessment guide, also based on family systems theory, can be used in any setting. The major elements of this guide are:
• individual subsystems
• interaction
• unique characteristics of the family
• synchrony with the environment.

Each of its major categories offers an opportunity to explore family and individual histories, both in equilibrium and under stress, as well as to assess the current situation.

The validity of standardized instruments assessing child development, family systems, and family interaction is usually destroyed by the trauma associated with burn injury, although their results might be useful as baselines from which to assess post-traumatic change over time. In any case, standardized instruments should, at best, supplement less rigid assessment guides.

Finally, the nurse must consider assessment as an ongoing process; the accuracy of the initial assessment and need for modification become clear only over time. The assessment tool must allow correction of discrepancies as they are identified.

Most of the literature on families of burn victims has been developed by social workers, psychologists, and psychiatrists. While a few have reported the use of standardized instruments, scant mention has been made of either theoretical models or assessment instruments. These disciplines do not traditionally use formal printed assessment guides, relying more on guides internalized through training. While the validity of these assessments is not questioned, an inherent weakness may lie in their limited accessibility and usefulness to other team members. A major value of a printed assessment guide and recording format, such as that proposed by Talabere and Graves (1976), is that organized family information can be centrally maintained, used, and updated by all team members.

Planning

Care planning in burn injury must address both long- and short-term needs. Because of the time involved and the commitment to qualitative as well as quantitative aspects of care, planning can also extend beyond burn-specific problems to noninjury-related needs. To be effective, it requires knowledge of the adjustment process, appropriate interventive timing, and realistic expectations for recovery. Finally, planning requires an awareness of all available resources: team, hospital, and community.

Family educational/informational needs and financial concerns require immediate attention. Consultation with community services may be more appropriate in a long-range plan, so that help will be available when needed.

As the time spent in the hospital increases, the past seems more distant, and the future seems brighter. Many families forget that past problems will probably recur after discharge. Such problems can be identified at initial assessment and are often amenable to direct and indirect intervention. For example, assessment may indicate that a mother has had difficulty setting limits for her children. Such a situation will only be exacerbated by the injury, but a care plan that addresses this specific problem can, through the use of modeling and discussion, greatly assist the mother. The skills she acquires may then be applied to the child at home as well as to his siblings. Long-standing marital/ family problems probably cannot be resolved or even addressed during hospitalization, but families can learn new problem-solving behaviors, and the nursing relationship might allow long-range monitoring and referral when difficulties arise. Additional areas of exploration are suggested in Table 11.2.

Discharge planning is a team process that should begin at admission. In the latter stages of hospitalization, it is difficult to determine accurately family resources and preinjury functioning, due to changes that have taken place since the injury and the anxiety that accompanies the anticipated discharge. For instance, previously well-functioning elderly persons may remain disoriented throughout most of the hospitalization but return to preinjury awareness levels in the home. Previously

Table 11.2 Suggested Areas of Assessment for Families of Burn-Injured Children

- Has the child reached appropriate developmental landmarks?
- How knowledgeable do parents seem about age-appropriate behaviors?
- Are parental expectations appropriate to the child's development?
- How aware do family members seem to be of environmental safety factors?
- What family roles and responsibilities will be altered by hospitalization?
- Who seems to make major family decisions?
- Who disciplines the child? How? Is there one thing for which the child is disciplined most often?
- Do the parents seem to know how to comfort the child?
- Is there another nonparent member of the household who has a particularly close relationship with the child?
- What have siblings been or what will they be told about what has happened to the injured child? How can contact be maintained with siblings?
- Is another family member being held responsible for the injury? How will this person's needs be addressed?
- Is there evidence of conflict between family members?
- Is there any suggestion of abuse or serious neglect? Are family members consistent in their accounts of what happened? Is the account consistent with the distribution of the burn? Is the account consistent with actions that could be taken by this child at the reported developmental level?

ambulatory elderly persons can often be ambulated or given exercises allowing them to regain mobility by discharge; early assessment in such cases might prevent a move to a nursing home. Additional areas of exploration for early discharge planning are suggested in Table 11.3. Other discharge concerns or needs, such as financial assistance for obtaining outpatient services and supplies, can be anticipated and addressed early in the hospitalization. Finally, early attention to discharge planning can be psychologically advantageous, allowing families to adjust to home care responsibilities in advance. A weekly call from the burn unit nurse to the school nurse, for example, will not only update the child's progress, but will make it less likely that in-school care responsibilities will be rejected (as is often the case when first contact is made at discharge). It may be possible to establish similar early expectations with employers.

In response to the pressure for shorter hospitalizations, some burn care facilities have developed innovative outpatient or home care services (Zuchelli, 1981). However, such measures are not always feasible when the patient lives a considerable distance from the hospital.

Even after lengthy hospitalization, continuing home care is important. Exercise and other therapy is required to protect fragile skin and prevent joint contractures. Family care, based on in-hospital training, is

Table 11.3   Suggested Areas of Family Assessment for Early Discharge Planning

- What does the patient's history suggest about postdischarge mental, physical, and social functioning?

- How knowledgeable do family members seem about the patient's preinjury functioning? Do they seem to know about the patient's daily routine? Can they provide detailed information? Which family members seem to be the most knowledgeable? Could a neighbor or friend provide more accurate information?

- Has there been previous concern about the patient's safety? Does the patient have dangerous habits?

- Which of the patient's former responsibilities will have to be assumed by others? Who will assume them?

- How committed do family members seem to be to the patient's continued independence? Are there barriers—for example, poor health, lack of transportation, distance, or work responsibilities—to family assistance?

- Who has helped the patient in the past? Who will be available to assist, if necessary, after discharge?

- Do family members seem willing to share responsibility?

- Do family members seem willing to alter their lives if the patient requires assistance?

- Is there interfamily conflict about what should have been done in the past (in relation to responsibility for injury prevention) or what would be best for the patient in the future?

preferred, but the trend toward early discharge may necessitate more home care than many families can manage.

Community resources are no longer a major problem, given the rapid expansion of home care agencies. There is, however, a shortage of nurses and therapists comfortable with and/or experienced in burn care. One improperly cleaned wound, for instance, can result in considerable skin loss in the week between home care visits. Hospital nurses and therapists may need to provide more education, construct teaching guides for home care personnel, or otherwise develop innovative home care aids to meet families' physical and emotional needs more effectively.

CASE STUDY

Assessment

Bob, 32, sustained second- and third-degree flame injuries over 40% of his body surface, primarily on his head, face, arms, hands, and chest. Although questions remained about the circumstances, it appeared that he had fallen asleep in his car and was burned when a lit cigarette ignited the upholstery and then his clothes.

Based on his age and the size and depth of his burns, Bob's estimated survival probability might have been as high as 85%. However, because he sustained inhalation injury from being burned in a closed space, the estimate was significantly lower. In addition, the depth of injury to his hands indicated potential functional limitations and possible digit loss.

Bob's family first visited on the afternoon following his admission and was shocked by his appearance. His face was massively swollen (to the point that his eyes were occluded) and he could barely move his lips. Both hands were splinted and elevated, and an endotracheal tube was in place. The undamaged parts of his body were covered. He appeared to be alert and oriented and could follow directions and respond to yes or no questions.

An initial assessment interview with Bob's wife, Janet, and his mother and stepfather, Mr. and Mrs. Beacham, was scheduled to follow the visit. A family systems model was used to obtain information about the individual family members and their preinjury functioning and interaction with the patient, both as individuals and as a family. Their current functioning, needs, and concerns were also queried. No formal instrument or tool was used. The assessing nurse prepared a brief interview summary and a list of family strengths, weaknesses, concerns, and plans for the hospital record. Further notes on identified problems and care planning were added by the social worker, the nurses, or the rehabilitation therapists to the daily progress chart.

Although the original intention was to meet with all family members together, the nurse asked the social worker to meet with Janet separately from Bob's parents. Janet had a problem. The nurse had shown her how to communicate through yes or no questions, but Janet had persisted in trying to ask Bob complicated questions. As a result, both were frustrated by her inability to understand his answers. She was interviewed in a private office adjacent to the patient care area.

Janet was in tears. She desperately needed answers to the questions she had been asking Bob, and she felt that he had been trying to ask her questions as well. She acknowledged feeling helpless and frustrated by her inability to think clearly and to frame answerable questions. At that moment, she needed reassurance that her feelings of helplessness were normal. She also needed simple decision-making guides to help her regain control. When the social worker demonstrated some examples of specific yes or no questions, Janet was able to think of some on her own. The social worker explained that patients often dissociate from information about their condition immediately after trauma, and that Bob's concerns, for the moment, were probably superficial. He might have wanted to know about his car, for instance, or if Janet had notified his employer of the accident. It was suggested that Janet tell Bob these things to spare him the frustration of trying to ask.

One of Janet's concerns required further exploration. She had just received notice of loan approval for a house they planned to buy and wanted to ask Bob if she should cancel it. She was told that he could not be expected to make that decision, and that she should put that aside for the moment. From an assessment standpoint, Janet's concern raised important functional questions. Did she always rely on Bob to make decisions? In her effort to take action, did she not recognize that this decision could wait? Or was she unconsciously trying to add to his burden?

Janet was open and willing to share information about herself and her relationship with Bob; indeed, asking her to do so gave her an easily accomplished task. They had been married for 3 years and had a 2-year-old daughter. Bob had been married before and had a son with whom he did not maintain contact. He had shared little with Janet about this aspect of his life. While he enjoyed his daughter, he spent little time alone with her. The family lived about 60 miles from the hospital in the rural community where Janet had grown up and in which her mother still lived. While each had friends, they did not have friends as a couple.

Both were employed in secure jobs of relatively long duration. Janet expressed pride in her job-related responsibilities and her move up the career ladder. She felt competent in her work role and enjoyed a good relationship with her employer and co-workers. She reported that Bob, in contrast, found the demands of responsibility stress producing.

She thought Bob had good health care benefits through his work. She had already initiated a claim but did not know when its income might begin. Their primary health insurance was provided by her employer; she thought it was comprehensive but planned to discuss it with her company.

Bob and Janet had had marital problems. The conflict centered around his heavy drinking; she had threatened to leave him 4 months earlier if he did not get help. Despite his attendance at a few group sessions for alcoholics, Janet believed Bob had not acknowledged his problem, but had only responded to her ultimatum. Although it was unconfirmed, she was certain he had been drinking before the fire.

Janet wanted to share the information about Bob's drinking privately because it would only upset his mother to hear it. Overall, she felt she had a good relationship with her in-laws; her only negative comment was that they tended to "sweep their problems under the rug." Janet and Bob's decision to relocate near their parents was, in part, based on Bob's belief that the rural environment would provide wholesome outlets and help curb his drinking. As Janet spoke, she realized that she was very angry with Bob and that she blamed him not only for injuring himself but for complicating her life and ruining their plans.

Janet joined Mr. and Mrs. Beacham for the second part of the assessment interview, which centered around their needs, their support system, and their ability to work together as a family. Additional information about Bob was also gathered. Mrs. Beacham began by saying that she had no questions. She said she had been told that everything possible was being done, and she realized that Bob was very fortunate. To consider Bob fortunate after having seen him was not a realistic appraisal of the situation. Her response, however, was common; it has been described in the literature as an attempt to establish an affirmative basis for coping. Unfortunately, such a reaction does not allay family fears and can block expression of concerns. In this case, the nurse's adopted response was threefold: it tempered the affirmative basis for coping by stating worst-case fears about how bad the accident might have been, gave the family permission to express concerns openly, and recognized that Bob had sustained a serious injury and that the experience was new and difficult for all of them. All of them described their reactions when they first heard the news. None had ever thought something like this would happen to him, and none had any previous experience with burn injury. Gradually, they began to formulate and articulate questions. Mrs. Beacham admitted that it was hard for her to look at Bob in his present condition; she felt reassured after speaking to him, but preferred to leave the rest of the day's visit to Janet and Mr. Beacham.

The family members provided additional assessment information when they realized it would help in planning Bob's care and rehabilitation. Bob's natural parents had divorced when he was 14, and he had had no further contact with his father. His stepfather had joined the family 3 years later, in the self-perceived role of friend rather than father substitute. Bob and Janet saw the Beachams three or four times a month, often spending the weekends with them during the summer. The family seemed to lose their sense of time and place when discussing their common love for boating and the pleasant experiences they had shared.

Janet also contributed throughout the interview, asking questions and adding information about how Bob acted when, for example, he was sick or angry. About Bob himself, the Beachams indicated that he tended to keep his concerns to himself. Although they thought they knew when he was worried, they left it to him to decide whether or not to tell them about it.

During the course of the interview, the family's informational needs became obvious. Since Bob's admission, they had had only brief, hurried contact with physicians and nurses, obtaining only fragmented information. Once advised of this, Bob's nurse was able to arrange a meeting of the family, the physician, the social worker, and herself. Although relatively brief, this meeting not only communicated necessary care-related information, but also reinforced team cooperation. It helped establish a trusting relationship and affirmed staff concern for the relatives as well as the patient.

After the initial family interview, central assessment elements were identified.

Individual subsystems. Janet saw herself as competent in several roles. Her acknowledgment of anger at this stage was unusual but beneficial, making the issue more easily addressed in the future if it was not resolved. Janet needed to feel in control and was beginning to regain this sense by focusing on the concrete tasks ahead of her.

Mr. Beacham had a history of peptic ulcer disease; he had no recent symptoms, however, and he was careful about his diet. Mrs. Beacham presented herself as a self-effacing woman. She was the least likely member of the group to express her own needs and repeatedly stated that she did not wish to "interfere." Indeed, both she and Mr. Beacham emphasized that, although they would visit every day, they did not want to intrude, and they expected Janet's needs to take precedence over theirs.

Bob's frame of mind could not be completely assessed until his condition improved, but certain information had been presented to him that needed to be explored further. For instance, it had been suggested that he had difficulty bearing responsibility; that he may have used alcohol as a coping strategy; and that the additional responsibility of purchasing a new home, combined with Janet's ultimatum about his drinking, might have contributed to the accident.

Family interaction. The entire family found it difficult to discuss painful subjects or express feelings. This suggested that they might have difficulty working together to resolve burn-related issues. Although Janet thought she could be more open than the others, she only contributed to this difficulty by restraining herself. The three could communicate clearly when they chose and seemed attached to each other as well as to Bob and Janet's daughter. Their roles were clearly defined and complementary. Although they had not previously managed a crisis as a group, Janet had assumed the leadership role in the crisis that she had with Bob and seemed to be assuming that role for the whole family during the present situation.

Unique family characteristics. The Beacham family was expected to remain stable, at least until Bob regained his independence. Despite their problems, both Janet and Bob had indicated a desire to preserve their marriage. There did not seem to be any previous, intensifiable conflicts between the noninjured relatives. Within their marriage, Janet seemed to be the stronger, more goal-oriented member, and the family accepted her as such. There was some concern that Bob and Janet's child might feel neglected since both parents would be absent for long periods. The family responded appropriately and expressed feelings indicative of a group trying to regain its equilibrium.

Synchrony with the environment. Janet enjoyed a strong social support system through both her community of origin and her work. The Beachams, too, reported a network of friends in their community. Since all worked in or near the city, the only hardship of visiting would be in terms of time spent away from home. Finances were adequate to meet major needs.

Planning

A complete assessment led to the following plan. Continuing patient assessment, periodic reassessment of family responses to changing conditions, and use of support systems were all required. Mrs. Beacham's overprotectiveness and Janet's potential for punitive anger against Bob required special monitoring. Predischarge consultation with an alcoholism treatment service was indicated, as was a plan for reintegrating the daughter into the family system when Bob's condition permitted. The need for education was ongoing, with information actively offered to Mrs. Beacham, since she was the least likely to ask for it.

Family reassessment was intended to be an ongoing process; further planning would be required as problems were identified. Although space does not permit detailed description of this process, the accuracy of the initial assessment was confirmed. Family functional patterns initially identified as strengths continued to contribute positively; identified weaknesses obstructed recovery, but, having been anticipated, they were more easily recognized and dealt with. Mrs. Beacham, for example, persisted in helping Bob feed himself even after the importance of his maintaining joint function had been explained. The planned intervention was to help her recognize that he was exhibiting regressed behavior and saying that he could not be relied upon to act responsibly in his own behalf. She was reassured that her helpless feelings were normal; nurses identified appropriate helping behavior and convinced her that it was all right to take a break when she felt overwhelmed.

One of the family's greatest strengths was its complementary definition of roles. Because of this, when members began to doubt the adequacy of the discharge plan and Mrs. Beacham was forced to consider retiring from her job as a solution, Mr. Beacham suddenly provided leadership. Throughout the crisis, he had shown himself to be more distant and objective; he pointed out to his wife that they could better assist their son financially if she continued to work, and he arranged for a retired friend to spend time with Bob during his first weeks at home.

Finally, continued assessment of Bob and Janet revealed that both acted on what they thought the other might be thinking, thus impeding effective communication. For instance, after a few months at home, both thought it would be nice to go out to dinner, but neither suggested it. Each assumed that the other was bothered by Bob's appearance and interpreted the other's failure to speak up as confirmation of that assumption. Based on early assessment, it was known that controlling her feelings was very important to Janet. The problem was not her reluctance to be seen in public with him. Also, in facing a difficult step, his pattern was to look to her for leadership. They could not check out their thoughts with each other. This was pointed out to them whenever it was observed. The decision-making pattern was pointed out to them in an effort to help them recognize it themselves.

Outcome

Janet and Bob's long-term outcome was considered favorable. Two years later, she contacted the social worker and asked her to tell staff members who remembered Bob that he was doing well. He was no longer drinking, and she felt good about their relationship. The fact that she called after such a long time indicated the lasting impact that hospital staff can have on a patient's family. Whether the family's involvement in this crisis contributed to the positive outcome or whether the crisis alone led the Beachams to rethink their direction in life cannot be determined. However, early assessment undoubtedly made well-planned interventions for both injury-specific and long-term issues possible.

CONCLUSIONS

Burn injury can provide a unique opportunity for nurses to affect family outcome because of the relatively long and intense care involvement and the good chance of survival. Timing may be the key to maximizing effectiveness. Early assessment captures the clearest history of pre-injury functioning. During a crisis, family members often volunteer information and establish relationships that facilitate discussion of broader family issues. Questions on these issues might be viewed as interference if initiated later.

Thus, optimal timing for family assessment coincides with the moment of highest demand for physical care of the injured family member. For the critically injured, interdisciplinary sharing of this responsibility is vital. If the assessment information is maintained in a usable manner consistent with team goals, family care need not remain the exclusive domain of a single discipline or team member. Early demonstration that family-focused care is a team commitment will pave the way for an integrated effort in ongoing assessment and planning.

REFERENCES

Abramson, M. "Group Treatment of Families of Burn-Injured Patients," *Social Casework* 56, 235–41, 1973.

Ahrons, C.R., and Arnn, S. "When Children from Divorced Families Are Hospitalized: Issues for Staff," *Health and Social Work* 6:21–28, 1981.

American Burn Association. *Directory of Burn Care Services—1985.* Phoenix, Ariz.: American Burn Association, 1985.

Andreasen, N.J.C., et al. "Factors Influencing Adjustment of Burn Patients During Hospitalization," *Psychosomatic Medicine* 34:517–25, 1972.

Andreasen, N.J.C., et al. "Incidence of Long Term Psychiatric Complications in Severely Burned Adults," *Annals of Surgery* 174:785–93, 1977.

Bernstein, N.R. *Emotional Care of the Facially Burned and Disfigured.* Boston: Little, Brown & Co., 1976.

Blades, B.C., et al. "Quality of Life after Major Burns," *Journal of Trauma* 19:556–58, 1979.

Bowden, M.L., and Feller, I. "Family Reaction to a Severe Burn," *American Journal of Nursing* 73: 317–19, 1973.

Bowden, M.L., et al. *Psychosocial Aspects of a Severe Burn: A Review of the Literature.* Ann Arbor, Mich.: National Institute of Burn Medicine, 1979.

Brodland, G.A., and Andreasen, N.J.C. "Adjustment Problems of the Family of the Burn Patient," *Social Casework* 55:13–18, 1974.

Chang, F.C., and Herzog, B. "A Follow-Up Study of Physical and Psychological Disability," *Annals of Surgery* 183:34–37, 1976.

Daley, L. "The Perceived Immediate Needs of Families with Relatives in the Intensive Care Setting," *Heart & Lung* 13:231–37, 1984.

Davidson, T.N., et al. "Social Support and Postburn Adjustment," *Archives of Physical Medicine and Rehabilitation* 62:274–78, 1981.

Feck, G., et al. *An Epidemiologic Study of Burn Injuries and Strategies for Prevention.* Washington, D.C.: U.S. Department of Health, Education and Welfare, 1981.

Feller, I. "Introduction to the Burn Patient Problem in the United States," *Fire Journal* 64:52–53, 1970.

Feller, I., and Flanders, S. "Mortality Review Based on Profile Analysis," *Quality Review Bulletin* 30–35, October 1979.

Feller, I., et al. "Baseline Data on the Mortality of Burn Patients," *Quality Review Bulletin* 3–7, July 1979.

Fleming, S., et al. "A Multidimensional Analysis of the Impact of High Cost Hospitalization," *Inquiry* 12:178–87, 1985.

Gladston, R. "The Burning and Healing of Children," *Psychiatry* 35:57–66, 1972.

Goodstein, R.K. "Burns: An Overview of Clinical Consequences Affecting Patients, Staff, and Family," *Comprehensive Psychiatry* 26:43–57, 1985.

Knudson-Cooper, M.S. "Adjustment to Visible Stigma: The Case of the Severely Burned," *Social Science and Medicine* 15:31–41, 1981.

Libber, S.M., and Stayton, D.J. "Childhood Burns Reconsidered: The Child, the Family, and the Burn Injury," *Journal of Trauma* 24:245–52, 1984.

MacArthur, J.D., and Moore, F.D. "Epidemiology of Burns: The Burn-Prone Patient," *Journal of the American Medical Association* 231:259–63, 1975.

Martin, H.L. "Antecedents of Burns and Scalds in Children," *British Journal of Medical Psychology* 43:39–47, 1970.

Noyes, R., et al. "Stressful Life Events and Burn Injuries," *Journal of Trauma* 19:141–43, 1979.

Parry, J.K., and Young, A.K. "The Family as a System in Hospital-Based Social Work," *Health and Social Work* 3:55–69, 1978.

Steiner, H., and Clark, W.R. "Psychiatric Complications of Burned Adults: A Classification," *Journal of Trauma* 17:134–43, 1977.

Talabere, L., and Graves, P. "A Tool for Assessing Families of Burned Children," *American Journal of Nursing* 76:225–27, 1976.

Wahl, A.L. "Nursing Theory and the Assessment of Families," *Journal of Psychiatric Nursing* 19:30–36, 1981.

Wilkins, T.J., and Campbell, J.L. "Psychosocial Concerns in the Pediatric Burn Unit," *Burns* 7:208–10, 1980.

Zuchelli, S. "The Burn Rehabilitation Program at Bothin Burn Center," *Journal of Burn Care and Rehabilitation* 2:111–16, 1981.

SECTION III

Intervening with Families with Life-Threatening Illness

12 Intervening with young married couples and cervical cancer

Kathleen M. O'Laughlin, RN, MS
Oncology Clinical Nurse Specialist
University of Chicago Hospital
Chicago, Illinois

OVERVIEW

The diagnosis of cervical cancer in a young married woman precipitates a developmental crisis for both her and her husband. Individual developmental tasks and family roles alike are affected by the disease and its treatment. Therapy commonly causes infertility and may affect sexual responsiveness and, while early-stage disease is rarely life threatening, families often perceive it to be. The nurse can best intervene with this family by providing support and accurate information.

CASE STUDY

Alice Grant, a 24-year-old black female, was diagnosed as having probable Stage Ia cervical cancer and admitted to the hospital for definitive staging and treatment. The oncology clinical nurse specialist (OCNS) interviewed Alice on admission. This interview determined that Alice was employed as an accountant and had been married for 6 months to John, age 27, a lawyer. Alice and John had hoped to start a family; her carcinoma had been found during a routine gynecologic examination. Alice was anxious and tearful during the initial interview.

The OCNS determined that Alice was going through a developmental crisis precipitated by both the diagnosis of life-threatening disease and the potential impairment of her ability to function in the roles of wife and mother. In Alice's case, the OCNS determined that the initial nursing role should be supportive. The nurse also identified the need to interview John and to assist the couple in resolving family role issues arising from Alice's illness.

John expressed great concern over Alice's health, verbalizing his fears regarding the spread of the disease and the loss of his wife. He also wondered how this had happened and whether he might be to blame. John affirmed the couple's desire to have children but felt that this issue was peripheral to the immediate crisis. The OCNS assured John that the cause of the disease was not known, and that he should not feel responsible. The OCNS decided, with their consent, to help the couple resolve the crisis.

After the staging workup was completed, having identified Alice's disease as Stage Ia, the medical treatment plan called for an abdominal hysterectomy.

The OCNS, with the physician, informed John and Alice of the findings and proposed treatment, including the effect of the surgery on Alice's ability to have children. They told the couple that the prognosis was good, but that Alice would require frequent follow-up to ensure early detection of any recurrence. The OCNS said that Alice's ovaries would be conserved in order to prevent the onset of menopausal symptoms. Alice was concerned about the impact of the hysterectomy on their sexual relationship. The OCNS assured her that normal sexual activity could continue after recovery, although gratification might be diminished because of the absence of the uterus.

After the hysterectomy, the OCNS helped John and Alice cope with their inability to bear children. They discussed such alternatives as adopting a child or remaining childless.

Realizing that John and Alice might need additional counseling after assimilating the initial information, the OCNS scheduled an appointment for 3 weeks after discharge. At that time, the couple verbalized optimism about the future and felt that the experience had drawn them closer. Though they had not yet resumed sexual relations, they were confident that they could cope with any changes. They had not yet decided what to do about the issue of children, but exhibited open communication. The OCNS terminated the relationship at this point but offered to be available if further help was needed.

NURSING PROCESS

Assessment

The health problem: Cervical cancer. Cervical cancer is a leading cause of neoplastic deaths in women. Although widespread use of the Pap smear has increased early-stage diagnosis of cervical cancers by 20% (Wilson et al., 1981), the test is still underutilized. It has been estimated that up to 30% of rural women have never had a Pap smear (van Nagel et al., 1983).

Presentation and etiology. Most cervical cancer patients present to the physician with abnormal vaginal bleeding (Morrow and Townsend, 1981), characterized by a continuous, thin, watery, blood-tinged discharge or by painless intermittent bleeding following intercourse or douching. Symptoms of more advanced cervical cancer include flank pain and changed bowel or bladder habits.

The cause of cervical cancer is unknown, but theories have been developed. Cervical cancer occurs more commonly in women who began sexual activity at an early age, who have had more than one sexual partner, who experienced their first pregnancy at an early age, and who are multiparous (Labrum, 1977). The adolescent cervix is believed more susceptible to carcinogens because of its high rate of metaplasia as columnar epithelium is converted to squamous epithelium (Morrow and Townsend, 1981). A long latency period is common, however, and most malignancies develop between the ages of 45 and 55. Cervical cancer diagnosed in younger families, which most often represents early-stage disease, is the focus of discussion in this chapter.

Treatment and sequelae. Treatment of early-stage cervical cancer may involve surgery, radiation, or a combination of the two (see Table 12.1); they are often combined for optimal results. The advantages of surgery include shorter treatment time, removal of the primary lesion, and reduced normal tissue injury; however, its use is limited to early-stage lesions. Radiation therapy, on the other hand, can treat all pelvic tissues, with limited damage to bladder, rectal, and/or coital function (Morrow and Townsend, 1981). Surgery is preferred in early-stage disease because of radiation's adverse long-term effects, including vaginal fibrosis, which may cause painful intercourse and drying of the vaginal mucosa; changes in gastrointestinal function; and pelvic fibrosis.

Surgical options include cervical conization and simple or radical hysterectomy. Conization involves the incision of a cone-shaped wedge of cervical tissue, which removes not only the lesion but also an adequate margin around it. This procedure is appropriate only for Stage 0 cervical cancer (carcinoma in situ). Conization does preserve fertility, making it the preferred option for families who desire children. Simple hysterectomy involves removal of the uterus only and is appropriate for Stage 0 and Ia cervical cancers. Radical hysterectomy entails removal of the uterus along with adjacent portions of the vagina, cardinal ligaments, and rectal and bladder pillars, as well as pelvic lymphadenectomy; it is used in Stage Ib and IIa cervical cancers.

Therapeutic radiation may be administered by intracavitary or external beam routes. Generally, use of intracavitary radiation alone is reserved for early-stage (Stage I) disease. It is combined with external beam radiation to the pelvis for Stage II tumors; external radiation by itself is given to patients with Stage III and IV disease (Morrow and Townsend, 1981). Chemotherapy may also be added to late-stage regimens.

Impact on the young married couple. The diagnosis of cervical cancer precipitates a developmental crisis for the young married family, whether the disease is immediately life threatening or not. Gotay (1984) demonstrated that, regardless of disease stage or cure potential, both cancer victims and their spouses were afraid of the diagnosis, of the possibility of disease progression and recurrence, and/or of potential infertility after treatment. Much of this fear can be traced to cultural perceptions of cancer. The very word, though it represents a number of very different diseases, brings to the public mind images of slow, painful death. The nurse can help the cervical cancer patient and her family develop realistic expectations regarding the disease course and treatment. Encouraging the family to develop coping mechanisms for the changes initiated by the diagnosis is another important aspect of the nurse's role.

Table 12.1   Cervical Cancer Therapies and Programs

Stage	Extent of Disease	Primary Therapy	5-Year Survival Rate*
0	Carcinoma in situ (noninvasive)	Therapeutic conization, cryotherapy, laser surgery, or simple hysterectomy	95% to 100%
Ia	Carcinoma confined to cervix (invasion < 3 mm)	Simple hysterectomy	72% to 91%
Ib	(invasion > 3 mm)	Radical hysterectomy or radiation	
IIa	Carcinoma extends beyond cervix but not to pelvic wall or lower third of vagina; no obvious parametrial involvement	Radical hysterectomy or radiation	51% to 75%
IIb	Obvious parametrial involvement	Radiation	
IIIa	No extension to pelvic wall	Radiation	20% to 43%
IIIb	Extension to one or both pelvic walls, or presence of ureteral obstruction	Radiation	
IVa	Extension beyond true pelvis, or invasion of bladder or rectum; metastasis to adjacent organs	Radiation and/or chemotherapy	0% to 17%
IVb	Metastasis to distant organs	Chemotherapy	

*Sources: Einhorn et al., 1985; Inoue and Okumura, 1984; Morrow and Townsend, 1981; Noguchi et al., 1983; and van Nagel et al., 1983.

Assessment of the family facing cervical cancer must include exploration of the family structure to identify developmental strengths and weaknesses. The Calgary Family Assessment Model provides a framework for such assessment; family structure (internal and external), development (stages, tasks, attachments, and alterations), and functioning (instrumental and expressive) all enable the nurse to conceptualize how individual members function within the family constellation (Wright and Leahey, 1984).

The diagnosis of cancer affects the young family's ability to complete the following important developmental tasks (Wright and Leahey, 1984):
• establishment of identity as a couple
• realignment of extended family relationships
• decisions about parenthood.

In addition to making the short-term adjustments required by cancer treatment, the couple may have to reconsider long-term family plans. Adoption or childlessness as alternatives should be explored. Normal realignment of relationships with the extended family may be complicated by the need to care for the wife—for example, to provide transportation to the hospital for daily radiation treatments or housekeeping assistance if she is fatigued from the treatment and/or disease. Finally, the physio- and psychological effects of hysterectomy, particularly radical hysterectomy, may alter the marital relationship itself.

The assessing nurse must evaluate family functioning both before and after cervical cancer diagnosis in order to recognize which changes result from the disease process, treatment, or efforts to cope with new life stresses. In this context, the nurse can determine whether the family's coping mechanisms are therapeutic and effectual.

Defining problems. Following initial assessment, the nurse should outline the family's strengths and problems. She should then attempt to determine which problems are within the scope of her expertise and which may require referral to another professional. In the typical client family, these problems will need to be addressed:
• the family's need for information
   —about the disease and its treatment
   —about fertility and sexuality
   —about supportive resources (institutional, community)
• the need to cope with a potentially life-threatening illness
• the need to redefine relationships with the extended family so the nuclear family can cope with its present problem.

Identified problems can then be labeled, using nursing diagnostic terms. Potential diagnoses for the early-stage cervical cancer patient and her family include:

• *knowledge deficit* about the disease, therapy, and associated life-style changes. High initial anxiety levels may contribute to knowledge deficits by making the patient and her family unreceptive to needed information.

• *moderate anxiety,* or increased arousal associated with a threat to the self or a significant other (Gordon, 1982). Characteristics include expressions of unfocused apprehension, nervousness or concern, restlessness, increased verbalization, pacing, hand tremors, narrowed focus of attention, diaphoresis, increased heart and respiratory rates, and sleeping or eating disturbances. Moderate anxiety is characteristic of cervical cancer patients and families during the diagnostic phase; uncertainty about the diagnosis, treatment, and prognosis all contribute to tension.

• *body image disturbance:* negative feelings or perceptions about physical characteristics, functions, or limitations (Gordon, 1982), often seen in the woman who undergoes hysterectomy for cervical cancer. Symptoms include actual or perceived changes in bodily structure or function, life-style changes because of these perceptions, fears of rejection or reaction by others, and verbalization regarding past strength, function, or appearance.

• *sexual dysfunction,* a perceived problem in achieving sexual satisfaction (Gordon, 1982). After hysterectomy and/or radiation therapy, either physiological or psychological factors—or a combination of the two—can cause sexual dysfunction in the patient and/or her significant other. Characteristics include verbalization of a sexual problem, actual or perceived limitations imposed by the disease and/or therapy, alterations in ability to achieve sexual satisfaction, and changes in the relationship with the significant other.

• *decreased activity tolerance:* insufficient energy to complete required or desired activities due to physiologic or therapeutic limitations (Gordon, 1982). Patients with cervical cancer undergoing either radiation or surgical therapy will experience a decreased activity tolerance for varying periods of time; patients and their families may have to adjust role expectations to the situation until recovery is complete.

• *an altered urinary elimination pattern;* characteristics include hesitancy, retention, incontinence, and decreased sensation of the need to void. This problem is experienced by cervical cancer patients who undergo radical hysterectomy. Changes in elimination may require continuous or intermittent catheterization on a long-term basis, which affects both the woman and her family.

Planning

Once a clear concept of the family's development, method of functioning, and constellation of problems is established, the care plan must be developed. Initially, or until the extent of the disease and requirements for therapy are defined, supportive functions may be sufficient. Later, the nurse's role will be primarily educative; she will provide the family with accurate information about the disease itself, the prescribed treatment plan, and any life-style changes that may be precipitated by treatment.

Intervention

Kooser and Marino (1981) conceptualize cancer as an inherent family experience—one that requires major adjustments by both patients and those close to them. The nurse can guide an affected family through the diagnostic and treatment phases of the disease by enabling members to verbalize their feelings and concerns and by providing accurate information.

Determining the meaning of the illness to the patient and her family will help the nurse plan further interventions. The nurse may explore this issue by asking these questions:
• What do you understand about your/your wife's condition?
• What have you been told about treatments? What has your spouse been told?
• What do you expect will happen during treatment?
• Do you and your partner have different expectations of the illness or of life after therapy? If so, how do your ideas differ?
• Do you anticipate any changes in your family's life-style as a result of the disease or treatment?

A family's reaction to the crisis of cancer diagnosis depends on members' individual and collective life experiences, their feelings about themselves and one another, and their expectations of family relationships. For some patients and/or family members, fertility loss may be the focal point; others may be most concerned about the potential loss of the ill relative.

The nurse must be aware of opportunities to make secondary gains that might amend some of the negative aspects of the disease for the ill individual. For example, a woman who does not enjoy sexual activity may use a cancer diagnosis as a reason to discontinue sexual relations with her significant other, regardless of whether there is a physiological reason for doing so. Allowing the patient and family to discuss their concerns and to reveal the rationales behind their coping strategies is an important initial nursing intervention.

The family also must be informed about cervical cancer physiology and treatment. When hysterectomy is planned, the couple will need to know its effect on their sexual functioning and fertility and why such a traumatic intervention was chosen. If the couple have planned additional childbearing and the patient's condition allows, the option of therapeutic conization should be discussed.

The nurse should explore the couple's feelings about lost fertility, particularly when children were planned but not conceived at the time of diagnosis. Women whose sense of identity is grounded in the child-bearing function may be devastated by the loss of the uterus. Many patients grieve as they adapt to their changing self-image and family role. Partners may feel that a woman who cannot bear children is less of a wife, or they may be unable to accept the loss of their potential fatherhood. The nurse may approach this issue by saying: "People who face a hysterectomy are often concerned about the fact that they will be unable to bear children. Is this one of your concerns?" This kind of question reassures the woman and her partner that their concerns are not unusual and "gives permission" for the topic to be discussed.

The diagnosis of cancer may even force the couple to postpone adoption as an alternative to childbirth, since some agencies refuse to consider such cases until the family can show that the wife is "cured." Adaptation to the idea of not having children may be very difficult.

Couples often worry about the effects of hysterectomy on their sexual relationship, a concern often fueled by misconceptions about the reproductive system. For instance, patients often ascribe to the uterus such functions as reproduction, excretion, regulation and control of body processes, sexuality, strength and vitality, and maintenance of youth and attractiveness (Edlund, 1982).

Numerous studies have tried, with varying results, to determine the psychosexual sequelae of hysterectomy. Rejection by male partners, hot flashes (after conservation of ovarian tissue), severe hot flashes (after ovariectomy), long-term psychourinary problems, weight changes, lingering fatigue, painful intercourse, depression, sleep disturbance, decreased sexual enjoyment, and change in the quality of the orgasm have all been noted (Edlund, 1982). Some researchers report little or no change in sexual or psychological functioning (Coppen et al., 1981; Novotna and Tuchova, 1979). Of those who do identify changes, some believe the changes are purely psychosomatic (Kuczynski, 1982) and others believe there are physiologic explanations for them (Newton and Baron, 1976; Newton, 1979; Zussman et al., 1981). Well-controlled studies in this area are still needed.

In sum, hysterectomy may change both the patient's and her partner's attitudes about their sexuality. Open discussion about postsurgical sexual relations, possibly facilitated by the nurse, can help eliminate misunderstandings or misconceptions. The type of question discussed above can be used to address this issue, for example, "Many women who undergo a hysterectomy are concerned about its effect on their sexual relationships. Is this one of your concerns?" Women and their partners need to know that the woman's sexual responsiveness may be altered by the surgery, but they should also know sexual relations may be resumed within 6 weeks, if healing is adequate. A booklet often provides the family with basic information and can be a starting point for discussion.

In regard to cervical cancer in particular, many couples are reluctant to resume the sexual relationship for fear that cancer is transmissible. If the patient has received radiation, the partner may also be concerned about exposure to X-rays through intercourse. The nurse should anticipate and address these concerns, since they may not be verbalized voluntarily by the partner. Fears of radiation could even complicate treatment for the patient receiving external beam radiation, when frequent intercourse is often recommended to avoid vaginal strictures or fibrosis (Krant, 1981). Obturators might be recommended if, because of the partner's anxiety or any other reason, intercourse is not feasible (Donaghue and Knapp, 1977).

After radical hysterectomy, the vaginal vault may be significantly shortened, resulting in discomfort or pain during sexual penetration. The nurse may need to suggest comfortable sexual positions (Donaghue and Knapp, 1977). She might also reassure the couple that regular intercourse will eventually stretch the vaginal vault, increasing both partners' comfort (Savage, 1982).

Because radical hysterectomy involves some bladder denervation, it also causes bladder dysfunction, some degree of which is permanent in approximately 50% of the women who undergo the procedure (Kristensen et al., 1984). This dysfunction may vary from mild retention requiring no therapy to major problems with urinary retention, incontinence, and infection. Long-term continuous or intermittent catheterization may be required. Patients and families must be aware of these possibilities and must learn how to minimize the risk of long-term dysfunction. Typical home care requirements include frequent emptying of the bladder (if a catheter is not in place), followed in some cases by intermittent catheterization for residual urine. The need to carry out this type of care for several months after surgery may be an additional stressor to the young family that might already be required to make major role adjustments.

Evaluation

Interventions for the cervical cancer patient and her family may be evaluated by assessing the clients' understanding of disease principles, treatment, and sequelae. Questions pertaining to these factors might include:

• What is your understanding of the disease and treatment?
• What effects do you expect may result from the medical treatment?
• What are your long-term expectations regarding the disease and its effect on your lives?

Evidence of open family communication regarding disease-related issues is another encouraging sign of effective intervention.

At times, the nurse will be unequipped to deal with certain family problems or issues. Family referral to another practitioner is appropriate in these situations and should not be viewed as evidence of failure.

Patients without complications for early-stage cervical carcinoma will usually not require home nursing intervention for their physical needs. Psychosocial adaptation may not, however, be achieved as readily; a home nurse may facilitate this process. The home health nurse should evaluate understanding of the disease and treatment, correct misconceptions, and promote open communication within the family constellation. Techniques used by the hospital nurse may be adapted to the home situation.

CONCLUSIONS

The young family facing cervical cancer presents a challenge to the professional nurse. Patients and their families require intensive physical and psychosocial care over varying periods of time. Information and counseling about actual and potential changes in the patient's physical and emotional status are needed. Family roles are often affected by these alterations, resulting in the need for effective coping by each family member. The nurse can be instrumental in assisting the family through this developmental crisis.

REFERENCES

Coppen, A., et al. "Hysterectomy, Hormones and Behavior," *Lancet* 1(8212): 126–28, 1981.

Donaghue, V.C., and Knapp, R.C. "Sexual Rehabilitation of Gynecologic Cancer Patients," *Obstetrics and Gynecology* 4(1):118–21, 1977.

Edlund, B.J. "Needs of Women with Gynecologic Malignancies," *Nursing Clinics of North America* 17(1):165–77, 1982.

Einhorn, N., et al. "Outcome of Different Treatment Modalities in Cervix Carcinoma Stage IB & IIA," *Cancer* 55(5):949–55, 1985.

Gordon, M. *Manual of Nursing Diagnoses.* New York: McGraw-Hill Book Co., 1982.

Gotay, C.C. "Experience of Cancer During Early and Advanced Stages: The Views of Patients and Their Mates," *Social Science Medicine* 18(7):605–13, 1984.

Inoue, T., and Okumura, M. "Prognostic Significance of Parametrial Extension in Patients with Cervical Carcinoma Stages IB, IIA and IIB," *Cancer* 54(8):1714–19, 1984.

Kooser, J., and Marino, L.B. "Psychosocial Care of Cancer Clients and Their Families: Periods of High Risk," in *Cancer Nursing.* Edited by Marino, L.B. St. Louis: C.V. Mosby Co., 1981.

Krant, M.J. "Psychosocial Impact of Gynecologic Cancer," *Cancer* 48:608–12, 1981.

Kristensen, G.B., et al. "Persistent Bladder Dysfunction after Surgical and Combination Therapy of Cancer of the Cervix Uteri Stages IB and IIA," *Gynecologic Oncology* 18:38–42, 1984.

Kuczynski, H.J. "After the Hysterectomy," *Nursing Mirror* 155:42–46, 1982.

Labrum, A.H. "Psychologic Factors in Gynecologic Cancer," *Primary Care* 3(4):47–52, 1977.

Morrow, C.P., and Townsend, D.E. *Synopsis of Gynecologic Oncology.* New York: John Wiley & Sons, 1981.

Newton, M. "Quality of Life for the Gynecologic Oncology Patient," *American Journal of Obstetrics and Gynecology* 13:866–69, 1979.

Newton, N., and Baron, E. "Reactions to Hysterectomy: Fact or Fiction," *Primary Care* 3(4):781–801, 1976.

Noguchi, H., et al. "Postoperative Classification for Uterine Cervical Cancer and Its Clinical Evaluation," *Gynecologic Oncology* 16(2):219–31, 1983.

Novotna, J., and Tuchova, H. "Mental Changes in Women with Gynecologic Cancer," *Neoplasma* 26(5):629–34, 1979.

Savage, J. "No Sex, Please, Mrs. Smith," *Nursing Mirror* 154(7):28–32, 1982.

van Nagel, J.R., et al. "Evaluation and Therapy of Carcinoma of Uterine Cervix," *Current Problems in Cancer* 8(5):1–41, 1983.

Wilson, J.K.V., et al. "Current Status of Therapeutic Modalities for Treatment of Gynecologic Malignancies with Emphasis on Chemotherapy," *Journal of Obstetrics and Gynecology* 141(1):81–98, 1981.

Wright, L., and Leahey, M. *Nurses and Families: A Guide to Family Assessment and Intervention.* Philadelphia: F.A. Davis Co., 1984.

Zussman, L., et al. "Sexual Response after Hysterectomy-Oophorectomy: Recent Studies and Reconsideration of Psychogenesis," *American Journal of Obstetrics and Gynecology* 140:725–29, 1981.

13 Intervening with families of infants with apnea

Judith M. MacDonald, RN, MSN
Associate Professor
McGill University School of Nursing
Nursing Consultant
Montreal Children's Hospital
Montreal, Quebec, Canada

OVERVIEW

This chapter describes appropriate nursing interventions for families with children experiencing infant apnea. The nursing process provides a framework for organizing care; the key concepts of family, health, learning, and development are discussed. The family's work and the nurse's actions are outlined. Care is collaborative, with active family participation encouraged. A brief description of infant apnea, as well as its diagnosis and treatment, is also included, as are studies of the disorder's impact on family life.

CASE STUDY

The Allen family is composed of Donald, age 30, Margaret, age 25, John, 2½, and Robert, 9 weeks. Margaret and Donald have been married for 4 years and are both high school graduates. Donald works in a local machine tool factory; Margaret, a former clerk, is now at home. Robert was admitted to a large children's hospital for investigation of an apneic episode following an upper respiratory infection. Two more periods of apnea were recorded on the day of his hospitalization, the first while he was asleep in his crib at home, and the second in the emergency department. On both occasions he was observed to be gray, limp when picked up, and responsive only after being shaken. Infant apnea was diagnosed after continued episodes of bradycardia and periodic breathing. Upon discharge, monitoring was recommended until the infant could tolerate respiratory stress without an apneic response, had not experienced apnea for 2 months, and presented with a normal respirogram.

Assessment

Once Robert was settled in the inpatient unit, Margaret and Donald were interviewed by the primary care nurse. The initial family assessment used the MacDonald Family Assessment Guide (Table 13.1). Questions elicited information about family resources (for example, support persons, money, health, housing, and transportation) as well as about function and organization. The Allens' understanding of the events surrounding Robert's admission was also assessed.

Table 13.1 MacDonald Family Assessment Guide—
A Guide for Teaching and Practice

- General resources
  —People, finances, housing, health, transportation

- Specific family dimensions
  —Boundaries, communication, roles, problem solving/decision making

- Individual within the family
  —Characteristics of the client(s) experiencing the problem; include self-concept, role function within the family, problem-solving strategies, relationships with others

- Additional data
  —Ideas, feelings, or concerns the family wishes to share as the interview ends

Source: J. MacDonald, 1983.

Assessment revealed that the parents were reacting with disbelief to Robert's diagnosis and were concerned about the home monitoring plan. Financial hardship had recently forced the Allens to move to a small, low-rent apartment, which meant less space for recreation and privacy. The baby shared a room with his parents, while John occupied a small second bedroom. The couple reported family health as generally satisfactory. They reported feeling "upset" and "fearful." Margaret owned a car and would be able to keep the clinic appointments with her mother, Mrs. Grey, who intended to assist with Robert's care. Mrs. Grey was a key family figure; she actively participated in family decisions, and her daughter expected her to learn cardiopulmonary resuscitation (CPR) and help use the apnea monitor. Donald was a quiet person whose major concern was providing an adequate income for the family. His own family was not in the city; he had few friends outside of work and, since marriage, had become even less involved with extrafamilial activities. Margaret, the couple's spokesperson, was an articulate, energetic woman who described herself as the family boss. She actively sought information and considered herself the person who would be most responsible for Robert's welfare in the months ahead.

Planning

Care planning for the Allen family was a multistep process, beginning with an effort to help the family accept the diagnosis of infant apnea. The implication of this diagnosis for their son's future was a major family concern. The second step was initiated as soon as family members demonstrated interest and a willingness to learn CPR. Before beginning CPR and monitor education, the nurse had to be sensitive to the family's present sense of crisis. Teaching had to be paced to fit the family's readiness for new information.

The third step was to help the family plan the reorganization of its home routine necessary to effectively monitor Robert's breathing after discharge. The posthospitalization care plan would include both daily telephone contact and a home visit to assess the family's establishment of the new life pattern and ensure that initial fears had been overcome. During a visit to the Allen home within the first week of discharge, the nurse planned to evaluate the apnea monitor setup and to demonstrate, if necessary, monitor lead application. Weekly clinic appointments would allow assessment of Robert's growth and development, a review of monitor data, and an evaluation of family coping through discussion of day-to-day events and description of concerns.

Intervention

Margaret spent each day of Robert's 2-week hospital stay on the unit, sleeping on a cot beside him each night. Her husband joined her for several hours each evening after visiting John, who was staying with his grandmother. Ongoing discussion of the diagnosis and treatment plan with the medical and nursing staff contributed to an understanding and acknowledgment of the apnea diagnosis. The parents' questions were answered during planned daily meetings with their primary care nurse; they were introduced to the idea of infant apnea as a developmental immaturity that would improve over time. Robert's normal developmental progress was pointed out frequently and the parents' knowledge of normal growth and development assessed regularly; information was provided as necessary.

By the end of the first week, CPR teaching had begun. After discussion of the rationale and procedure, the resuscitation routine was modeled. Both parents participated, at first by practicing on a lifelike doll. On several occasions each parent was asked to describe the CPR process verbally before working with the doll. After assessing both parents' previous opportunity and perceived ability to handle electrical equipment, an experienced staff member demonstrated the apnea monitor.

In addition to practicing these home care skills, the parents were encouraged to consider the implications of becoming a "monitoring family"—for instance, the need to control vacuum cleaner, dishwasher, and shower noise, lest they mask the sound of the monitor alarm, and the need to ensure that a second person was always present in the car to observe the baby. The Allens were also made aware of 2½-year-old John's increased need for parental contact after the 2-week hospital separation and of the normal anger, jealousy, and regressive behavior he might display after Robert's return.

When the nurse asked her to identify people whom the family could rely on for aid, Margaret became aware of her potential for isolation. Her mother was her closest ally, and Margaret expected her assistance during the daytime; Mrs. Grey was therefore involved in the home care training, coming to the unit to learn CPR and monitor use.

The nurse also instructed the Allens—as she would any monitoring family—to notify their local emergency services of the possible need for future assistance. The family was also advised to place emergency numbers on the telephones and to purchase or rent an intercom system to make the alarm easier to hear. The hospital provided the home monitor and required leads.

Evaluation

Ongoing evaluation marked each phase of the Allens' hospital care. Donald and Margaret gradually became more comfortable with Robert's diagnosis and began to talk about his condition as a transitory phenomenon that would be outgrown. Hospitalization was uneventful; Robert experienced no further apneic episodes.

Margaret was much more anxious than her husband about their son's return home; she verbalized fears and needed additional time to review CPR and monitoring skills. Demonstrating proper CPR procedure to her mother seemed to give her confidence in her own ability. Donald stayed overnight once, and both he and his wife responded appropriately when a monitor lead loosened and the alarm sounded. Both parents could identify Robert's developmental landmarks and, while concerned about the implications of apnea for his future progress, remained hopeful in their own assessment of their son.

Within 10 days after discharge, the family had settled into a home care routine. Through daily phone contact, the clinic nurse learned that for several sleepless nights *both* parents had been guarding the monitor! After a period without any apneic episodes, the Allens adjusted. Daily events were carefully planned; the period turned out to be less stressful than they had anticipated.

Robert's brother, John, initially demanded attention, but the family plan, which gave him a specific block of time with his father each evening, seemed helpful. Mrs. Grey rehearsed CPR with her daughter and felt more comfortable in her role as babysitter. A home visit revealed a well-placed and correctly set up monitor. At the first clinic appointment, Robert's height, weight, and head circumference were measured; these concrete indications of development were important to a family still seeking reassurance that their child was maturing normally. The family members' competence at home care was assessed and their abilities, perceived by the nurse as positive, were described to them. The Allens felt that they had mastered the hospital phase and had begun to reestablish themselves at home. They looked forward to the time when Robert would be off the monitor and life would return to normal. Although they readily acknowledged that life would never be quite the same as before Robert's diagnosis, they suggested that this crisis had brought them closer and had made them value their life together.

NURSING PROCESS

Assessment

The health problem: Infant apnea. Infant apnea has been defined by Brooks (1980, p. 136) as "an unexplained and frightening episode of cessation of breathing for 20 seconds or longer or a shorter respiratory pause associated with bradycardia, cyanosis, or pallor." Infant apnea is an established clinical syndrome that has been closely associated with the diagnosis of sudden infant death syndrome (SIDS). During the past 10 years, there has been much research into both the syndrome itself and families whose children might be at risk (Brooks, 1982).

Steinschneider (1972) made an important contribution to the idea of a relationship between the clinical phenomenon of infant apnea and the occurrence of sudden infant death syndrome. His findings suggest that infants with prolonged apneic periods may be at risk for SIDS and support the idea of a premorbid, clinically evident indicator for the heretofore mysterious syndrome. These and similar findings have made the assessment and diagnosis of apneic infants with bradycardia a subject of much interest.

The link between infant apnea and sudden infant death is further evidenced by descriptions of infant apnea as "near-miss" or "aborted" SIDS. Brooks (1982) calls these terms undesirable since they suggest a more definite association between the two conditions then can currently be proven. He points out that while an infant experiencing prolonged apnea may approach death, it cannot be proven that the child would not have corrected its own cardiorespiratory function without assistance. Indeed, the ability to self-correct becomes increasingly evident as the infant approaches 6 months of age.

Four groups of infants are at risk for sudden infant death syndrome:
- premature infants with frequent apneic episodes
- previously healthy full-term infants found to be cyanotic and apneic during sleep
- siblings of SIDS infants
- apparently healthy infants with hidden abnormalities detected on polygraph recordings during SIDS research.

Hospital assessment and diagnosis of the apneic infant focus on identifying such key mechanisms and disease processes as seizure disorder, upper airway or tracheal obstruction, automatic ventilation failure, sepsis and meningitis, apnea of prematurity, and respiratory infection (Brooks, 1982). Brief hospitalization for observation and evaluation offers an opportunity to identify treatable contributing disease processes; a complete clinical workup is accompanied by continuous monitoring of the child for periods of bradycardia (heart rate below 50 beats per minute) or apnea for longer than 15 to 20 seconds. Gould and Jones (1979) suggest that infant apnea treatment be directed toward preventing life-threatening apnea episodes and toward helping the family members deal with the stresses of having an infant who they believe may die at any time.

Infant apnea and family development. Families coping with infant apnea cut across all segments of the developmental cycle. Families with their first child, middle-aged parents of teenagers who choose to begin a second family, and young couples having their second or third child are all typically found. Single parents are not immune to this experience, nor has infant apnea been associated with any one ethnic or socioeconomic group.

Couples whose first child is apneic are doubly afflicted by their own lack of child care experience and grief over the perceived loss of a "perfect baby." Home monitoring may be more restrictive—and intrusive—than the new parents imagined. At this phase of family life, the hospitalization of an infant, often during the first weeks of life, can be devastating. The assessment of infant apnea can delay a family's progress toward achieving perceived competence and skill in infant care and can keep them from redefining their new roles within an expanded family.

Families of preschool, school-age, or teenage children must also master the complex tasks associated with managing infant apnea. Reorganizing family roles, distributing child care among friends and relatives, and maintaining communication among parents and children can be particularly difficult. Fortunately, this stage of the family life cycle is marked by an abundance of social resources, with other family members available to assume household and child care tasks. In such families, a newborn's hospitalization may not affect all individuals equally. Teenagers, for instance, might welcome the opportunity for greater responsibility and a greater sense of freedom and control. School-age children, when supported by friends or relatives, may adapt without apparent distress, although Wasserman (1984) noted sibling difficulties nearly 2 years after monitor discontinuation. Among the siblings interviewed, he noted anxiety, decreased attention span, and generalized behavioral problems. Family life stage is clearly an important determinant of adaptation to the crisis of infant apnea.

Theoretical framework: The McGill Model. The McGill Model of Nursing is a family-focused framework centered around the belief that individuals, families, and communities aspire to improved health status and have the capacity to achieve this goal (Allen, 1977). Its three major components are individual, family, and collaborative nursing care.

Individual health. Audy (1971, p. 142) has described health as "a continuing property potentially measurable by the individual's ability to rally from insults, whether chemical, physical, infectious, psychological, or social." These insults, he notes, have the potential to train the body to a higher level of health after recovery. Mastery of situational, maturational, or developmental crisis is believed to improve individual or family health; in short, health and illness coexist within the model. These ideas—of learning from health crisis and developing to a higher level of health—form the basis of most nursing interventions (Warner, 1981).

Family health. The family is a primary unit of nursing concern, because it is the context in which individuals learn to improve health. The family is affected by the health of each member, and each member is influenced by the health of the system as a whole. Family strengths, abilities, and other resources can all enhance problem-solving capabilities; by filtering individual members' concerns through the family framework, the nurse helps clients recognize that their problem-solving and goal-attainment processes are influenced by their significant others.

The MacDonald Family Assessment Guide was designed to provide nurses with the broad family data base necessary to plan care using the McGill Model (MacDonald, 1983). The tool presupposes that the family is an open, dynamic system best understood through its resources, its structure and function, its communication patterns, and its beliefs and values (see Table 13.1).

Collaborative nursing care. A collaborative health care relationship depends on mutual goal setting among nurse and family members, with the nurse serving as role model, stimulator, and facilitator (Gottlieb, 1981). The nurse tailors ideas to fit family needs; the pace of work is dictated by the family's progress. The nursing process is neither setting nor situation specific. The nurse pairs her knowledge and skills with the client family's resources. Together they plan, execute, and evaluate ideas. The McGill Model emphasizes this nurse/family interdependence as a way of building health potential through shared problem solving and learning.

In most cases, infant apnea is usually a transitory crisis that occurs early in the lives of both infant and, in many cases, family. The family's ability to cope with this event will be shaped by many factors; the nurse must talk openly with family members in order to plan care that responds to their unique characteristics. This is an important feature of the McGill Model of Nursing.

Planning

In infant apnea, nursing care must be planned for every stage of the family's experience:
• *beginning phase* (from the initial apneic episode to the establishment of home monitoring)
• *midphase* (the first 2 to 6 months of monitoring, during which the family adapts to caring for the apneic child)
• *end phase* (from the initial planning through the actual discontinuation of monitoring and the period of readjustment to life without the machine).

During the beginning phase, the family members must master the body of knowledge regarding their infant's diagnosis; they must learn to accept the condition's implications and subsequently must master technical resuscitation and monitoring skills. This education takes place within an acute care setting, often during a time of family disorganization and high stress; it may take several weeks to accomplish, depending on the infant's behavior and the family's readiness to assimilate new knowledge and skills. The nurse must plan for frequent family contact in order to assess learning readiness, comprehension, and effective information use.

The second phase, or midphase, takes place outside the acute care setting. The nurse's function is to provide continuity of care. Before discharge, primary care and clinic nurses should share family assessment data and progress evaluations. During this phase, frequent contact with the family must be maintained. Daily telephone calls, a home visit in the first week, and weekly clinic appointments are all helpful. The primary nurse must plan for ongoing evaluation of the family members' individual and systemic adjustment to a new home life, one that is reorganized around the need to monitor their infant's respiration during all periods of sleep. Concerns regarding siblings, marital relations, and accomplishment of activities of daily living should be noted.

Planning for the termination or end phase of monitoring involves increased family stress and reorganization; nursing contact in this stage should resemble that of the beginning phase in intensity. Frequent contact with the family allows members to share plans and concerns and to evaluate outcomes.

In each of the above-described phases, successful care planning depends upon an ongoing assessment of the family's coping abilities. Apnea severity and frequency will determine the course of family health management, so the nurse's plan should anticipate variations in family experience.

In infant apnea, most nursing care is provided outside the hospital setting and must be planned for accordingly. The nurse who plans community care must be aware not only of the family's own support system, but of community resources as well. Social service agencies, parental support groups, and emergency services can all augment nursing services during the infant's illness.

Intervention

The entire family system is involved in the crisis of infant apnea. Lives are reorganized to provide effective monitoring; the infant's crib is generally moved to the parent's bedroom; the monitor is moved from room to room throughout the infant's day; and a second person is recruited to assist when the infant is transported. Such adjustments cause both systemic and individual stress. Black et al. (1978) and Wasserman (1984) have noted effects on marital relations and siblings. Such studies suggest care without whole-family involvement.

To be sure, most researchers note that a single caretaker, usually the mother, assumes primary responsibility for the apneic infant. According to Wasserman, such women experience feelings of overwhelming responsibility, of social limitation due to the perceived lack of competent caretakers, and of inability to return to work due to lack of alternate caretakers. From the nurse's viewpoint, mothers are most likely to be seen in clinics, although other family members participate during home visits and telephone contacts. On acute care units, both parents are taught the required skills; in the case of a single parent, a second person must also learn CPR and home monitoring. The pace and timing of education depend on an ongoing assessment of the above (see Table 13.2).

Gottlieb (1981) has described the nurse's role in apnea care as stimulator, awareness raiser, and role model. As **stimulator,** the nurse should ask provocative questions that force the family to reflect on the situation.

Example:

Nurse (to mother): You say your husband seems to avoid touching or being near the baby. Sometimes by avoiding contact one protects oneself from becoming emotionally involved in case the baby dies. What would you think about that idea?

In asking this question, the nurse places the situation in a new light and suggests a pattern that the family might not have considered.

Table 13.2 Family Work and Nursing Interventions in Infant Apnea

PHASE: Beginning (from diagnosis to hospital discharge)
GOAL: Successful coping in a stressful period

Family Work	Nursing Interventions
Cope with impact of diagnosis and care plan.	• Assess family members' perception of event. • Listen to their ideas. • Assist to express feelings. • Give information as required.
Master knowledge about diagnosis, CPR, and monitoring.	• Assess readiness to learn. • Plan teaching program to fit unique characteristics. • Carry out plan, pacing to fit family style. • Evaluate learning.
Master technical skills of CPR and use of apnea monitor.	• Same as above. • Model skills of CPR and use of monitor.
Respond to periods of apnea.	• Listen to feelings and concerns. • Set up trial situation. • Evaluate ability to respond. • Discuss progress. • Plan future work.
Accept responsibility for home monitoring.	• Assess family members' perception of their competence. • Share evaluation of their abilities. • Discuss home preparations. • Plan home visit.

(continued)

Table 13.2 Family Work and Nursing Interventions in Infant Apnea *(continued)*

PHASE: Mid (home monitoring)
GOAL: Family competence at monitoring

Family Work	Nursing Interventions
Adjust to home monitoring.	*Daily phone contact:* • Listen to concerns. • Discuss strategies, offer ideas. • Reframe experiences to highlight strengths. • Provide source of understanding of their experience. • Review knowledge and skills as requested. *Home visit within first week:* • Evaluate monitor setup. • Meet with family to provide support, as listed above.
Teach caretakers to use monitor and administer CPR.	• Suggest demonstration of alarm and CPR. • Suggest setting guidelines for behavior in emergency. • Assist in teaching plan and evaluation if required.
Help all family members adjust to reorganization of family life.	• Monitor individuals' adaptation. • Listen to concerns. • Provide suggestions. • Discuss problem solving and results.
Normalize relations between infant and family.	• Encourage normal handling of infant. • Empathize with expressed concerns. • Model appropriate techniques or behaviors if necessary.
Monitor infant's growth and development.	• Measure growth, weight, and head circumference at clinic visits. • Do Denver Development Test for 2 to 3 months. • Observe for indicators of normal and abnormal behavior.
Deal with fears (inside and outside family) that infant may be developmentally delayed.	• Help parents express concerns. • Listen to ideas. • Focus on infant's attainment of developmental milestones. • Suggest joining parent group to find forum, support, and discussion. • Evaluate ability to deal with concerns. • Offer information as requested.

PHASE: *Mid (home monitoring)*
GOAL: *Family competence at monitoring (continued)*

Family Work	Nursing Interventions
Cope with chief caretaker's feelings of heavy responsibility and isolation.	• Encourage expression of feelings. • Explore current situations. • Suggest alternatives. • Link with other monitoring families if desired. • Evaluate problem solving.

PHASE: *End*
GOAL: *Return to normal (precrisis) life; integration of health crisis into family's perceptions of positive growth*

Family Work	Nursing Interventions
Plan to discontinue monitor (in accordance with decision of health care team).	• Encourage expression of feelings and concerns. • Discuss plans for discontinuation ("cold turkey" or gradual).
Discontinue monitor.	• Make a daily phone call to discuss problem solving and outcomes. • Offer suggestions as appropriate. • Monitor effects of stress on individuals and whole family (e.g., is family sleeping through the night?).
Reorganize family life.	• Note changes in roles and relationships. • Listen to concerns. • Offer suggestions as appropriate.
Integrate this experience into family life.	• Encourage discussion of experience. • Frame events as a growth experience. • Discuss evaluation of problem solving and goal attainment. • Offer ongoing health and family management care (e.g., issues of discipline, communication, knowledge of child development).

The nurse can strengthen the family's problem-solving skills by encouraging members to analyze their situation. As **awareness raiser,** the nurse helps the family members bring what they have learned about their situation from an intuitive to a more conscious level.

Example:

(Mother explains that she cannot plan ahead, that she feels isolated and overwhelmed by the responsibility of caring for her apneic child.)

Nurse: You are now able to describe your plans to take your other child to the neighbors' and to keep a suitcase ready in case of emergency. You have correctly rehearsed the CPR with me, and your mother has offered to babysit next week. I see that you are learning to anticipate events and are becoming quite resourceful at obtaining help. Your CPR knowledge is good.

The nurse here summarizes what the client has told her, highlighting positive signs of adaptation and ability. This intervention does not deny the mother's concerns but attempts to alleviate them by reframing the actions she has taken.

The nurse as **role model** demonstrates both technical and problem-solving skills. Nurse-client collaboration leads to shared insights into past accomplishments as well as plans for the future.

Example:

Nurse (to father): I have studied my notes from the past weeks and I notice an improved problem-solving pattern. You needed the homemaker's aide when you first began monitoring, but now you have assumed responsibility for grocery shopping and weekend meals. Your wife has established a network of friends and doesn't feel so isolated. We'll need to plan for the day when you discontinue monitoring, since that is always a stressful time. Among other things, you'll need to decide whether to reduce monitoring gradually or suddenly. In the past, family meetings have been effective—perhaps it's time for another one?

This analysis and review of past effective strategies provides a model for the family's future use.

Throughout the period of care both direct and indirect interventions are used. Nurses can offer specific information as well as reframe ideas and behavior. This nursing model assumes that, by working together to develop goals and problem-solving strategies, a family can weather its current crisis successfully and rise to a higher level of functioning in the future.

Additional resources. Sometimes the family of an apneic child is overwhelmed and cannot manage its health crisis. In such cases, other health professionals may be needed. Many social service agencies can provide trained personnel to assist with homemaking or financial problems. The nurse can, by sharing her insights and observations, nurture a trusting relationship between the family and other health professionals. The medical plan to discontinue monitoring, for example, will be based on the infant's clinical progress. But the family's plan to do the same will be based on members' perceived ability to do so. The nurse can assess family readiness by asking, "What are your feelings about discontinuing the monitor? Do you have concerns as a family? As individuals? What are your plans for this next phase?" and by exploring feelings, specific concerns, and possible solutions. She can thus help the family prepare for this next critical stage. At the same time, the nurse can help the medical team schedule the discontinuation to fit the family's needs.

Evaluation

A few months after the resumption of normal life, nurse follow-up becomes important. It helps the family understand the process of change it has been through, the changes themselves, and the individual and familywide outcomes. Questions might include, "How has the experience of being 'a monitoring family' affected you as a group? As individuals? What would you say has been the most important result of this experience for each of you? For you all?" The coping strategies, problem resolution, and mastery of fear should also be reviewed.

In short, it is important to acknowledge the family impact of the apneic crisis. The fact that negative aspects will take time to resolve must be confronted, and efforts toward that resolution should be supported and encouraged. The nurse can help the family perceive the crisis period as a period of learning and attainment of new problem-solving skills.

The need for ongoing nursing contact with apnea families has been clearly pointed out by Wasserman (1984). She interviewed families on five occasions, two of them on follow-up, over a 5-year period. The follow-up, at approximately 21 months and 2½ years after discontinuation, was used to collect data on the monitored infant, siblings, and parents. By the second follow-up interview, 9 of the 14 monitored children showed evidence of speech, learning, and motor problems. (Five of the 9 had required resuscitation during the initial episode.) This study also describes parental concerns about siblings at the time of the first follow-up interview, but most of these had been resolved by the final interview.

CONCLUSIONS

Infant apnea is a life-threatening event involving the whole family, but it is a time-limited crisis that can be mastered at each phase through hard work. The event occurs early in the infant's life and sometimes that of the family of origin, and its implications for future growth and development are unknown; they may be detrimental. It is also thought that infant apnea is related to the occurrence of sudden infant death syndrome (SIDS). Attainment of the infant's and family's developmental goals may be slowed or accelerated by these events. Families describe a period of increased togetherness during the early phase, but the strain over time can cause breakdown (Wasserman, 1984).

The nurse can be an important factor in enabling a family to cope with an apneic crisis and its aftermath. Ongoing use of the nursing process to make assessments, plan care, and evaluate outcomes is critical, as is an organized approach to intervention. Family involvement at each stage ensures that the ideas of involved health professionals will be tailored to the family's own pace and style. Successful nursing care helps families attain a higher level of group well-being and enables individuals to achieve a higher level of functioning.

REFERENCES

Allen, F.M. "Comparative Theories of the Expanded Role and Implication for Nursing Practice," *Nursing Papers* 9(2):38–55, 1977.

Audy, J.R. "Measurement and Diagnosis of Health," in *Environmental Essays on the Planet as Home*. Edited by Shepard, P., and McKinley, D. Boston: Houghton-Mifflin, 1971.

Black, L., et al. "Impact of the Apnea Monitor on Family Life," *Pediatrics* 62(5):681–85, 1978.

Brooks, J.G. "Apnea of Infancy and Sudden Infant Death Syndrome," *American Journal of Disease of Children* 136(11):1012–23, 1982.

Brooks, J.R. "Respiratory Tract and Mediastinum," in *Pediatric Diagnosis and Treatment*. Edited by Kempe, C.H., et al. Los Altos, Calif.: Lange Medical Pubns., 1980.

Gottlieb, L. "Nursing Clients Toward Health: An Analysis of Nursing Interventions," *Nursing Papers* 13(1):24–31, 1981.

Gould, J.B., and Jones, O. "Management of the Near-Miss Infant: A Personal Perspective," *Pediatric Clinics of North America* 26:857–65, 1979.

MacDonald, J. *Family Assessment—A Way to More Effective Care. A Guide for Teaching and Practice*. Montreal: McGill University School of Nursing, 1983.

Steinschneider, A. "Prolonged Apnea and Sudden Infant Death Syndrome: Clinical and Laboratory Observations," *Pediatrics* 50:646–54, 1972.

Warner, M. "Health and Nursing: Evolving One Concept by Involving the Other," *Nursing Papers* 13(1):10–17, 1981.

Wasserman, A. "A Prospective Study on the Impact of Home Monitoring on the Family," *Pediatrics* 74(3):323–29, 1984.

14 Intervening with families of children with congenital heart disease

Jacqueline N. Ventura, RN, PhD
Assistant Professor
Department of Family Health Care
School of Nursing
University of California, San Francisco
San Francisco, California

OVERVIEW

The family's responses to the first hospitalization of their child with congenital heart defects are examined. Nursing assessments and interventions used to ease the family through a life-threatening crisis are described. The chapter will show that nursing plans, when formulated with the aid of the family and other health professionals, can help the family resume normal functioning. Postcrisis nursing processes are explored; interventions of support, coordination of care, and anticipatory care that balance the child's needs with the family's needs are presented.

CASE STUDY

Sixteen-year-old Gloria Johnson, her 17-year-old husband, Dale, and their 4-week-old son, Cally, were driven 100 miles to the University Hospital by Gloria's parents for evaluation of Cally's failure to thrive and cleft lip and palate. The Johnsons, a Protestant family of Norwegian ancestry and lower-middle-class socioeconomic status, live on a dairy farm in a small rural community. The young couple had been married 4 months before the infant's birth.

The local physician reported that, despite the coordinated efforts of hospital and community nurses to teach Gloria and her mother special feeding techniques, Cally had not gained weight. Gloria was anxious, fearful, and unwilling to look at or hold her baby. When hospitalized for the first time, Cally became cyanotic during feeding and crying episodes. Physical examination, chest X-rays, and laboratory tests indicated congenital heart disease. Given the combination of a severe cardiac condition and a cleft lip and palate, and considering his parents' age and lack of parenting skills, the infant's prognosis was guarded.

Cally was hospitalized again at 6 months for Z-plasty lip repair and at 18 months for first-stage cleft palate repair; his mother stayed with him each time.

Following Cally's third hospital stay, Gloria delivered a healthy infant son. At 22 and 30 months, Cally was seen at three clinics—plastic surgery; ear, nose and throat; and cardiology—to evaluate the palate repair, assess growth, and determine readiness for cardiac surgery.

In the hospital, the family clinical nurse specialist, staff nurses, medical staff, surgeons, and social workers provided Cally with team-based care. The family nurse specialist interviewed the family during hospitalizations and clinic visits and maintained communication among specialists, community health providers, and the family. The community health nurse and physicians monitored Cally's progress, provided routine care, and assisted the family with day-to-day child care issues. As Cally grew, the speech therapist, audiologist, and otolaryngologist became active team members.

Family functioning was assessed during the initial hospitalization and reassessed during later visits. Instrumental functioning remained constant. Howard worked at a local dairy, and Gloria's parents provided financial assistance despite their own limited budget. The grandparents also drove the family to and from the hospital and clinic and provided child care. The family's expressive functioning changed during Cally's illness; although mother-infant interactions increased, spousal and father-infant interactions decreased.

This discussion focuses on the family's responses and adaptation to Cally's first hospitalization; it will show how nurses can help a family through a life-threatening crisis during the 6 weeks following an infant's birth. Nursing plans, formulated with the family and with health professionals during the initial hospitalization, can accommodate a family's needs and help its members resume normal functions after the crisis.

NURSING PROCESS

Assessment

The health problem: Congenital heart disease. Congenital heart disease occurs in 8 or 9 of every 1,000 children. Forty-one percent of the most severely affected infants die during their first year, while others require cardiac catheterization and surgery. Sixty-five percent of the children born with heart disease survive to age 20 (Waechter et al., 1985, pp. 784–836). Congenital heart disease is classified by its effect on blood flow (normal, increased, or decreased) and on the presence or absence of cyanosis. In cases of increased pulmonary blood flow due to atrial septal or ventricular septal defect, or patent ductus arteriosus, the infant is prone to episodes of congestive heart failure and/or pneumonia. Decreased pulmonary blood flow is evidenced by cyanosis, fatigue, and delayed motor development. In defects causing increased pulmonary blood flow, cardiac medications (for example, digitalis, diuretics, and vasodilators) are used to prevent congestive heart failure. Surgery is the treatment of choice for all major cardiac defects (Pediatric Cardiology, 1985).

Cardiac defects often occur simultaneously with cleft lip and palate, the other two most common congenital defects; all three result from genetic and environmental factors. Cleft lip is reported once in every 1,000 Caucasian births, occurs more commonly in boys (63%) than girls (37%), and is most often found on the left lip (Waechter et al.,1985, pp. 857–863). Although cleft palate occurs once in every 2,500 births—usually in families where a parent or sibling has had the defect—the Johnson family genogram did not reveal any similarly affected member. Surgical lip repair can occur at 10 weeks of age, but hard and soft palate repair is postponed until 18 to 24 months after birth (Day, 1984).

Adolescent parents and congenital defects. When Cally was born, Gloria and Dale were trying to manage two family developmental stages (stage one, marriage, and stage two, families with new babies), as well as their own individual adolescent development. During her pregnancy, Gloria had physically sustained the two highest growth rates observed in humans—those of the fetus and those of the adolescent (Ross Laboratories, 1984). These developmental tasks and the couple's age at first parenthood contributed significantly to the stress of Cally's congenital defects.

Although the stresses of adolescent parenthood have been associated with poor birth outcomes, there is little evidence that the adolescent mother's physical immaturity leads to maternal and infant birth problems (Mercer et al., 1984). Gloria said that she had dieted and not sought prenatal care in hopes that her pregnancy would not be discovered. She was now concerned that this may have caused Cally's defects. Such poor outcomes as low birth weight and prematurity are more closely associated with inadequate nutrition (Neeson et al., 1983), low socioeconomic status, and fatherless homes (Ross Laboratories, 1984).

Studies of the normal transition to parenthood show that parents function less effectively when they report symptoms of psychological distress (for example, depression, anxiety, and somatic complaints) and perceive their infant as having a difficult temperament or being "fussy" (Ventura, 1982; Ventura and Boss, 1983; Ventura, 1986; Ventura and Stevenson, 1986). Cally's congenital defects significantly increased his parents' depression, anxiety, and perceptions of difficult infant behavior. Their psychological responses to and perceptions of Cally's behavior were associated more with their loss of the fantasized image of their baby (Mercer, 1974) than with the normal issues of new parenthood.

Gonzalez and Reiss (1980) suggest that families with a member who has a chronic, life-threatening illness mobilize in order to cope with the severe condition. But as the crisis passes, they tend either to focus on the ill member or ignore him, in relation to the rest of the family.

These dysfunctional coping patterns reflect unrealistic perceptions of the situation and an inability to overcome old psychological responses and to develop new coping patterns.

Developmentally, Cally was like most children with congenital defects: similar to normal children of his age, but subject to growth delays. By comparison, the developmental impact on Dale and Gloria was far more pronounced. Both confronted two major, identity-changing maturational crises: adolescence and parenthood. Unplanned pregnancy limited the Johnsons' ability to complete the first family developmental stage—establishing an identity as a couple, forming attachments and relationships with their new extended families—and hindered their efforts to assume the tasks of new parenthood and the second family developmental stage (Duvall, 1977).

The double ABCX model. The double ABCX family stress model allows the nurse to monitor family adaptation to multiple stressors (Patterson and McCubbin, 1984). The interaction of the stressors (a) with existing resources (b) and family perceptions (c) is a useful indicator of family functioning (Hill, 1958).

Stressor pileup (aA), however, can occur in families of children with serious defects. Management of the illness strains the family's finances, adds caretaking tasks, and increases conflict between the child's and the family's needs. These stressors can be offset by resources (bB), which are defined as the family's social, interpersonal, and material characteristics. While Gloria's parents provided affection and financial help, community and hospital health professionals also helped reduce the family's stress. Perceptions (cC) are the family's definition of the stressors it encounters; such perceptions can affect the family's belief in its own ability to handle the crisis. Confidence can be shaken as members face the unpredictable course of congenital heart disease, or it may be strengthened if they view the condition as a challenge that requires constructive effort to manage.

Planning

Planning care with families whose infant has a life-threatening congenital defect relies on the nurse's knowledge of developmental stages and the phases of family response to illness. It also requires an established therapeutic relationship (Leavitt, 1982), assessment of family resources and changing perceptions over time, and collaboration with the health care staff to achieve care that balances medical management with strategies to preserve family function.

Changes in health care delivery. Early patient discharge, home care, and new technology combine to increase the need for advanced family nursing skills. Given these major changes in health care, planning must address three categories of care:

Support. When an infant is hospitalized for a life-threatening congenital condition, nurses must make sure the family continues its accustomed home care patterns. Feeding, bathing, elimination, and comfort activities regularly provided by the family should be continued. Health professionals familiar with the family can serve as surrogate parents for part of the child's hospital stay, offering relief from the family's heavy responsibilities. Community and social resources, including helping agencies, church members, friends, and neighbors, can assist the family during and after hospitalization.

Family nurses should foster health policies that support families of congenitally ill children. For example, such families could function more effectively if respite services were available. Such services could provide skilled day care or short-term respite care with direct reimbursement to participating nurses.

Coordination. Initially, families of children with life-threatening conditions need concrete medical explanations. As later episodes occur, they need up-to-date, detailed information about proposed surgical and noninvasive interventions. They need to assist staff members in making decisions (Ferraro and Longo, 1985).

Before home care begins, community professionals such as hospital nurses, physicians, surgeons, and others involved in the child's care should communicate through face-to-face conferences with the family, telephone contact, and the sharing of chart summaries. A hospital nurse and/or physician should remain in touch with the family, using telephone calls or letters to request information or to express concerns. This coordinator should also make referrals to other specialists.

Anticipatory care and problem solving. The anxiety, depression, and helplessness experienced by some families during the crisis stage make it inappropriate to educate the family about all aspects of infant care at the time of initial diagnosis. Rather, priorities must be set so that health teaching becomes an ongoing part of home, community, hospital, and clinic services.

Anticipated problems: Developmental deficits/speech impediments. The nurse predicted that, because of his defect, Cally would never be as large or as active as other children his age. The cleft palate would produce speech impediments; it also meant that, throughout childhood, Cally would have more acute illnesses—especially colds and ear infections—which are prevalent in children with this defect.

Questions to assist in planning nursing care. How can the nurse help parents deal with play activities and socialization as the patient becomes a toddler? What suggestions will reduce the risks of acute illness for patient and family? How can nursing, medical, and surgical personnel prepare child and family for surgery and minimize their anxiety? How can nurses help these families deal with younger and older siblings? What strategies can promote both handicapped and normal children's growth and development? How can nurses help families celebrate events and rituals (holidays, birthdays, weddings) in light of the need for specialized child care?

Interventions

Indications and contraindications for family intervention. Data on families with life-threatening chronic illnesses (Gonzalez and Reiss, 1980) indicate a need on the part of nurses and other health professionals to help such families cope with disappointment, with the necessary corrective procedures, with their child's developmental delays, and with the maintenance of daily family life routines. Blake (1964) shows how nurses can combine theoretical knowledge and clinical expertise to move parent and child rapidly from crisis to recovery during hospitalization for open-heart surgery.

Intervention for these families is contraindicated, however, when nursing staff is limited or when family-oriented care is not supported by the administration and/or senior medical personnel. Because of the complexity of these families' problems and members' vulnerability, it is counterproductive for nurses to try to provide consistent care or establish therapeutic relationships when they cannot guarantee follow-up. Intervention is also contraindicated when the nurse is a novice (Benner, 1984) or has limited family care skills (Wright and Leahey, 1984).

Crisis intervention. Family stress theory indicates that a health crisis can produce up to 6 weeks of family disorganization as members attempt to cope with fear, guilt, and feelings of helplessness. Family functioning during this time can be improved by conceptually separating short-term family adjustment from long-term family functioning and by designing care to meet family needs at specific stages of the illness. Therefore, early interventions generally involve joint efforts by health professionals in hospital, community, and clinic settings to balance the child's needs with those of the family's.

Crisis interventions were initiated at the following three levels:

Individual in system. Cally's feeding response was one of the first activities monitored because it increased the physiological demand on his heart, was complicated by his facial defects, and was most problematic for the family. Alternative feeding techniques, comfort measures, and body positions were explored in hopes of reducing physiological demands and increasing Cally's rest periods. Nurses reported that Cally took 4 ounces of formula in 45 to 90 minutes; he gained little weight and cried frequently.

In Cally's case, the initial nursing goal was to provide adequate nutrition. Three measurement criteria were established to evaluate progress toward this goal: reduction of the infant's feeding period to 45 minutes, lengthened sleep periods and reduction of the number and length of crying episodes, and documented daily caloric increases with weight gain.

Interventions were directed toward positioning the infant and reducing environmental stimuli. For example, when Cally was placed in a sitting position for feeding (allowing a preemie nipple to be placed at the side of his mouth), he sucked normally. "Bubbling" him after each half ounce of formula prevented regurgitation. Rest and sleep were enhanced by placing Cally on his side in a knee-chest position. These actions were based on knowledge of physiological responses to cyanotic heart disease, in which increased oxygen needs lead to higher hemoglobin levels, thus increasing blood viscosity and decreasing peripheral blood flow. Sitting and knee-chest positions helped Cally's heart pump blood to his extremities. To conserve caloric intake, the nurse extended Cally's rest periods by modifying hospital care routines. Physicians' examinations and laboratory procedures, completed early in the morning, were followed by uninterrupted rest periods. The infant was allowed to sleep for 4 to 5 hours following his feedings. Bath and other care procedures were performed in late afternoon or evening to further accommodate the need for rest.

After a week, the three evaluation criteria had been met and a diagnosis of tetralogy of Fallot had been made. The nurse and health team began to balance Cally's physical needs with his parents' needs. His mother needed emotional support and instruction in caretaker skills, while his father needed information about his child's prognosis.

Parent-child system. Observations of early mother-infant interactions revealed Gloria to be an exhausted adolescent; she sat by her child's bedside but relinquished the infant to a nurse whenever he appeared distressed. Two nursing goals were established: developing Gloria's caretaking skills and increasing mother-infant attachment (Bowlby, 1969). The latter goal was to be evaluated by behavioral measures of attachment: for Cally, that meant crying, eye contact, and following his mother, among others (Robson, 1967); for Gloria, it meant approaching the infant in response to his cries and cues for feeding, diaper changing, and soothing (Ainsworth et al., 1970).

Interventions not only provided support and information, they also promoted problem-solving skills, while taking into account Gloria's age and need to establish her own identity. The nurse helped physicians explain Cally's diagnosis and treatment in ways that his young mother could understand. As the nurse praised Gloria for her new parenting skills, the mother became less anxious; she began to feed Cally and notice his behavioral cues.

These interventions were based on two concepts of family stress theory (Patterson and McCubbin, 1984). The first concept maintains that help (bB factor) from a professional enhances a family's problem-solving skills by acknowledging and appreciating each member's concerns, thus guiding them all through the stressful situation. The second concept attests that the health professional offers relatives greater perspective on the critical event (cC) by pointing out the positive aspects of their infant's behavior, rather than focusing on the defects and allowing the parents to interpret their child's problem as a reflection on their identity.

At the end of Cally's 2-week hospitalization, Gloria's ability to feed and comfort her infant and manage his symptoms signaled that evaluation criteria had been met. She was able to ask nurses and physicians for information and exhibited an understanding of Cally's medical condition.

Family system. After an examination of Cally's condition, of his family's resources and coping behaviors, as well as of other stressors, a strengths and problems list was formulated (see Table 14.1).

The overall nursing goal was to help the family function during the crisis and begin postcrisis adaptation. The criteria required to indicate family movement from crisis to adaptation included the ability to see Cally as a whole baby, with strengths as well as defects; to show him to others; and to solve problems regarding infant and family needs.

The family needed support during this period. Members needed to be reminded and encouraged to eat and to sleep, and they required directions to hospital washrooms, cafeterias, lounges, parking lots, and the chapel. They had to be reassured that it was all right to leave Cally's bedside; they also needed help in formulating questions for physicians and other health care providers.

Interventions designed to clarify the nature and causes of Cally's defects, as well as his diagnosis and prognosis, were provided to the Johnsons throughout the first hospitalization by all health care personnel. Nurses, a pediatrician, and a cardiologist conferred with the family 2 days prior to discharge to review management plans, anticipate developmental landmarks, formulate strategies for avoiding childhood

Table 14.1   Johnson Family Strengths and Problems List (Family assessment at first hospitalization)

System	Strengths	Problems
Whole Family	• Whole family comes for interview. • Grandmother holds, cuddles, and talks to infant.	• Infant's congenital defects • Low family income and educational level • Lack of information about diagnosis, treatment, prognosis • Round trip from home to hospital of 200 miles, with grandparents as main source of transportation
Marital/Parental	• Grief reactions related to infant's defects is evident. • Concern about being capable parents is evident. • Father present at hospital.	• Lack of touch among members, except with infant • Lack of verbal communication between Gloria and Dale • Impact of unplanned pregnancy and birth of infant with defects

illnesses, and advise about projected surgical procedures, dental care, and speech therapy.

Staff members also encouraged the couple to discuss spousal and family conflicts that might arise as they dealt with Cally's ongoing care. For example, their dependence on Gloria's parents for housing, financial assistance, and child care was an ongoing strain. This situation was especially difficult for Dale, who had left school and taken a full-time job before Cally's birth in order to acquire separate housing for his family. At the time of hospitalization, the grandparents assisted in Cally's care and appeared supportive of the young family, but they had never openly discussed their feelings about the situation. Staff members encouraged the two generations to talk, and the grandparents informed Gloria and Dale of their willingness to help.

Staff members devised methods for the family to report Cally's and/or the family's problems. While at the hospital, Gloria had begun to write down her questions for staff members, and she was encouraged to continue doing so at home. It was decided that the public health nurse would visit on the day after discharge, and the family nurse would call daily for a few weeks thereafter until daily care routines were established.

The community nurse and local physician were subsequently notified of Cally's hospital course, of the family's responses to his condition, and of the care plan. Written summaries were compiled for local care providers and the hospital record.

This intervention strategy is based on recent research indicating that a child's chronic illness generates less family conflict if external assistance and support, effective problem-solving skills, physical and emotional health, and feelings of control over circumstances are provided or established (Patton, 1986; Patterson and McCubbin, 1984). Such families also appear to do better over time if they can learn not to be overwhelmed by their predicament and learn instead how to balance care of the ill child with the social and emotional development of all family members (Patterson and McCubbin, 1984).

Upon evaluation, behavioral changes indicated that intervention criteria had been met. Parents and grandparents became acquainted with other parents in the hospital and learned not only how to explain Cally's "lip problem" but to point out his wonderful attributes (for example, he was a cuddly baby, he ate and slept well). During the latter days of the first hospitalization, both generations huddled to discuss christening plans.

The christening and a traditional party to introduce the new baby to extended family and community were held 2 weeks after discharge. As the immediate family became more familiar with Cally and observed others' responses to him, they became less anxious. The party itself was a success, opening up new lines of social support for the young family. Thereafter the Johnsons invited friends to their home and took Cally to public places. The child remained free from illness during his first 6 months of life.

Postcrisis interventions. Family functioning is enhanced when the family reframes its perceptions after the life-threatening situation has been resolved (Patterson and McCubbin, 1984). As members adapt to the ill child's condition, they become knowledgeable and skillful in providing care that was once the nurse's domain.

When subsequent hospitalization is required for life-threatening events and/or surgical intervention, staff members usually assume that the family is in crisis. However, hospitalization does not always precipitate a crisis for the family of a congenitally ill child. Indeed, many of these families manage better when included in decision making and care planning (Ferraro and Longo, 1985). Research studies also indicate that such families adapt positively at home when caregiving tasks are divided among all members (Anderson, 1981; Ventner, 1981). Given the Johnsons' Norwegian heritage, caretaking tasks were shared primarily by Gloria and her mother, although Dale and his father-in-law were able to feed, change, and comfort Cally.

Family interventions thereafter encouraged affection and support between Gloria and Dale, since research indicates that spousal support facilitates adaptive parenting, spousal interactions, and positive perceptions of the infant (Ventura, 1986). Long-term nursing goals were established to help the family anticipate surgical procedures and to address their concerns about delays in the infant's growth and ambiguities about the extent of his heart defect. Table 14.2 summarizes family interventions during Cally's postcrisis hospitalizations and clinic visits. Clinical and research findings show that the child does better if the parent is present during hospitalization and if parents and child have the support of health professionals (Blake, 1964; Waechter et al., 1985).

Evaluation

At discharge, Cally had gained weight, and both Gloria and her mother had learned to feed him and to provide comfort measures that reduced his crying and cyanosis. Hospital and home care had been coordinated and a tentative schedule of surgical repair procedures formulated.

The staff had worked consistently to provide family care; Dale, however, had not been included. Staff members quickly pointed out his disinterest—he usually sat in the lobby or smoked cigarettes in the stairwell while Gloria was being instructed. But he had also hitchhiked to the hospital alone on two occasions to see his son. He had expressed his need to be independent of his in-laws and voiced his frustration at having to rely on them. Because of Cally's need for skilled care and perhaps due to staff members' limited repertoire for involving young fathers in care, the nursing focus leaned toward mother-infant interactions and mothering skills. It was a serious oversight to leave Dale on the periphery of care and not to involve the grandfather more in helping the young man.

To prevent similar deficits in delivering family care to families with a child with a life-threatening condition, nurses might ask these questions:

- How can we help the father provide child care?
- What care tasks has he performed before?
- What are his concerns?
- Does the father share his concerns more easily with male members of the health team?
- Are there other fathers available to provide support and practical assistance?
- Do men in the family and community (father-in-law, brothers, uncles, friends, colleagues, clergymen) meet for recreation and help?
- What strategies can provide mother and father respite and privacy?
- How can we help grandparents manage their grief and concern for their children and grandchildren?

Table 14.2   Family Interventions During the Postcrisis Period

Child's Age	Purpose of Hospitalization or Clinic Visits	Summary of Family Health Interventions
6 months	Z-plasty lip repair	• Rooming-in of mother • Visits from father and grandparents on weekends • Financial counseling
18 months	Cleft palate repair (first stage)	• Rooming-in of mother • Play therapy to prepare child for surgery • Family visits • Family preparation for new infant's arrival (including discussion of prenatal care, the parents' fears about having a second child with defects, and Cally's reaction to a new sibling) • Referral to dentist and speech therapist following discharge
22 months	*Monitoring of lip and palate repairs; reevaluation of cardiac defects; planning for cardiac surgery	• Coordination of physicians • Organization of chart information • Discussions with community physician, nurse, speech therapist, and dentist • Anticipatory care of infant (growth and development) and family (adaptation to new infant) • Encouragement of father's participation in care conferences
35 months	Cardiac catheterization; open-heart surgery for shunt repair	• Rooming-in of mother and grandmother • Help for family dealing with anxiety over long surgical procedure

*Clinic visits

CONCLUSIONS

A particular format has been presented for helping families of children with congenital heart defects; it examines family coping behaviors, resources, and definition of the situation in relation to the phases of illness. The concept of providing family care over time requires that nurses make a commitment to family care, work in collaboration with other professionals, and take responsibility for devising interventions that balance the child's and the family's needs. Support, service coordination, and anticipatory care and problem solving are particularly important.

REFERENCES

Ainsworth, M., et al. *Patterns of Attachment.* Hillsdale, N.J.: Lawrence Associates, 1970.

Anderson, J. "The Social Construction of Illness Experience: Families with a Chronically Ill Child," *Journal of Advanced Nursing* 2:427–34, 1981.

Benner, P. *From Novice to Expert.* Menlo Park, Calif.: Addison-Wesley Publishing Co., 1984.

Blake, F. "Open Heart Surgery in Children: A Study in Nursing Care," *in United States Department of Health, Education and Welfare Children's Bureau Monograph.* Washington, D.C.: U.S. Government Printing Office, 1964.

Bowlby, J. *Attachment and Loss,* vol. 1. New York: Basic Books, 1969.

Day, D. "Genetics of Congenital Lip Defects," *Clinics in Plastic Surgery* 11(4):693–700, 1984.

Duvall, E. *Marriage and Family Development,* revised ed. Philadelphia: J.B. Lippincott Co., 1977.

Ferraro, A., and Longo, D. "Nursing Care of the Family with a Chronically Ill, Hospitalized Child: An Alternative Approach," *Image: The Journal of Nursing Scholarship* 17(3):77–81, 1985.

Gonzalez, S., and Reiss, D. "The Family and Chronic Illness: Technical Difficulties in Assessing Adjustment." Milwaukee: Paper presented at the meeting of the National Council of Family Relations, 1980.

Hill, R. "Generic Features of Families under Stress," *Social Casework* 49:139–50, 1958.

Leavitt, M. *Families at Risk: Primary Prevention in Nursing Practice.* Boston: Little, Brown & Co., 1982.

Mercer, R. "Mothers' Responses to Their Infants with Defects," *Nursing Research* 23(2):133–37, 1974.

Mercer, R., et al. "Adolescent Motherhood Comparison of Outcome with Older Mothers," *Journal of Adolescent Health Care* 5(1):7–13, 1984.

Neeson, J., et al. "Pregnancy Outcomes for Adolescents Receiving Prenatal Care by Nurse Practitioners in Extended Roles," *Journal of Adolescent Health Care* 4:94–99, 1983.

Patterson, J., and McCubbin, H. "Chronic Illness: Family Stress and Coping," in *Stress and the Family: Vol. II, Coping with Catastrophic Stress.* Edited by McCubbin, H., and Figley, C. New York: Brunner-Mazel, 1984.

Patton, A., et al. "Stress and Coping Responses: Adolescents with Cystic Fibrosis," *Children's Health Care* 14(3):77-80, 1986.

"Pediatric Cardiology," *Maryland Medical Journal* 34(5), 1985.

Robson, K. "The Role of Eye-to-Eye Contact in Maternal-Infant Attachment," *Journal of Child Psychology and Psychiatry* 8:13–25, 1967.

Ross Laboratories. *The Adolescent Family: Report of the Fifteenth Ross Roundtable on Critical Approaches to Common Pediatric Problems.* Columbus, Ohio: Ross Laboratories, 1984.

Ventner, M. "Familial Coping with Chronic and Severe Childhood Illness: The Case of Cystic Fibrosis," *Social Science and Medicine* 15A:187–97, 1981.

Ventura, J. "Parent Coping Behaviors, Parent Functioning and Infant Temperament Characteristics," *Nursing Research* 31:268–73, 1982.

Ventura, J. "Parent Coping—A Replication," *Nursing Research* 35:77-80, 1986.

Ventura, J., and Boss, P. "The Family Coping Inventory Applied to Parents with New Babies," *Journal of Marriage and the Family* 45:867–75, 1983.

Ventura, J., and Stevenson, M. "Relations of Mothers' and Fathers' Reports of Infant Temperament, Psychological Responses and Demographic Characteristics," *Merrill-Palmer Quarterly* 32(3):225-89, 1986.

Waechter, E., et al., eds. *Nursing Care of Children.* Philadelphia: J.B. Lippincott Co., 1985.

Wochrer, C. "Expanding the Circumplex Model: *What Can the Study of Ethnic Families Contribute to Family Theory?"* Dallas: Paper presented at the Annual Meeting of the National Council of Family Relations, 1985.

Wright, L., and Leahey, M. *Nurses and Families: A Guide to Family Assessment and Intervention.* Philadelphia: F.A. Davis Co., 1984.

15 Intervening with families of school-aged children with cancer

Marilyn M. Friedman, RN, PhD
Professor of Nursing
Department of Nursing
California State University
Los Angeles, California

OVERVIEW

This chapter will help nurses understand and support the family who has a school-aged child with cancer. The family stress and coping theory is discussed, following by suggested assessment and intervention strategies the nurse can use to provide family psychosocial care. A case example illustrates how the theory applies to the family in crisis. The chapter also assists the nurse in setting goals that will help the family cope with the child's cancer.

The following vignette describes a family who has a 10-year-old boy with acute lymphoblastic leukemia (ALL) in first remission and on chemotherapy. It illustrates some of the more common problems a family in this situation can experience. The case study also shows how one pediatric oncology clinic nurse worked with the family members to help them cope more effectively with the stress and demands of their situation.

CASE STUDY

The Thomas family is a white, middle-class family living in a large urban community. Son John was diagnosed as having leukemia 6 months ago. The Thomases experienced enormous frustration in obtaining an accurate diagnosis. Their family physician on three occasions told them that their son had a simple case of the flu, with residual fatigue and enlarged lymph nodes. When blood tests were finally performed, he was quickly hospitalized at a nearby medical center and the final diagnosis was made. Although John was seriously ill at the time of diagnosis, he had a positive and rapid response to chemotherapy. Since his first hospitalization, however, he has been readmitted because of very low blood cell counts and fevers of unknown cause.

Although the parents were told that John's chances of surviving were good (over 50%), the boy's grandfather, a retired physician, remembered the cases of leukemia he had seen and prepared John's father for the worst. The parents read literature on leukemia (which was somewhat out-of-date) and appeared intellectually to have accepted their son's illness. Yet they were hesitant to discuss the illness with John or his two brothers, who were 7 and 9 years old.

Mr. Thomas works as a sales representative for a large corporation, while Mrs. Thomas is a busy homemaker. She is responsible for all decisions and tasks regarding the home and family when her husband is traveling on business (approximately two to three 3-day trips a month). Since John's diagnosis, his father has worked longer hours in addition to being "on the road," thus leaving Mrs. Thomas not only greater household and child care responsibilities, but also the caretaker tasks related to John's illness and treatment.

At present, John is seen weekly at the pediatric oncology clinic for follow-up care and treatment. This involves almost a whole day every week for both Mrs. Thomas and John; the medical center is more than an hour's drive from their home, and waiting in the laboratory and to see the physician is common. In addition, John has frequently missed school because of fatigue, colds, or other infections. Making arrangements for the other two children on clinic days is also a problem for John's mother.

During clinic visits, the pediatric oncology primary nurse has noticed that Mrs. Thomas looks tired and has difficulty getting John to behave while they wait to be seen. During a regular nursing visit, the mother expresses her feelings of being overburdened and describes the discipline problems she is having at home with her boys. She says that her husband does not discipline John, which makes his brothers angry and jealous of his special status. With no discipline from the father, John is difficult to manage; consequently, he "acts out" whenever he wants his way. His friends at school and at the clinic and hospital do not like to play with him because they say he is "selfish and bossy."

In talks with the mother, the nurse discovers that husband and wife do not share their feelings about John's illness with each other. Mrs. Thomas says she wants to talk and express her concerns (her way of coping), while the father tries to avoid "even thinking about it since it's so depressing." Thus, he works harder to keep his mind off things (his way of coping). Since Mr. Thomas is not involved with daily child care and trips to the clinic, his perceptions are different from his wife's. According to Mrs. Thomas, the couple has made no effort to sit down with the other two children and talk about John's illness and treatment.

The thrust of the nurse's role with the Thomas family during this period of time has been threefold—assessment, collaboration, and psychosocial intervention. First, through the evaluation of both child and family, she has completed patient and family assessments on an ongoing basis. These assessments form the basis for communicating and collaborating with the health team (physician, other nurses, psychologist, social worker, play therapist, and so on). The nurse has also encouraged both parents to attend clinic visits; when the father did attend, she and the other health team members emphasized the importance of open, honest communication among all family members about John's illness and care and of meeting the individual, developmentally based needs of all of their children including John.

In a meeting with the nurse alone, the father related his pessimistic view of John's prognosis and his feeling that, since John would probably die, "why try disciplining him?" Later, Mrs. Thomas expressed her empathy towards her husband's feelings but explained that John needed to be treated "like a boy his age." With little discipline, his obnoxious behavior was making everyone miserable, including himself. With further dialogue, Mr. Thomas gained a fuller appreciation of his wife's perspective and the negative consequences of his refusal to discipline John.

After several joint visits, the nurse observed that the parents could now share concerns and be supportive of one another. Nevertheless, since the couple's relationship had not been a close one before John's illness, their pattern of minimal support continued. Mrs. Thomas turned to her own support network of women friends. The nurse helped her to confide in old friends and encouraged her to join a parent support group in the community to better meet her emotional needs.

One positive result of the close collaboration between nurse and physician occurred when the nurse explained to the Thomases' primary physician the father's feelings of hopelessness. The physician then showed the father some new research on ALL that revealed an improved prognosis. By showing his confidence in new methods of treatment, the physician helped Mr. Thomas become more optimistic.

From this case study, several family problem areas were identified:
• the work overload that John's illness created for his mother and the father's lack of participation in the family
• poor communication between parents and children about John's illness
• lack of communication between Mr. and Mrs. Thomas and their discrepant coping styles in dealing with John's illness
• Mr. Thomas's infrequent discipline of the boys and their resulting behavior problems
• anger and resentment among the boys
• Mr. Thomas's sense of futility and lack of hope.

Each of these problem areas was addressed by the nurse and/or other health care team members as the family and John were cared for in both the clinic and hospital areas.

NURSING PROCESS

Assessment

The health problem: Childhood cancer. Childhood cancer refers to a multiple number of cancers in children; the most common is acute lymphoblastic leukemia. Cancer ranks second only to accidents as a cause of death in children between the ages of 5 and 14. Nevertheless, it occurs rarely. The incidence of newly diagnosed cases of childhood cancer in the United States was estimated to be 6,000 in 1985 (American Cancer Society, 1985). Common childhood cancer sites include the blood (bone marrow), bone, brain, nervous system, kidneys, and soft tissues.

Recent statistics on all forms of childhood cancer confirm that it is not necessarily fatal. Approximately 45% to 88% of all children with cancer will survive 5 years or more from the date of diagnosis, depending on the site of the cancer (American Cancer Society, 1985). The increased survival stems from the application of high-dose-concentration radiation and chemotherapy treatment. These medically aggressive regimens last an average of 2 to 3 years and, in spite of their effectiveness, have many side effects and complications, such as loss of hair, nausea, vomiting, fatigue, and lowered resistance to infection. The medical problems that these families face are compounded by continual uncertainty and fear of death (Camaroff and Maguire, 1981; Blumberg et al., 1980).

The extended life expectancy of the child with cancer demands a shift in the family's priorities, an adoption of the philosophy to live "one day at a time," and the making of realistic plans for the future. The family's quality of life directly affects the quality of life of the sick child, thus being of special importance.

Families with school-aged children. One important goal of nursing care is to help the family and its members move toward completion of individual and family developmental tasks while living with childhood cancer (Gray-Price and Szczesny, 1985). Family developmental theory is useful in helping us understand the characteristics of the family with school-aged children, including the family developmental tasks of that stage, and the way these dovetail or mesh with each individual's needs. Particularly important is the school-aged child and his developmental tasks. With a description of the family's and the child's development during this life cycle stage, we can better evaluate a given family and compare developmental norms with the family's and individual's behaviors.

According to Duvall (1977), the family life cycle stage with school-aged children commences when the eldest is 6 years old and starts elementary school. This stage ends when the eldest reaches age 13 and begins adolescence. At that point, the nuclear family has usually reached its maximum number of members and, because of the many activities the children engage in, these years are busy ones. The family developmental tasks during this life cycle stage are described in Table 15.1.

Table 15.1 Developmental Tasks of the Family with School-Aged Children

- Continuing to communicate effectively within the family
- Cooperating with respect to family tasks and activities to achieve family goals
- Maintaining economic stability
- Providing both adequate space and privacy for family members' activities
- Maintaining close ties with extended family
- Becoming involved in community activities and programs
- Promoting children's school achievement
- Maintaining a satisfying marital relationship
- Continuing to validate family norms and values

Source: Duvall, 1971, 1977.

Concomitant with the family unit's attempts to meet its developmental tasks, each family member works on his own developmental tasks. According to Erikson (1963), parents are struggling with the dual demands of their children's upbringing and their own growth as individuals and as a couple. School-aged children, at the same time, are developing responsible attitudes towards school, building relationships with their peers, and maintaining their self-esteem (Erikson, 1963).

The prime parental responsibility at this time is learning to "let the child go"; that is, separating from the child (Friedman, 1957). Increasingly, peer relationships and outside activities play larger roles in school-aged children's lives, gradually pushing them to separate from the family in preparation for adolescence.

Cancer has a pronounced impact on families with school-age children. From literature and professional observations, childhood cancer produces strains and hardships in the family that make the successful completion of the family's developmental tasks much more difficult. Observing the preceding list of family developmental tasks, we see that some tasks are affected more by cancer than others. Family communication is often strained and inadequate (although, with help, it is often strengthened). A shift in roles and responsibilities typically occurs, as well as a tendency to let the sick child be less responsible and less involved in the daily tasks of family life. Also, high health care expenses strain the family's finances.

The sick child intrudes in the parents' relationship, and finding time to be alone may be almost impossible. Maintaining close ties with extended family can be a problem. Some extended families draw closer and offer a lot of support; in other cases, the parents of the sick child find that their families want support themselves (and become a further stressor) or pull away because of their refusal to face the child's illness. Families often become so involved in the sick child's care that participation in community activities suffers. Furthermore, the parents' ability to encourage any of their children's school achievement deteriorates because of the parents' involvement with the sick child's care.

Maintaining a satisfying marital relationship during this life cycle stage poses a problem for many couples (Locke and Wallace, 1959), and childhood cancer typically acts as another stressor on the marriage. The validation of family values and norms may be altered. Families may question their values even more because of the uncertainty of their situation; they may decide to live "one day at a time" and become less materialistic and more child centered. Hence, some families, faced with a profound problem such as childhood cancer, make positive value changes.

Cancer, of course, affects not only the family as a whole, but also the sick child. Work on age-specific developmental tasks is often deferred during the diagnostic and early treatment stages of the illness. Yet, the sick child is still growing and developing and has needs similar to those of his healthy peers. During the prolonged treatment phase, these needs can no longer be ignored. In many cases, the sick child shows regressive behaviors more characteristic of a preschooler and becomes egocentric and dependent. The sick school-aged child's peer and school relationships are often problematic. Difficulties in disciplining the child stem from the child's developmental regression and the parents' tendency to indulge him, to lower their expectations of him, and to overprotect him.

Too much closeness between the mother and the sick child often exists. This intensity leaves inadequate space for the child to grow and separate from his parents. In a circular fashion, the child's failure to advance successfully through the usual psychosocial developmental milestones intensifies the family's—usually the mother's—tendency to focus too much on the child.

Family stress and coping theory. One of the most widely used tools in treating the psychosocial aspects of disease is the family stress and coping theory (Spinetta and Deasey-Spinetta, 1981; Folkman and Lazarus, 1984). Family crisis intervention, a popular strategy, is based largely on this theory. Along with family developmental theory, this framework can guide the nurse in her work with families who have a school-age child with cancer or another life-threatening illness. A theoretical framework or model is vital in helping the nurse spot the areas she should focus on. Hence, a model will aid her in deciding what questions and observations to ask or make during the family assessment. Equally important, theory explains how and why people and groups do what they do. In other words, it gives meaning to her observations. A good theory should convincingly explain what happens under certain circumstances. The stress and coping theory can be a powerful explanatory and prescriptive theory in pediatric oncology family nursing practice.

In family stress and coping theory, as well as in family crisis intervention theory, strong emphasis is placed on perceiving the illness in the context of its environment (Mailick, 1979). The theoretical writings of Hill (1949) and McCubbin and Patterson (1983) suggest that life stressors and family stressors are inversely proportional to each family member's health and the family unit's health and functioning. Moreover, the family's definition of its situation—whether it be realistic or distorted—affects family functioning and adaptation. Conversely, family coping efforts are responses to family stressors which, if comprehensive and appropriate, can facilitate family functioning. According to Hill's family stress theory (1949), the interaction of three primary factors (stressors, family's definition of its situation, and family coping efforts) determines whether a family will descend into crisis or successfully weather the cancer experience.

Using family stress and coping theory as a guide, the nurse's assessment of family stressors, the family's definition of their situation (cognitive appraisal), and the family coping efforts and resources will indicate the ability to function. Family stressors are events in the family's or its members' lives that produce stress or tension and remain unmanaged. Family coping efforts are the behaviors or responses made by the family and its members to reduce stress and to resolve the problem. The type of coping depends on the problem. The family's ability to cope also depends on the backlog of stressors existing when the child becomes ill, the members' definition of their situation (the way they perceive or interpret their circumstances), and the resources they possess. The ways in which families cope depend on the stage of the cancer experience; parents will cope differently during the early diagnosis and treatment stage than they will during the remission and therapy stage or relapse stage.

Using the family stress and coping model, a family-focused nurse should also look for evidence of the family's level of health or functioning. Some authors say that the level of family tension and conflict indicates how well the family is functioning (McCubbin et al., 1982; Friedman, 1985).

Consistent with family stress and coping theory, family nursing interventions should help the family reduce or eliminate stressors and tension. The nurse should encourage the family to utilize familiar or new coping strategies as needed. Helping family members see their sick child's dilemma in a more hopeful light is also consistent with family stress and coping theory. Also, supporting the family members' efforts to care for themselves is vital.

Knowledge of common family stressors and effective coping patterns used by families with childhood cancer provides the basis for applying the above theoretical framework. The subsequent sections review these areas.

Family stressors associated with childhood cancer. The intensive and extensive treatment of cancer has an unquestionably stressful impact on the family. Individual members of the family and members' personal relationships with one another are bound to change. Because of the severe stress precipitated by the disease, families who have a child with cancer are a high-risk group for family dysfunction. If a family was troubled prior to the child's illness, the illness only exacerbates the existing strains (Lansky and Gendel, 1978) and makes the risk of dysfunction even greater.

Understanding the nature of family stressors during a child's treatment for cancer is a prerequisite for empathetic and sensitive assessments and interventions. Slavin (1981, p. 16) perceptively describes parental stressors:

> It is clear that treatment for childhood cancer involves major emotional stresses for parents. In addition to the grief reactions and emotional pain involved in the threat of the loss of the child, there are substantial practical stresses in day-to-day living which affect the whole family....

Coupled with the often exhausting disease-related demands of transportation and frequent medical visits, the child's symptom management and distress (fatigue, hair loss, nausea and vomiting, weight loss, etc.) and major medical complications (infections, low blood cell counts, relapses, etc.) are most worrisome to parents (Friedman, 1985).

Kalnans et al. (1976), in a study of 45 families of children with leukemia, observed that the majority of these families also experienced one or more of the following:
• a death of another leukemic child, family member, or friend
• an illness requiring hospitalization, surgery, or ongoing medical care in a family member other than the leukemic child
• one or more occupational changes
• financial problems
• other major family events, such as a move or a change in recreational or social life.

At the same time, healthy siblings continue to need parental care as well as help in understanding their brother's or sister's illness. They often become sources of worry and concern to parents because of their difficulty in adjusting to the changes. Furthermore, parents can create stress by not openly communicating with their children or each other. Closed communication only escalates and compounds the other stressors.

Dealing with the ever-present state of uncertainty regarding the sick child's death may also be a problem. Camaroff and Maguire's (1981) study of the psychological and social implications of leukemia reported that the most striking feature of leukemia was the unpredictability of its course and its final outcome. Foster et al. (1981), in their interviews with parents whose children were long-term survivors (in remission 5 years or longer), noted that fear of recurrence was ever present, regardless of how many years had elapsed.

Assessing a family's ability to cope with childhood cancer. Assessing family coping patterns and resources will provide a further foundation for helping families adapt. It is helpful to classify family coping as either intrafamilial (among members) or extrafamilial (external to the nuclear family). Internal family coping strategies identified in the research literature include:
- maintaining or creating family cohesion (Foster et al., 1981; Friedman, 1985)
- maintaining a close, supportive relationship between spouses (Foster et al., 1981; Friedman, 1985)
- employing cognitive coping methods, including the use of religious beliefs (Friedman, 1985; Schulman, 1976)
- maintaining optimism and hope (Friedman et al., 1963; Friedman, 1985; Guillory, 1982)
- partially denying the prognosis/implications (Lazarus, 1981)
- endowing the child's illness with meaning (Friedman et al., 1963)
- maintaining a sense of humor in the family (Foster et al., 1981)
- communicating openly and honestly among family members (Foster et al., 1981; Friedman, 1985)
- keeping things "normal"—maintaining normal routines (Schulman, 1976; Futterman and Hoffman, 1971).

The author (Friedman, 1985) interviewed 55 Anglo and Latino families who had children with cancer in first remission and on therapy. Two types of family coping strategies were associated with families who were functioning at a more healthy level (as measured by the extent that parents reported family conflicts). These were support between spouses and optimistic beliefs. Both the qualitative field notes and quantitative measures demonstrated the positive effects of these two strategies. By comparison, some of the most troubled families (those scoring high on the family conflict instrument) displayed very unsupportive spousal relationships and a negative, overwhelming view of their situation.

Since the parents are the "architects" of the family (Satir, 1967), their mutual support and nurturing of each other are crucial for keeping up morale and regulating family tensions. The degree to which spousal support was present often depended on whether or not the spouses were congruent in their coping strategies (Koocher and O'Malley, 1981). Many wives remarked that they coped with their child's illness by talking about it and openly expressing their concerns and feelings, while their husbands coped by hiding feelings and acting strong or stoic.

Although internal family coping strategies are indispensable, most of the recent literature emphasizes the necessity for families under stress to seek greater external support. This would include informational support, or emotional support from such people as friends, relatives, and clergy. Families who are more cognitively grounded will seek knowledge and information concerning the stressors, and nurses can be instrumental in providing it. This may include information on parenting, child development, caregiving, and family adjustment—in addition to medical information.

Families also cope by linking up with community groups. Parents who have participated in self-help or support groups have reported them to be very important (Friedman, 1985). Informal social support systems are equally important. Extended families, friends, neighbors, co-workers, and other parents who have children with cancer can provide emotional support, as well as information, child care, transportation, or financial assistance.

Parents need to establish good lines of communication with pediatric oncology team members so that they will feel free to ask the necessary questions and seek the care they need. Other sources of professional or formal support are social workers and counselors, clergy, school nurses, school teachers, and family physicians.

Seeking spiritual support from a family's church/temple can serve both as an internal cognitive coping strategy and an extrafamilial one. In the author's study of Anglo and Latino families with childhood cancer (Friedman, 1985), belief in God and prayer were identified by the greatest number of families as the most important coping strategy employed since their child became ill. This response was especially common among Latino families.

Unfortunately, families also choose unhealthy ways of adapting (coping is a positive way of responding to a stressor). Denial of the child's illness (that is, of the full implications and prognosis), shifting of the burden of medical care, scapegoating, abuse, and lack of effective or open communication are general family maladaptive patterns. Lansky and Gendel (1978) note that two other common family dysfunctional sequelae of childhood cancer are the formation and persistence of a symbiotic, enmeshed relationship between mother and sick child and school phobia—by both the child and mother.

Family assessment questions to ask. Early assessment of the family's stressors and potential coping resources is encouraged by practitioners and researchers in pediatric oncology (Kaplan et al., 1976; Kupst et al., 1983). Mailick (1979) also emphasizes the significance of contextual and emotional stressors. She recommends a search of the family members' physical, social, and emotional environment for obstacles that might prevent them and their sick child from coping as effectively as possible. Table 15.2 outlines the assessment areas and questions the author has found helpful in working with families dealing with childhood cancer.

Table 15.2   Assessment Questions

- What family and family member stressors (both short- and long-term) have been experienced in the family?
- What is the family's definition of its situation relative to the sick child? Do family members have a realistic and objective appraisal of their circumstances?
- What strategies has the family employed to help it cope with the sick child and concomitant hardships?
- Do family members differ in their ways of coping with the child's illness? If so, how?
- Is the family using any dysfunctional adaptive strategies? If so, describe.
- What coping resources does the family or its members have available?
- How is the family functioning? To what extent are the family members' needs being met and family tensions regulated?

Partially adapted from Friedman, M. *Family Nursing: Theory and Assessment*, 2nd ed. East Norwalk, Conn.: Appleton-Century-Crofts, 1986.

Planning

After having identified the strains the family is experiencing and the way it is coping, a nurse needs to establish general and specific long- and short-term goals. These should be discussed with family members and mutually agreed upon. The most important goal will be the achievement of a higher level of family functioning. To help the family reach this abstract goal, the family nurse should help them eliminate or reduce strains and stressors. Secondly, by identifying coping tasks and behaviors, she should support effective coping strategies. Essential to the achievement of these two primary goals is cooperation among the health team members. Also, in setting goals, the parents should take as active a role in the sick child's care as possible. Parents need to be presented with acceptable options. Reinforcing parents when they are assertive in asking about choices helps them become better informed and hence more effective participants.

Several more specific areas for setting goals come to mind. The first entails helping parents to be aware and responsive to all family members' needs. Since siblings of the sick child are profoundly affected by the cancer experience (Koocher and O'Malley, 1981), "the family must find a way of balancing the demands made upon them for rearranging their lives, so as to be able to provide special care to the patient as well as ensure that the needs of other family members for continued growth and differentiation are met" (Mailick, 1979, p. 124).

The nurse must also assist the parents in managing role shifts. Role shifts require a delicate exchange of caretaking responsibilities and a division of labor that compensates for the loss of the sick child's functions without shutting him out of family life.

Open and honest family communication patterns constitute a core psychosocial goal in these circumstances. Isolation of the sick child and distancing of relationships within the family will result from closed, dysfunctional family communication.

Helping families deal with uncertainty and maintain hope is another significant psychosocial goal. When the sick child is on therapy and in remission, family members may enter a phase of partial denial, where they focus on the positive aspects of the situation and minimize the likelihood of a relapse. This helps them replenish their hope and emotional and physical resources, while giving them the energy to sustain the aggressive and demanding medical treatment regimen (Lazarus, 1981).

Intervention

General strategies. After mutual goals have been set, the next step in the nursing process is to generate alternative approaches to achieving the stated goals and then to identify available resources. Resources include prior coping strategies not yet tapped, family and individual strengths, the family social support system, and physical and community sources of assistance outside the family's present system.

Actual intervention may be carried out by the nurse, by the members of the health team, or by the family itself. The collaboration of the sick child, family, health team members, and other significant persons promotes and enhances the fullest possible adaptation of the family (Mailick, 1979). Accepting the family members as partners in the decision-making process throughout the cancer experience can encourage family adaptation (Blumberg et al., 1980).

Because the medical treatment and follow-up care of the child with cancer may continue over a period of years, continual reassessments are made. Updated interventions based on what the family and nurse and other team members believe to be important within the present context must then follow. Since the course of the sick child's cancer is characterized by vacillating periods of stress ("ups and downs"), the supportive strategies will correspondingly vary.

Specific strategies. Several more interventions that are geared to the family with a sick child in remission are listed below. These should correspond to the goals mutually set.

Promote open communication. Strategies to promote open, honest communication are essential. The nurse can act as a communication role model and encourage parents to share information, feelings, and perceptions with other family members, while encouraging their children to do likewise. For example, the nurse could meet with the whole family and ask the various members to express their understanding of the sick child's illness and treatment.

Open family communication leads to shared family support, mutual consolidation, and working through of losses. "Members of the family need to find comfort and solace in each other in their grief" (Kaplan et al., 1976, pp. 87-88).

Deal with uncertainty. The nurse should also help parents deal with their uncertainty and strengthen their hope. In remission, partial denial helps families replenish their hope and personal resources. Yet to completely deny the possibility of relapse and negative consequences will leave a family vulnerable to great despair if relapse occurs. Hence, a balancing of partial self-deception (healthy illusion) and hope with a realization of the possibility of relapse characterizes the optimum state of mind. For the family who is stoic and cheerful, the family nurse should encourage the expression of emotions. As Kupst et al. (1983) found, the intervenor's mere recognition that the diagnosis and treatment of cancer is indeed a hardship for everyone encourages family members to open up. Responding empathetically to parents who express their fears and worries is vital; it lets them know that they are not alone and shows them that you recognize and validate their anxiety. Encouraging parents to vent their fears and uncertainty, while supporting their optimism and hope, helps families adopt a more balanced perspective.

One way to relieve uncertainty and correct misconceptions is to provide the family members with detailed supportive information about the disease, including therapy, untoward effects, and practical advice on care. This activates their cognitive resources and relieves anxiety (Moos and Tsu, 1977). Anticipatory guidance, such as preparing family members for stressful future experiences (for example, treatment, possible adverse reactions, or sibling reactions), helps reduce stress and promote healthy coping skills when the event occurs.

Foster family and individual development. One of the major functions of families is to meet the psychological needs of their members. When young and school-age children are in the family, this is largely the parents' job. Fostering the development of each family member includes minimizing the detrimental effects of the cancer on the development of the sick child, the siblings, and/or the parents. The family nurse may help promote the parents' understanding of growth and development and of the importance of treating the sick child as normally as possible with respect to discipline and age-appropriate expectations. The nurse may also encourage parents to recognize siblings' developmental needs, as well as their own. Counseling parents to take time out for themselves is often sage advice (Blumberg et al., 1980). This not only helps parents meet their own needs for recreation and companionship, but also reduces the fatigue and "burnout" that result from chronic caretaker responsibilities.

Evaluation

Evaluation consists of looking for evidence that the goals the nurse and the family mutually agreed upon have been met. This fact emphasizes the importance of having clear, behaviorally measurable goals. The central question is: how did the family respond to the nurse's planned interventions? Evaluation should occur each time a nurse updates her nursing care plan. Since the amount of stress childhood cancer and its treatment cause a family is unpredictable, and because the family's coping responses constantly change in response to new situational demands, ongoing evaluation and modification of goals is essential. Observation of family members and their interactions is a useful strategy for gathering information for evaluation.

CONCLUSIONS

Intervening with families who have school-age children with cancer primarily involves a nurse's support and counseling. The nature of the psychosocial support and counseling will differ, however, from the psychotherapy services that mental health practitioners typically provide. There will be no delving into motives or subconscious sources of emotional stress (Koocher and O'Malley, 1981). Since family members face great stress and uncertainty, "giving patients and families the opportunity to talk about their concerns and receive information about their experiences is critically important. Being able to anticipate stressful events—such as hair loss, drops in blood counts associated with chemotherapy—can lessen the emotional drain even though the actual experience has not been altered" (Koocher and O'Malley, 1981, p. 175). Acknowledging the family's difficult situation, empathizing with members' perceptions and concerns, and yet encouraging hope and optimism are basic interventive approaches.

REFERENCES

Adams, D. *Childhood Malignancy: The Psychological Care of the Child and His Family.* Springfield, Ill.: Charles C. Thomas, 1979.

American Cancer Society. *1985 Cancer Facts and Figures.* New York: American Cancer Society, 1985.

Blumberg, B., et al., eds. *Coping with Cancer.* Washington, D.C.: National Institutes of Health, National Cancer Institute, 1980.

Camaroff, J., and Maguire, P. "Ambiguity and the Search for Meaning: Childhood Leukemia in the Medical and Clinical Context," *Social Sciences and Medicine* 15B:115–23, 1981.

Duvall, E. *Family Development,* 4th ed. Philadelphia: J.B. Lippincott Co., 1971.

Duvall, E. *Marriage and Family Relationships,* 5th ed. Philadelphia: J.B. Lippincott Co., 1977.

Erikson, E. *Childhood and Society,* 2nd ed. New York: W.W. Norton, 1963.

Folkman, S., and Lazarus, R. *Stress, Appraisal, and Coping.* New York: Springer Publishing Co., 1984.

Foster, D.J., et al. "The Parent Interviews," in *The Damocles Syndrome.* Edited by Koocher, G.P., and O'Malley, J.E. New York: McGraw-Hill Book Co., 1981.

Friedman, D.B. "Parent Development," *California Medicine* 86:25, 1957.

Friedman, M. *Family Nursing: Theory and Assessment,* 2nd ed. East Norwalk, Conn.: Appleton-Century-Crofts, 1986.

Friedman, M. "Family Stress and Coping among Anglo and Latino Families with Childhood Cancer," Unpublished doctoral dissertation. Los Angeles: University of Southern California, 1985.

Friedman, S.B., et al. "Behavioral Observations on Parents Anticipating the Death of a Child," *Pediatrics* 32:609–15, 1963.

Futterman, E.H., and Hoffman, I. "Crisis and Adaptation in the Families of Fatally Ill Children," in *The Child and His Family: The Impact of Disease and Death,* vol. 2. Edited by Anthony, E.S., and Koupernik, C. New York: John Wiley & Sons, 1971.

Gray-Price, H., and Szczesny, S. "Crisis Intervention with Families of Cancer Patients: A Developmental Approach," *Topics in Clinical Nursing* 7(1):58–70, 1985.

Guillory, P.A. "Impact of Cancer on Adolescents and Their Families: An Exploration of Coping Responses," Unpublished doctoral dissertation. Los Angeles: University of Southern California, 1982.

Hill, R. *Families under Stress.* New York: Harper & Row, 1949.

Kalnans, I., et al. "Concurrent Stresses in Families with a Leukemic Child," *Journal of Pediatric Psychology* 1(5):81–91, 1976.

Kaplan, D.M., et al. "Predicting the Impact of Severe Illness in Families," *Health and Social Work* 1(3):72–82, 1976.

Klopovich, P., and Trueworthy, R. "Adherence to Chemotherapy Regimens among Children with Cancer," *Topics in Clinical Nursing* 7(1):19–25, 1985.

Koocher, G.P., and O'Malley, J.E. "Implications for Patient Care," in *The Damocles Syndrome.* Edited by Koocher, G.P., and O'Malley, J.E. New York: McGraw-Hill Book Co., 1981.

Kupst, M.J., et al. "Strategies of Intervention with Families of Pediatric Leukemia Patients: A Longitudinal Perspective," *Social Work in Health Care* 8(2):31–47, 1983.

Lansky, S.B., and Gendel, M. "Symbiotic Regressive Behavior Patterns in Childhood Malignancy," *Clinical Pediatrics* 17(2):133–38, 1978.

Lazarus, R. "The Costs and Benefits of Denial," in *Living with Childhood Cancer.* Edited by Spinetta, J.J., and Deasy-Spinetta, P. St. Louis: C.V. Mosby Co., 1981.

Locke, H.J., and Wallace, K.M. "Short Marital Adjustment Tests: Their Reliability and Validity," *Marriage and Family Living* 21:251–55, 1959.

Mailick, M. "The Impact of Severe Illness on the Individual and Family: An Overview," *Social Work in Health Care* 5(2):117-28, 1979.

McCubbin, H.I., and Patterson, J.M. "The Family Stress Process: The Double ABCX Model of Adjustment and Adaptation," *Marriage and Family Review* 1(2):7–37, 1983.

McCubbin, H.I., et al. "Family Coping with Chronic Illness: The Case of Cerebral Palsy," in *Family Stress, Coping and Social Support.* Edited by McCubbin, H.I., et al. Springfield, Ill.: Charles C. Thomas, 1982.

Moos, R.H., and Tsu, V.D. "The Crisis of Physical Illness: An Overview," in *Coping with Physical Illness.* Edited by Moos, R.H. New York: Plenum Pubs., 1977.

Satir, V. *Conjoint Family Therapy.* Palo Alto, Calif.: Behavior and Science Books, 1967.

Schulman, J.L. *Coping with Tragedy: Successfully Facing the Problem of a Seriously Ill Child.* Chicago: Follett Publishing Co., 1976.

Slavin, L.A. "Evolving Psychosocial Issues in the Treatment of Childhood Cancer: A Review," in *The Damocles Syndrome.* Edited by Koocher, G.P., and O'Malley, J.E. New York: McGraw-Hill Book Co., 1981.

Spinetta, J.J., and Deasy-Spinetta, P. *Living with Childhood Cancer.* St. Louis: C.V. Mosby Co., 1981.

U.S. Department of Health, Education and Welfare, Public Health Service. *Facts of Life and Death.* Washington, D.C.: U.S. Government Printing Office, 1978.

16 Intervening with families of adolescents with burns

Loree Stout, RN, MN
Family Clinical Nurse Specialist
Mental Health Services
Holy Cross Hospital
Calgary, Alberta, Canada

OVERVIEW

This chapter examines the impact of severe burns on an adolescent, his family, and the professional health care system. It also explores the impact of the patient, family, and clinical systems on the course of the adolescent's illness. The most salient concepts necessary for the assessment and planning processes are briefly outlined. Possible direct interventions for all three systems are discussed.

CASE STUDY

The Wilson family was referred by a staff nurse to a family clinical nurse specialist in a large general hospital. The following details about family structure, reason for hospitalization, and reason for consultation were discussed.

The family includes Mr. Wilson, age 45, a bus driver, and Mrs. Wilson, age 43, a salesperson at a major department store. Married 20 years, they have four children: Brian, age 18, who plans to attend a university in the United States this fall; Brad, age 15; Todd, age 12; and Susie, age 4 (see Figure 16.1). The paternal grandfather died 5 years ago. The paternal grandmother and maternal grandparents all live in Canada.

Three weeks ago, 12-year-old Todd accidentally set Brad afire with gasoline as the two played in their backyard. The details of the accident were not clear to the nurse at the time of referral. Brad suffered third-degree burns on his arms, chest, thighs, and legs. Todd escaped with only a few singed hairs.

For the first 10 days of hospitalization, only Brad's parents visited; Mr. and Mrs. Wilson did not want Brad's brothers to see him in this condition. At the urging of the nursing staff and at the request of Brian, Mr. and Mrs. Wilson agreed to have the brothers visit. Brian has visited three times and has been temporarily successful in elevating Brad's mood. Todd has visited once during the 3 weeks and was withdrawn during the visit. The staff nurses report that the father has been angry and upset at the nursing staff regarding Brad's care, whereas the mother has appreciated the nurses' efforts. The nurses have seen Mrs. Wilson frequently crying when she leaves Brad's room.

Brad has been in the hospital for 3 weeks. He has been "a difficult patient" for the entire period, resisting efforts by the nursing staff to perform procedures to hasten his recovery. During the past few days his "stubborn stance" has escalated, along with physical difficulties. Brad is refusing meals and has become dehydrated, enuretic, and encopretic. His deteriorating physical status is a great concern to the nursing staff and Brad's family. The family is putting more pressure on the nursing staff to "do something to help Brad get better."

Figure 16.1 Genogram—The Wilson Family

The Wilson family was referred by a staff nurse to a family clinical nurse specialist (FCNS) in a large general hospital. The following details about family structure, reason for hospitalization, and reason for consultation were discussed.

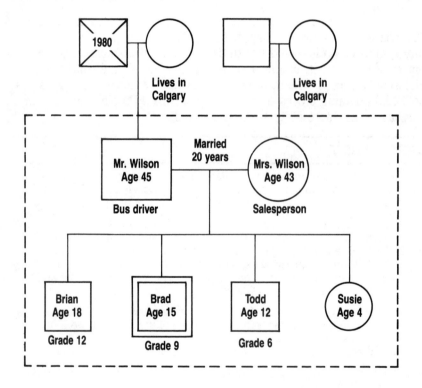

NURSING PROCESS

Assessment

The health problem: Burns. In order to understand how burns affect the patient and the family, we need to characterize the illness in language that is meaningful for individuals and families. Rolland (1984) proposes a model that translates biomedical diagnosis into psychosocial diagnosis by developing a category system that groups diseases according to characteristics that are psychosocially meaningful. Within the broad distinctions of onset, course, outcome, and degree of incapacitation of illness (Rolland, 1984), Brad's burns can be classified as acute, constant, nonfatal, and incapacitating. (Additional information about burns is contained in Section II, Chapter 11, in this volume.)

The injury that results from severe burns is initially acute, followed by stages of systemic complications and, in many cases, chronic disability. For acute-onset diseases, there is relatively greater strain on the family members to juggle their energy between protecting the patient from further disintegration, damage, or death and restructuring their lives and solving problems (Adams and Lindemann, 1974).

Other problems the burn trauma patient and his family must cope with include:
* pain
* multiple physical treatments for the sites of injury and subsequent complications
* overwhelmingly large numbers of health care professionals rendering treatment
* a long treatment period with enforced dependency necessary for survival
* helplessness
* separation from family
* lower self-esteem due to physical loss and personal meaning of the loss
* a feeling of vulnerability
* fears of death and uncertain prognosis (Goodstein, 1985).

Family systems approach. Family systems theory offers not only new forms of treatment that focus on the family as a unit, but also new ways of thinking about an individual's relationships to others. The key concepts of systems theory are wholeness, organization, and patterning (Papp, 1983). Applying these concepts to the medical context, systems theory takes individually oriented, linear, biomedical approaches and expands them to include another level of analysis; this level of analysis explores how symptoms, illness, and interpersonal relationships are embedded in an interactive, contextual system (McDaniel and Amos, 1983).

While serious illness or injury obviously has a powerful impact on the patient, the changes in his health and behavior also reverberate within the whole family unit as it adjusts to or resists the change (Doherty, 1985). The family's response also affects the patient and the course of the disease. Because the health care provider, the patient, and the family become parts of one system, the provider's interventions affect the family, and the family affects the provider (Doherty, 1985).

A burn victim's admission to the hospital activates three distinct systems: the patient system, the family system, and the clinical system providing care. In assessing the Wilson family, therefore, it is necessary to consider the nature of the illness, the impact that severe burns can have on Brad and his family at this particular time in the family life cycle, and the impact on the health professionals involved in his care.

Adolescent patient system. In assessing the impact of the injury on Brad and the meaning that it has for him, the nurse must be familiar with a 15-year-old boy's normal behavior; many of Brad's needs evolve from the tasks of this stage of human development. He will be struggling with the specific developmental tasks of early and middle adolescence, which include:
- becoming comfortable with his own body
- striving for independence
- building relationships with both the same and opposite sex
- learning to verbalize conceptually
- developing a value system (Adams, 1983, Hoffman et al., 1976).

Development of body image is a major step in adolescence and is closely associated with the individual's self-concept. Adolescents are hypersensitive to any change in their bodies and perceive any anatomical or biophysical insult in a heightened and exaggerated manner (Hoffman et al., 1976). A severe burn inflicts obvious skin wounds that require continual debridement and extensive skin grafting, which may result in significant scarring. In addition to disfigurement, immediate immobility, major metabolic complications, and pain, severe burns to the arms and legs may cause contractures leading to permanent disability. Thus, burns pose a major threat to the integrity of body image, and the adolescent may respond to this with denial, anger, or depression (Tull and Goldberg, 1984).

Striving for independence from his parents and other adults, the adolescent is experiencing struggles with dependence/independence. He vascillates between adult and childlike behavior as he is less involved with his family. At the same time, he still needs love and family stability (Adams, 1983). The functional and mobility-limiting nature of burns, combined with long-term treatment and hospitalization, greatly affect this developmental task. Among the few options available to the seriously ill adolescent to challenge and differentiate from adults are, paradoxically, noncompliance with medical procedures and treatments and depressive or provocative behavior. These expressions of frustrated autonomy often increase adults' surveillance of the adolescent, thus escalating the crisis (Libow, 1985). The sick adolescent may face ambivalence regarding the need for autonomy and the temptation to abdicate responsibilities and regress to a state of infantile dependency (Hoffman et al., 1976).

During early and middle adolescence, a teenager's interactions with his peer group help to bring about self-understanding and self-acceptance (Daniel, 1977). Also, an adolescent's sense of independence and self-determination tend to be developed through his social network (Tull and Goldberg, 1984). Thus, the isolating effect of hospitalization and absence from school creates fear, anxiety, and withdrawn behavior (Goldberg, 1984). Exacerbating the loneliness are long periods of isolation to prevent infection.

Changes in cognitive functioning—which are evident in middle adolescence—involve movement along a continuum from concrete thinking to formal operational thought (Adams, 1983). The nurse must assess Brad's understanding of his injury and treatment, as well as their personal meanings for him. It is important to remember that adolescents see their illness in terms of its effects on their body image and feelings, rather than in terms of its physical effects.

Brad's severe burns and subsequent hospitalization will interfere with his quest for independence, his confidence, his feelings about his body, and his involvement with peers. The nurse must remember this when assessing Brad and his family.

Questions to ask the adolescent. In assessing the impact of burns on adolescents, a nurse must remember that her attentiveness, listening, and honesty are important to them. If the interview is hurried or fragmented by interruptions, the adolescent will interpret this as lack of interest (Adams, 1983). Questions that the nurse could ask include: "What is the worst or most difficult part of being hospitalized? What could be changed that would make it better? What do you think or worry about the most? Who in your family is most concerned? What do you think he or she is concerned about? What do you think your friends would say if I asked them what they think is your biggest problem?" Because adolescents often have difficulty expressing their thoughts, the nurse can obtain more useful information by asking what they think others might think or feel.

Family system. Within a family systems view, stress in any one member of the family affects other members. In addition to an increased likelihood of at least transitory behavioral problems with Brad, his parents and siblings are also affected emotionally. Illness in a family often causes its members to undergo behavioral changes and develop coping strategies to accept and deal with the disruption the illness creates.

Emergency admission of a child to the hospital constitutes a greater stress for parents than an elective admission (Eberly et al., 1985). When an accident occurs, family members experience disbelief, denial, and shock, but they do not have to deal with the patient's physical pain and overstimulation of the senses.

> Initial fears for the victim's life, sorting out what caused the accident from often fragmented facts, trying to involve significant people, making decisions, and denying uncontrollable affective responses often turn the otherwise normal family members into a disorganized, unworkable system (Ragiel, 1984, p. 74).

The circumstances surrounding an accident may also intensify stress. Regardless of whether the parents were at the scene of the fire, feelings of responsibility and guilt often surface (Eberly et al., 1985; Goodstein, 1985; Ragiel, 1984).

The family is afraid of many things: its member's appearance, loss of function, and pain. Family members often block their emotions, lest the patient will think they are unsupportive or weak. The family's responses to the patient's first questions regarding his functioning and body image may be insincere. Thus the family can unconsciously reinforce the patient's lowered self-image.

Benjamin (1978) describes the psychological sequelae that families experience in coping with potentially fatal accidents or initially acute illnesses. The eight children whose case histories form the basis of her observations were between 7 and 11 years old when they became acutely ill. Although all of the children made good medical recoveries, family adjustment problems were marked by incomplete mourning expressed through depression, preoccupation, and helplessness when children began to improve and a sense of helplessness and lack of control. Parental passivity and anxiety set the stage for hyperactivity and behavioral problems in the children and for fantasies that the sick child had died and returned from death. Several children spoke of themselves as if they were ghosts or freaks and viewed themselves as somehow tainted by this return from death. Several parents focused

on the horror of the idea that one could experience death and then return to tell about it; they believed that their child was pervasively
changed by the experience.

Through semistructured interviews, Velasco de Parro et al. (1983)
studied 10 families who had children with leukemia. They found that all
families had a similar pattern of organization, including:
• increased isolation from previous outside or social activities
• inclusion of the sick child in the parental subsystem, eliminating him
from the sibling subsystem, and overprotection of the sick child at
the expense of the other children in the family
• a rigid alliance between the mother and leukemic child, with the
father and siblings assuming a peripheral position
• a tendency to include the maternal grandmother and/or parental
daughter within the parental subsystem
• an inability among family members to express their feelings and
fears and to solve their conflicts.

Though the ages and illnesses of children in these studies are different from Brad's, some of the same dynamics may exist among his
family members and should be considered before assessing them.

When caring for a child with an acute traumatic injury, the nurse
must consider the family as the primary unit of care. Usually literature
presents siblings' adaptations and responses resulting from chronic
life-threatening illness in a brother or sister. Caution must be used in
applying these findings to families with acute severe injury. Since the
affected child demands a great deal of attention, needs of other family
members become secondary but important nonetheless.

A study conducted by Spinetta (1981) found that children's responses
to a sibling who was seriously ill included:
• a lower self-image (4- to 6-year-olds)
• a feeling that parents were psychologically distant (4- to 12-year-
olds)
• problems with anxiety, depression, and other maladaptive responses
(6- to 12-year-olds)
• a perception of their families having more conflict and less cohesion
(13- to 18-year-olds).

A major source of stress for siblings results from emotional realignment in the family. Many children described feelings of isolation or
rejection as they saw the parents and sick children as dyads that excluded them (Cairns et al., 1979; Taylor, 1980).

The structural shift of parental focus onto the ill child can induce
feelings of anger, jealousy, and resentment in the siblings (Cairns et al.,
1979; Kramer, 1984; Sourkes, 1981). Their reluctance to confront their

parents most likely stems from a fear that their complaints may worsen the situation (Cairns et al., 1979; Kramer, 1984). The healthy siblings often feel shame over these negative feelings, as well as guilt that they are the "healthy one" and that they have no right to complain (Kramer, 1984; Sourkes, 1981). These internalized feelings of anger, shame, and guilt can torment a child, especially when intensified by fears of the ailing sibling's possible death.

Studies indicate that separation from family members and the need to grapple with unanswered questions add to the healthy child's anxiety. Because of inadequate information, many children feared they would develop their sibling's illness, or that the sibling would die suddenly (Kramer, 1984; Sourkes, 1981; Taylor, 1980).

When the illness leads to dramatic physical or personality changes in the child, the sibling may wonder if the patient is still the same person. Siblings may perceive the hospital as a threatening place, and they may have difficulty understanding that dreadful or painful procedures can also help their sibling. In the absence of experience, an integrated understanding is difficult to achieve (Sourkes, 1981).

Questions to ask the family. As consultant to the various systems, the nurse's first step must be to develop a definition of the problem that is relevant to the setting and useful for the family and staff. From the referral, the nurse can hypothesize that the family will identify Brad's regressive behavior as the problem, but she should not assume that this is the only problem. Assuming what families will need without verifying those assumptions will only make the families feel more discounted, devalued, and disenfranchised by professional intervention (Spaniol et al., 1984). The nurse should, therefore, ask each member of the family what he perceives as the problem, how it affects him, and how he would explain the initial occurrence of the problem (how does he understand it?). She must find out, too, how members have attempted to solve the problem and what the results have been by asking: "Who have you discussed the problem with? Have you been given advice from other people about the problem? What do you think about the advice? How did you decide what to do? What solutions, if any, have been helpful? How do different members of the family react when the problem occurs?"

Answers to these questions help the nurse understand the situational and interactional nature of specific actions. It is also useful for her to know what solutions have been tried and which have been successful or unsuccessful, in order to avoid suggesting unsuccessful interventions.

The nurse will need a clear family assessment framework to help her explore and understand family dynamics. Many nurses have found the

Calgary Family Assessment Model (CFAM) useful; it consists of three major categories: structural, developmental, and functional assessment (Wright and Leahey, 1984). Each category consists of several subcategories. The nurse needs to decide which subcategories are relevant and appropriate to assess each family.

The structure of the Wilson family, its life cycle stage, and a knowledge of the effects that sudden traumatic injuries of an adolescent can have on the family will guide the nurse's decisions about relevant areas to assess. When interviewing the Wilson family, for example, the nurse focused on the category of functional assessment, including both instrumental and expressive functioning.

In the area of instrumental functioning, the nurse should briefly inquire how the family is managing its daily routines in terms of school, work, recreation, and social activities. She can gain a greater in-depth understanding by assessing roles.

The subcategories under the functional assessment that the nurse should explore are communication patterns, problem solving, roles, beliefs, and alliances.

A nurse can assess communication during the interview by noticing how family members respond to different questions; she may not need to ask the family directly about its communication. Possible questions include: "How do different people in the family show their worry, fear, or guilt? From whom has each family member received information about Brad's injuries and treatment?" Answers to these questions will reveal the family's problem-solving skills and the ways its members identify problems.

Initial questions to assess family roles, alliances, and possible structural changes since the accident could include: "What differences have you noticed in the family since Brad's accident? Whose life has changed the *most* since the fire? In what way has it changed? Which family member(s) has taken over parental responsibilities while the parent(s) is at the hospital with Brad? How are siblings involved in Brad's hospitalization? What has been the most difficult change for the siblings? What concerns do the siblings have about the relationship with their parents?"

The nurse must assess family beliefs, particularly the meaning that the illness has for the family and their cognitive understanding of both injury and treatment. Sample questions include: "Of all the families that this could have happened to, how do you understand (or make sense of) it happening to your family? What does each member understand about the injuries and treatment? What information has assisted you most in understanding Brad's condition? Who in the family still has questions about his injury and treatment? What are the questions?"

By pursuing this line of inquiry, the nurse will gain access to information that may assist both her and the family. Family members are often unaware of the impact of the illness on each other. When family members disclose information and make new connections among themselves, it commonly mobilizes them to change (Wright and Leahey, 1984).

Clinical system. Clinical staff members face the horrifying physical effects of burns and painful treatment procedures, yet they must overcome their natural sympathy to provide the necessary care. This denial of experience can tax the emotional and physical health of the staff if they are not provided with an outlet (Ragiel, 1984).

The closer the patient is in age or appearance to the caregivers, the greater the chance that the staff will identify with the victim. When this identification occurs and is consciously recognized, the staff must take care not to become overly engaged (Ragiel, 1984).

When a caregiver identifies too much with her role of healing the sick and the treatment fails, she often feels anger toward herself and the patient. Since it feels wrong to be angry at an innocent victim, she will often suppress her feelings. To avoid guilt, staff members often withdraw (Ragiel, 1984). They may appear defeated, demoralized, and immobilized by their perceived failure.

At every level of interprofessional collaboration there are issues of identity, economic well-being, and power (Doherty, 1985). These issues can result in power struggles between professionals about who knows best what the family/patient needs and who "owns" the family/patient. Territorial issues, plus the difficulties of coordinating the many health care professionals who will be involved in the patient's care, can make collaboration difficult. Just as child care depends on respectful collaboration between parents, optimal care for families rests on respectful collaboration among health professionals. The clinical system must be consistent in order for family systems interventions to succeed over the long run in health care settings (Doherty, 1985).

Questions to ask the health care providers. An initial step in the consultation calls for asking questions of the clinical system to clarify the nature, history, duration, and context of the behavioral problem. Similar questions as were asked of the family members might be asked; for example: "What do they each perceive as the problem? How is it a problem for them? How do they understand the problem? What, if any, solutions have worked?" If at all possible, these questions should be asked in the context of a multidisciplinary conference. This helps assess alliances (agreements and disagreements), problem solving, boundaries, and communication patterns among members of the health care team.

Planning

When planning strategies, the nurse must remember that families with a sick family member do not see themselves as patients, nor do they always request consultation. Nurses may have an advantage over other health care professionals in approaching such families, because their role is clearly understood as providing direct patient care and, as such, their presence does not introduce a potentially alienating psychological or psychiatric element. Families might attend a nursing care meeting more readily than a family therapy session (Wright and Leahey, in press). Specific statements to the family such as "At this hospital, it is considered part of comprehensive care that families are seen in consultation" or "We've been more successful with patients when families have been involved in their care" can be very reassuring to the family (Mandelbaum, 1984, p. 317).

The immediate goal of the family meeting is to evaluate family dynamics and involve the family in the patient's care. Other goals are to facilitate effective nursing and medical management of the patient and to maintain or marshal the continuity and support of the family (Minarik, 1984).

In planning family-focused care, the family clinical nurse specialist (FCNS) must join the clinical system. It is essential, therefore, that the FCNS appreciate that Brad's injuries cannot be treated by one profession alone and that each member of the health care team will contribute to his recovery. When the nurse acquires this philosophy, she can easily show respect for the contributions of all health care professionals.

A useful principle to remember when working within the medical system is neutrality (Selvini Palazolli et al., 1980). Neutrality refers to a nursing attitude (or general pattern of activity) that includes a sense of respect, acceptance, curiosity, fascination, and even admiration for the system. The nurse is not interested in blaming anyone or changing the system (Tomm, 1984). This acceptance allows the system freedom to organize itself.

Hypothesizing. Another important principle identified by Selvini Palazolli et al. (1980) is hypothesizing. Hypothesizing refers to the nurse's conceptual activity in generating suppositions, hunches, explanations, or alternative explanations about the family and the problem in its relational context. Hypotheses serve to organize available data and enable the nurse to connect the relevant behavior of all family members.

They also enable the nurse to ask the questions that may elicit information to either confirm or refute her hypothesis. The nature of the nurse's intervention will be guided by her hypothesis about the presenting problem.

The content of the following hypotheses is derived from information about the Wilson family's structure and behavior, previous clinical experience with patients and families in a hospital inpatient setting, and theory in general. It is important to remember that hypotheses are simply suppositions intended to guide the executive activity of the nurse. They are not "truths" about the family or clinical system. Hypotheses should always be evolving on the basis of feedback in the nurse-family system (Tomm, 1984).

The following hypotheses are generated to highlight the interrelationship of the various systems involved: 1) The stress of Brad's sudden and traumatic injuries altered the family members' capacity to articulate their thoughts and feelings about each other. Each member was locked into his feelings of guilt, anger, sadness, and fear. This kind of conspiracy of silence can have detrimental effects on family members.

Because of his serious injury, Brad became more egocentric and more sensitive to his family's nonverbal behavior. Unfortunately, when family members withhold their feelings or avoid answering a patient's questions directly, the patient's fantasies about the reason for the familial withdrawal can be more damaging than the truth (Ragiel, 1984).

Distorted communication in the family will also affect the siblings. Todd probably felt responsible for the accident and Brad's resulting injuries and may continue to feel guilty about escaping injuries himself. Internalized feelings of shame and guilt may cause him torment and explain his withdrawal. From a cognitive point of view, cause and effect is a difficult concept for young children to grasp; they may feel that they caused the accident. When combined with intense fear or guilt, a young sibling's imagination often produces "magical links" in order to make sense of what is overwhelming or incomprehensible. Although there is no information in the referral about Susie's response, the nurse should obtain her version of the cause of Brad's illness and hospitalization.

Brad's parents may have become angry and frustrated in response to Brad's regression. A parent's feeling of guilt regarding his own anger and resentment is often masked by overprotectiveness, which in turn may prevent the adolescent from utilizing his strengths and skills, foster dependence, and generate even more anger from the parents to the patient (Abrams and Kaslow, 1976). Brad's behavior, therefore, may be a response to the family's overprotectiveness and distorted communication.

Mr. Wilson's behavior may also be understood in light of the conspiracy of silence. Unable to express the anger he feels towards Brad, he redirected his anger, manifesting it in verbal attacks or complaints against the staff (Ragiel, 1984).

2) When a family member becomes critically ill, family life begins to revolve around the sick child, whose needs demand enormous amounts of nurturing from the parents. The structural shift and emotional realignment in the family can produce in siblings feelings of isolation and exclusion. The parents' overprotection can also lead to distancing Brad from siblings and friends.

Parents often respond to their increased demands at home by withdrawing from previous outside social activities. This can lead to decreased support from close friends and relatives.

3) The core therapeutic triangle consists of Brad, his family, and the clinical system.

> The clinical system maintains the most authority, with the family and patient systems alternating membership in a dyad. Since it is almost impossible for three systems to interrelate on an equal basis, one must relinquish power. The patient, being in the most vulnerable position, is often rendered powerless. Staff and family members frequently converse together about the patient, often making the patient feel powerless, unimportant, and uninformed (Ragiel, 1984, p. 76).

Brad's regressive behavior can be understood as a response to his feeling helpless and powerless, and as his way to shift the power in the triangle in his direction.

4) A variation of the third hypothesis suggests that Brad may be "triangulated," or caught in the middle of a conflict between his family and the staff. Communication between the family and clinical systems frequently lapses. The family, fearing that it might interfere with the staff's care of the patient, may withhold its concerns or questions. Staff may arbitrarily select information to share with the family or patient. Thus, all parties get bits and pieces of information and receive different data. Neither the family members nor the health care team feel they are "getting the whole story." The family members may question the staff's competence, feel abandoned by them, displace their own feelings onto the patient, and argue with staff on behalf of the patient (Goodstein, 1985).

Attempts by the family and staff to combine forces and support Brad may fail because of the guilt or covert struggles each system harbors towards the other (Ragiel, 1984).

Intervention

The very process of bringing the family together to discuss an issue for the first time can be the most dramatic intervention provided. This is particularly salient when the injuries are the result of an accident in which one of the other family members was involved. Many families experience an inability to communicate their feelings and thoughts about the events surrounding the accident. The nurse can help the family through interventions that open up the family emotional system (Herz, 1980). She can accomplish this by asking the family questions that the family members cannot ask each other. In interviewing the Wilson family, the nurse asked each family member to describe the events surrounding the accident: what happened, who did what, how each learned about the accident, and so on. To assess any possible guilt, a nurse can ask each person what regrets he has about that day, what he wishes he had done differently, or what he believes was the most and least helpful thing for him that other family members have done. Each family member's response to such questions provides data for the nurse in assessing the family's communication.

In the case of the Wilson family, the nurse initially assumed that its members' current behavior manifested their attempts to adjust to and cope with Brad's serious illness, which had disrupted their normal pattern of functioning.

Behavioral symptoms have different meanings in different contexts. Some are less vital to family equilibrium than others. If a symptom appears in response to a crisis, it will probably pass when the crisis passes, making it unnecessary for the nurse to become overly preoccupied with it (Papp, 1983). On the other hand, as in Brad's case, a stubborn stance may become embedded in a repetitious cycle of interaction that serves a stabilizing function in the family; at that point, intensive interventions will likely be necessary.

In assessing the Wilsons, the nurse's initial assumption was that Brad's stubborn stance was a response to changes in the family's functioning as it attempted to adjust to his serious illness. Working on this assumption, the nurse chose to define the problem, offer new information, and intervene directly at the family's cognitive, affective, and/or behavioral level.

Interventions directed at the cognitive level of family functioning supply new information or new ideas about a particular problem. Interventions directed at the affective level seek to modify intense emotions that might be blocking a family's problem-solving efforts. Those targeted at the behavioral level of family functioning can help family members interact and behave differently toward one another (Leahey and Wright, 1985).

Interventions that were directed at the cognitive, affective, and behavioral levels of functioning for Brad, the Wilson family, and the clinical system are described as follows.

Adolescent patient system: Cognitive. The quantity and relevance of medical information that professionals share with the adolescent patient largely determine his degree of adjustment. The nurse needs to listen carefully to Brad; his expressions and questions can indicate how much information he is ready to hear. The nurse must not evade his questions but give simple, straightforward, hopeful appraisals (Goodstein, 1985).

Adolescent patient system: Affective. The adolescent needs an objective and empathetic person who can listen to his expressions of fear and anger without making him feel guilt. If the nurse anticipates the anger and guilt that his forced dependency fosters in Brad, she will be more prepared to respond in an open, empathetic, and accepting manner.

The staff must arrange meetings each day with Brad, outside of his scheduled treatment periods, so that pain-free relationships will develop. It is important to try to limit the numbers of different professionals involved in his care and to give ample warnings of staff rotation.

Adolescent patient system: Behavioral. When working with adolescents, it is necessary to involve them as much as possible in their daily care. For instance, the nurse gave Brad as much responsibility and control over his care as possible. Devising creative ways of allowing the patient progressive increases in autonomy can counterbalance the unavoidable limitations imposed by serious injury and hospitalization (Libow, 1985).

Family system: Cognitive. Information about Brad's injuries, treatment, and anticipated progress can enhance the family's problem-solving skills. The nurse should answer questions and concerns and assist the family in obtaining information as necessary from professionals in the health care system. She should set an example by presenting information in a factual way to the family and the patient, letting them decide how to use the information. In this way, the nurse encourages the family, including the patient, to take maximum responsibility for life decisions (Herz, 1980).

The nurse can anticipate the possible reactions that a family may have to a sudden traumatic injury. She can provide information that will help members understand the changes in the adolescent's behavior and emotions. Parents also need to understand behavioral and emotional responses that siblings may exhibit in response to the hospitalization and changes in the family. In Brad's case, his parents could be helped to recognize their own need for respite by framing the idea as helpful to Brad. The parents might say, "As our stresses increase, we must take good care of ourselves so that we have the energy to take good care of you."

The nurse can teach the family that the patient's loss of emotional control is common in serious injury and may foster maladaptive behaviors. Helping an adolescent to maintain a high level of self-esteem and integrity throughout the experience can be an important task of the family. Verbal or nonverbal communication to the patient that he is loved provides major support. In addition, it was important to increase Brad's level of control over himself and his environment (Tull and Goldberg, 1984). The family can be helped to understand that despite potential problems with activity, the adolescent with a serious illness should continue peer and sibling involvement in order to promote self-esteem and diminish fear of rejection and isolation.

Family system: Affective. The nurse should create and maintain a relationship in which the family can better deal with the stresses, challenges, and supportive tasks involved in the care of a sick adolescent. The family needs a safe listener who can deal nondefensively with intense feelings, understand the reasons for negative behavior, and help channel feelings of helplessness, fear, sadness, anger, and guilt into constructive expressions (Ragiel, 1984). Families commonly have difficulty acknowledging their own feelings. One of the most useful interventions that a nurse can offer a family who has a seriously injured member is to validate the family's emotional responses. Confirmation of family members' affect can alleviate loneliness by helping family members connect the illness and their feelings of stress (Leahey and Wright, 1985).

The nurse should focus on family strengths as well as on areas of weakness. Family members' self-esteem and sense of competence are greatly enhanced by acknowledgment of their strengths. Too much emphasis on dysfunction can lead to overinvolvement and intrusion by the nurse and can foster the family's dependency (Wright and Leahey, 1984).

Family system: Behavioral. Direct and consistent communication helps a family adjust to serious illness (Olsen, 1970). The nurse can encourage the family to overcome interactional and informational difficulties and create new ways to solve problems. Questions that the nurse asks in the context of the family meeting can help the family practice open discussion. Such questions can also demonstrate that expressions of affect can reinforce a feeling of togetherness (Tull and Goldberg, 1984).

The nurse can help the family show its injured child that he is loved and valued without overprotecting him. In addition, parents can learn to set consistent, firm limits with the child. "Behavioral contracting" with the child may help to avoid control battles and provide him with clear expectations. If the nurse helps parents contribute toward their adolescent's comfort and eventual recovery, their feelings of helplessness may decrease.

> Fairly directive strategies including assignment of tasks in the session itself and homework assignments for individual family members can not only effect useful structural changes, but also provide a sense of control and nurturance to a family feeling powerless and endangered. Therapeutic interventions designed to join the nurse's authority with the parents and empower the parents in their caretaking role are particularly important because the parent of a critically ill child is already struggling to maintain some semblance of control and usefulness within the disempowering context of the hospital culture (Libow, 1985, p. 102).

Families may need the nurse's "permission" to set aside time for themselves. Designing a task that requires the parents to take a break may be helpful. The nature of the task will depend on information elicited from the family assessment. For example, the nurse may ask Brad's siblings to plan a "fun" evening for the family away from the hospital. Part of the children's task might be to ask grandparents to spend time with Brad at the hospital on that evening.

Clinical system: Cognitive. The staff needs information about the family and its concerns. The FCNS invited Brad's primary nurse to view the family session through a one-way mirror. By observing the family interview, the staff nurse shifted her focus from the patient to the entire family. The view of family interaction from this new position will place what was seen from the old position in perspective (Anderson, 1984). Brad's behavior can then be understood within his interrelational context.

If the staff has a clearer understanding of the interrelatedness of the three systems, of the process of triangulation whereby someone is caught between two conflicting parties, and of staff members' need to express their feelings, then the staff members in the clinical system can support each other. They will be more effective with the patients and their families (Ragiel, 1984).

Clinical system: Affective. The staff sometimes needs support from someone outside of the family and patient systems. The FCNS can meet with the nurses and allow them to release their anger, guilt, helplessness, or frustration. Sometimes staff members cannot recognize and contain their own anxieties and conflicts, and the emergence of behavior problems in the adolescent or family unit may signal a serious dysfunction in the larger system (Libow, 1985). The FCNS can also be effective in preventing emotional difficulties and in helping people reframe behaviors and emotions viewed as negative into behaviors and emotions viewed as normal and adaptive.

Clinical system: Behavioral. Because stress emanating from staff was listed as the third highest source of stress for parents of children with unplanned admissions, strategies that limit the number of people interacting with these families could reduce confusion and increase the parents' trust in the staff (Eberly et al., 1985). It would be helpful if the primary nurse served as spokesperson for daily communication with the family, to provide relevant information about the illness and a degree of support that is acceptable to the family.

The FCNS can organize or participate in conferences with all health care professionals. Multidisciplinary conferences provide a forum for collaboration; ideally, information and goals will be congruent and there will be feedback among the professionals involved. Without well-developed, problem-focused, and mutually respectful collaboration, the patient and family may be triangulated into a conflictual relationship with negative results. Weekly nurses' groups could provide the staff members with an opportunity to vent their feelings about difficult cases and to receive support from each other. The treatment system must be consistent in order for family systems interventions to be successful over the long run in health care settings.

Evaluation

Evaluation would require answers to two questions: Has behavior changed as planned? Has the complaint/symptom been relieved? Evaluation is a continual process that reviews the systems' responses to questions and interventions.

CONCLUSIONS

This chapter examined the impact of critical injury (burns) on the ill adolescent, his family, and the professional health care system, as well as the impact of the patient system, the family system, and the clinical system on the course of the illness. "This knowledge, combined with an understanding of the interrelationship of the three systems, can aid health care professionals in facilitating conjoint movement toward the goal of psychological survival for all victims of trauma—patient, family, and clinical" (Ragiel, 1984, p. 77).

REFERENCES

Abrams, J., and Kaslow, F. "Learning Disabilities and Family Dynamics: A Mutual Interaction," *Journal of Child Clinical Psychology* 5:35–40, 1976.

Adams, B. "Adolescent Health Care: Needs, Priorities and Services," *Nursing Clinics of North America* 18(2):237–47, 1983.

Adams, J., and Lindemann, E. "Coping with Long-Term Disability," in *Coping and Adaptation.* Edited by Goelko, G., et al. New York: Basic Books, 1974.

Anderson, T. "Consultation: Would You Like Co-Evolution Instead of Referral?" *Family Systems Medicine* 2(4):370–79, 1984.

Benjamin, P. "Psychological Problems Following Recovery from Acute Life-Threatening Illness," *American Journal of Orthopsychiatry* 48(2):284–90, 1978.

Cairns, N., et al. "Adaptation of Siblings to Childhood Malignancies," *Journal of Pediatrics* 95:484–87, 1979.

Daniel, W. *Adolescents in Health and Disease.* St. Louis: C.V. Mosby Co., 1977.

Doherty, W. "Family Interventions in Health Care," *Family Relations* 34:129–37, 1985.

Doherty, W., and Baird, M. *Family Therapy and Family Medicine: Toward the Primary Care of Families.* New York: Guilford Press, 1983.

Eberly, T., et al. "Parental Stress after the Unexpected Admission of a Child to the Intensive Care Unit," *Critical Care Quarterly* 8(1):57–65, 1985.

Goldberg, R. "Toward an Understanding of the Rehabilitation of the Disabled Adolescent," in *The Psychological and Social Impact of Physical Disability.* Edited by Marinelli, R., and Dell Orto, A. New York: Springer Publishing Co., 1984.

Goodstein, R. "Burns: An Overview of Clinical Consequences Affecting Patients, Staff and Family," *Comprehensive Psychiatry* 26:43–57, 1985.

Herz, F. "The Impact of Death and Serious Illness on the Family Life Cycle," in *The Family Life Cycle: A Framework for Family Therapy.* Edited by Carter, E., and Goldrick, M. New York: Gardner Press, 1980.

Hoffman, A., et al. *The Hospitalized Adolescent.* New York: Free Press, 1976.

Kramer, R. "Living with Childhood Cancer: Impact on the Healthy Sibling," *Oncology Nursing Forum* 11(1):44–51, 1984.

Leahey, M., and Wright, L. "Intervening with Families with Chronic Illness," *Family Systems Medicine* 3(1):60–69, 1985.

Libow, J. "The Care of Critically and Chronically Ill Adolescents in a Medical Setting," in *Handbook of Adolescent and Family Therapy.* Edited by Mirkin, M., and Koman, S. New York: Gardner Press, 1985.

Mandelbaum, E. "The Family Medicine Consultant: Reframing the Contribution of Medical Social Work," *Family Systems Medicine* 2(3):309–19, 1984.

McDaniel, S., and Amos, S. "The Risk of Change: Teaching the Family as the Unit of Medical Care," *Family Systems Medicine* 1(3):25–30, 1983.

Minarik, P. "The Psychiatric Liaison Nurse's Role with Families in Acute Care," *Nursing Clinics of North America* 19(1):161–71, 1984.

Olsen, E. "The Impact of Serious Illness in the Family System," *Postgraduate Medicine* 47:169–74, 1970.

Papp, P. *Process of Change.* New York: Guilford Press, 1983.

Ragiel, C. "The Impact of Critical Injury on Patient, Family and Clinical Systems," *Critical Care Quarterly* 7(3):73–79, 1984.

Rolland, J. "Toward a Psychosocial Typology of Chronic and Life-Threatening Illness," *Family Systems Medicine* 2(3):245–62, 1984.

Selvini, M.P., et al. "Hypothesizing-Circularity-Neutrality: Three Guidelines for the Conduction of the Session," *Family Process* 19(1):3–12, 1980.

Sourkes, B. "Siblings of the Pediatric Cancer Patient," in *Psychological Aspects of Childhood Cancer*. Edited by Kellerman, J. Springfield, Ill.: Charles C. Thomas, 1981.

Spaniol, L., et al. "How Professionals Can Share Power with Families: Practical Approaches to Working with Families of the Mentally Ill," *Psychosocial Rehabilitation Journal* 8(2):77–84, 1984.

Spinetta, J. "The Siblings of the Child with Cancer," in *Living with Childhood Cancer*. Edited by Spinetta, J., and Deasy-Spinetta, P. St. Louis: C.V. Mosby Co., 1981.

Taylor, S. "The Effect of Chronic Childhood Illness upon Well Siblings," *Maternal-Child Nursing Journal* 9:109–16, 1980.

Tomm, K. "One Perspective on the Milan Systemic Approach: Part II," *Journal of Marital and Family Therapy* 10(3):253–72, 1984.

Tull, R., and Goldberg, R. "Life-Threatening Illness in Youth," in *Death and Grief in the Family: Family Therapy Collections*. Edited by Frantz, T. Rockville, Md.: Aspen Systems Corp., 1984.

Velasco de Parro, M., et al. "The Adaptive Patterns of Families with a Leukemic Child," *Family Systems Medicine* 1(4):30–35, 1983.

Wright, L., and Leahey, M. "Family Therapy Training in Nursing," in *Handbook of Family Therapy Training and Supervision*. Edited by Liddle, H., et al. New York: Guilford Press (in press).

Wright, L., and Leahey, M. *Nurses and Families: A Guide to Family Assessment and Intervention*. Philadelphia: F.A. Davis Co., 1984.

17 Intervening with families of young adults with AIDS

Kay Tiblier, PhD
Associate Clinical Professor
School of Nursing
University of California
San Francisco, California

OVERVIEW

This chapter describes the international public health problem and life-threatening illness of acquired immune deficiency syndrome (AIDS). The social-psychological impact of AIDS on the patient and his family is presented, as well as the role of the family in the hospital. Specific intervention ideas such as dealing with the stigma of AIDS are discussed. A detailed case study highlights the challenges and problems of caring for AIDS patients, their lovers, and their families.

CASE STUDY

Greg Benson was a 26-year-old Ohio native who had lived in San Francisco for 6 years and worked as a bank clerk. For the past 3 years he had lived in a monogamous relationship with his lover, Andy. He came to the hospital complaining of shortness of breath that was becoming worse. He was admitted to the intensive care unit. Three months before this hospital admission, Greg had been treated as an outpatient for pneumocystis pneumonia, and diagnosed with AIDS. He had not told his parents that he was ill or gay. He had, however, told his only sibling, Steve, that he had AIDS. Steve already knew that his younger brother was gay.

During his hospitalization, Greg's visitors were so numerous that an envelope was placed outside his door for messages from friends. Andy was a nearly constant visitor at the bedside of the respirator-dependent Greg. Realizing the seriousness of his condition, Greg asked Andy to tell his parents that he was sick and to ask them to visit. Andy asked a mutual friend to call them. Andy and a male friend met Greg's parents, Barbara, a housewife, and Hank, a retired businessman, at the airport and provided them with a car and a place to stay. Greg's employer sent Hank and Barbara flowers and invited them to dinner.

Initially, the family members seemed to the staff to be especially friendly and well functioning, but they were referred to the clinical sociologist by a nurse who questioned their cheerfulness. The parents were seen during the following 5-week course of the disease, and Greg's brother Steve, a 19-year-old college sophomore, was included on his arrival. An interdisciplinary team (physician, nurse, and clinical sociologist) met with the family to discuss the diagnosis. On initial assessment, Barbara denied the possibility that her son could be fatally ill and often spoke for Hank. Both parents felt that Greg was "just going through a stage" regarding his sexuality. The nurse's intervention goals included encouraging the family to find housing nearby rather than to keep a constant hospital vigil; to accept the realities of the outcome of AIDS; to acknowledge the relationship between Greg and Andy; to encourage better intrafamily communication; to shift some concern to son Steve, who appeared to have been identified as the "bad child"; and to get Greg's personal affairs in order.

As Greg's condition worsened, the family's expressions of good nature were replaced by resentful comments. As their tension mounted, family members blamed physicians and nurses for Greg's decline. They reached a critical point when they disagreed about life-support measures. Although the patient had given power of attorney to Andy, his parents contended that they were legitimate next of kin and demanded a full code.

The argument between the AIDS patient's family and his lover as to who would serve as the patient's advocate reflects many of the unresolved conflicts and crises that occur with each diagnosis of AIDS. Although the family members abruptly terminated their sessions at Greg's death and felt unable to share his diagnosis with other family and friends, they had partially accepted the situation. Support by nursing personnel is paramount in resolving these myriad issues before the patient dies, so that the family can better deal with the stages of bereavement.

NURSING PROCESS

Assessment

The health problem: The acquired immune deficiency syndrome. AIDS is a major international public health problem. By the end of 1984, nearly 8,000 patients had been reported in the United States, and almost half had died (Jaffe et al., 1985). Epidemiologists reported 16,000 cases before the end of 1985 and predicted that that number would double each year for the forseeable future. Since 1977, when AIDS was first documented, the illness has been diagnosed with increasing frequency around the world.

A new human retrovirus, human immunodeficiency virus (HIV), also known as lymphadenopathy-associated virus, is the primary etiologic agent of the syndrome. Although infection with the AIDS virus does not necessarily result in AIDS or AIDS-related conditions, the virus must be present in the system for AIDS to occur.

AIDS represents an impairment of the body's ability to resist certain diseases that the healthy immune system combats without difficulty. People with AIDS are susceptible to many diseases labeled "opportunistic," since they occur rarely in individuals with normal immune functions. The two most common of these diseases are a rare form of cancer called Kaposi's sarcoma, involving lesions of the skin and other body organs, and Pneumocystis carinii pneumonia, a more common protozoan infection of the lungs. Other opportunistic infections include a variety of viral and fungal agents.

Presenting symptoms. Among the presenting symptoms associated with AIDS are minor illnesses such as colds or flu, but in AIDS these symptoms are usually persistent or recurrent. The symptoms may include unexplained, persistent fatigue; fever, chills, or night sweats that last for several weeks; unexplained weight loss; enlarged lymph nodes, usually in the neck, armpit, or groin; pink or purple flat or raised blotches on or under the skin; persistent white spots or blemishes in the mouth; persistent diarrhea or dry cough; and shortness of breath. Mood disturbance and cognitive dysfunction have been found to be pervasive clinical features of AIDS patients. Although at high risk for psychological problems, AIDS patients tend to be underdiagnosed and undertreated for neuropsychiatric symptoms (Perry and Tross, 1984). Sometimes the depressive symptoms are the first sign of central nervous system infections and, if monitored, can be an effective clue to a need for further intervention.

Transmission of the virus. AIDS can be transmitted through sexual contact in the same manner as other sexually transmitted diseases. It can also be spread through direct blood contact (as from sharing hypodermic needles) or transmitted to an unborn child by an infected mother. Transmission through blood transfusion should no longer occur where screening programs are in place.

Homosexual or bisexual men, intravenous drug users, and men with hemophilia have accounted for 94% of the cases of AIDS to date. There is increasing evidence of spread beyond the original high-risk groups. More infection in the general heterosexual population is expected (Echenberg, 1985).

AIDS as a social problem. As AIDS has spread and a greater number have become ill and died, the media have brought to the public's attention the implications of AIDS. Public fear and concern have increased (Wallis, 1985). The median age of AIDS patients has been 34 years; 92% are below the age of 50. The tragedy of the epidemic is intensified by the young age of the victims, the lack of proven treatment, the cost of treatment, and the prolonged, debilitating, and often fatal illnesses that occur. Many patients survive one illness only to suffer a fatal recurrence of another infection or to develop a fatal cancer. Once diagnosed, the average patient faces a life expectancy of only months, although death may come as early as within several weeks or as late as after 5 years or more. Despite the many medical interventions, no cure has been found to date, and death is almost certain.

As a new, contagious, and presently incurable disease, AIDS has received enormous public attention and evoked a broad range of professional and lay responses. As with other diseases, such as tuberculosis or cancer, these responses are colored not only by scientific data, but by myth, superstition, and stigma. Because the primary group at risk is gay men, attitudes, beliefs, and emotional reactions to homosexuality have influenced the early response to AIDS.

Because there are no completely satisfactory generic terms for describing people on the basis of sexual preference, the term "gay" is used; it is preferred by many gay people themselves (Jay and Young, 1979) and refers to life-style choice. The term "homosexual" is more precisely used in its literal meaning: of one sex. Gay men, composing an estimated 10% of the male population, are highly diverse in terms of age, race, ethnicity, personality, and socioeconomic status. Some are married and have children (Bell and Weinberg, 1978).

The incidence of AIDS has been highest in young gay men, and therefore the focus of this chapter is on gay male AIDS patients and their families. Many of the concepts presented, however, can be applied as well to the other groups contracting AIDS.

AIDS and care providers. The financial cost of an epidemic of this magnitude places an immense burden on the health care system, and the less tangible costs can be seen on any ward providing care to patients with the disease. The strain on patients, their friends and relatives, and the medical, nursing, and support staff is great. Several decades have passed since medical caregivers have had to face an epidemic of a fatal infectious disease among previously healthy persons (Landesman et al., 1985). Nurses must be willing to attempt to provide "competent and compassionate care in an area with more questions than answers" (Nichols, 1983, p. 1083).

AIDS poses a dilemma for health care workers: how to respond to a fatal disease that has no known cure, is transmissible, and is occurring in groups of people who are not well accepted into the mainstream of society (Lusby, 1985).

In many hospitals, special care units are being set up for AIDS patients to provide quality nursing care, to coordinate support services for the patient and his family, and to provide support as well for health care workers involved in the care of AIDS patients. Nursing care plans are best individualized to meet the needs of each patient. Good nursing management requires an interdisciplinary approach that addresses treatment of symptoms and of the psychological problems that come with a threatening illness. The nurse must also help the patient with the social stigma attached to being gay, with his fears of contaminating others, and with living with AIDS and perhaps dying after the hospital stay (Morin, 1984).

Ryan (1984) underscores the need for the nurse to approach the patient in a holistic manner, to address both strengths and weaknesses in assessment, and to avoid the tendency to stereotype. The nurse should be nonjudgmental, as she faces the common problems of anxiety, isolation, drain, and stress seen in those who care for persons suffering from terminal diseases (Simmons-Alling, 1984, p. 32).

Social-psychological impact of AIDS on the patient. The impact of AIDS on the patient is pervasive and characterized by catastrophic loss (Rubinow, 1984). These losses include health, employment, financial autonomy, life-style, self-esteem, privacy, self-control, and sometimes social support. Sociological variables that contribute to the devastating impact for the individual include his age, physical distance from family of origin, social stigma, employment disruption with resulting financial destitution, and potential alienation from significant others.

As AIDS progresses, the patient may experience loss of intellectual function, paralysis, or blindness. And ultimately, the patient will lose his life. The AIDS patient may be left with unresolved feelings about his sexual preference. He may experience guilt, anger, and self-blame. Socialized in a predominantly heterosexual culture, the patient may have internalized the shame that characterizes current social attitudes toward homosexuality (Malyon, 1982). The patient may abandon sexual activity or identify sex with transmission of illness. This in turn may lead to loss of perceived means of giving and receiving love and affection, leading to isolation and despair.

The impact of AIDS on the family. Although the tragedy of AIDS is now widely recognized as an epidemic, little attention has been given to the impact of the disease on the significant others who are affected by the diagnosis. "Significant others" for the homosexual patient may include lover and friends rather than, or besides, his family of origin. This expanded sociological definition of the "family" is the most helpful to health care providers caring for AIDS patients.

When a family member is diagnosed as having AIDS, catastrophic change within the family may occur. As Helmquist (1984) characterizes it, life may suddenly resemble a roller coaster ride. Family members have many questions concerning medical issues, as well as intense feelings of anger, fear, despair, uncertainty, and frustration.

Hill and Hansen (1964, p. 803) identified four factors that influence the family's ability to cope with illness. These included characteristics of the event (nature of the illness, disability, prognosis, and perception of the illness); perceived threat to family (relationships, status, and roles); available resources; and past experience with illness. The diagnosis of AIDS, as seen through this analytic framework, is devastating. It presents the family with multiple crises simultaneously, each one demanding immediate attention and intervention.

The role of the family in the hospital. Sociologists Anselm Strauss and associates (1984) have identified three types of "the work of kin in hospitals," each of which is affected by the nature of illness, the technology for managing it, and the organization features of that management. These types are:
• working with a sick relative "psychologically" (the sentimental work)
• performing necessary legal-administrative tasks
• making crucial decisions.

Other important new roles for the family include:
• acting as advocate for the patient
• monitoring his comfort.

The sentimental work of kin. A central role for kin is to help the patient endure his pain or discomfort or keep his composure, as well as handle any identity problems brought about by the illness. This "sentimental work" (Strauss et al., 1982) may alleviate the anxiety, fear, and depression accompanying illness by kin being present to touch and soothe. At times, the nurse can act as a role model for family members who are unsure how to respond. The empathetic and sympathetic caregiver who touches and handles the patient gently and demonstrates that she is comfortable with him and accepts him sets an example for a cautious relative. Sentimental work should be interwoven with the smooth flow of medical tasks; the nurse's style may include such symbolic gestures as mentioned above, allied with standard nursing roles.

Legal-administrative work. When the AIDS patient cannot act in his own behalf and has no family member acting as his agent, multiple problems may emerge for physicians, nurses, and others responsible for maintaining bureaucratic order. For example, proper documents must be signed, financial agreements made, and informed consent obtained. It is therefore helpful for someone to be designated to represent the patient in a legitimate manner. In California, it is possible for the patient to grant "durable power of attorney" to empower a significant other to make decisions regarding medical care (especially, for instance, artificial maintenance of life) for him if he becomes unable to represent himself. In such a circumstance, the kin serves as advocate for the patient and protects the physicians and hospital against legal action and charges of negligence. The work of kin becomes an important adjunct to formal hospital procedures. One trusted significant other can do much to relieve the patient's problems by filling out disability forms, making sure insurance is kept current, and looking after ongoing bills and other correspondence.

Making crucial decisions. Strauss and his associates speak of decision making as intellectually and emotionally demanding, difficult to pursue, fateful of outcome, yet little understood by hospital staff. As in other chronic illness trajectories, the following conditions tend to be present with AIDS:
• fragile trajectories prone to destabilization
• frequent and serious crises requiring close medical attention and intensive care
• complications and a cumulative pattern of debilitation
• increasingly problematic and/or experimental options for treatment.

The family members possess unique knowledge that may be utilized in the decision-making process. They are familiar with the structure and dynamics of the family, its social and financial resources, its ability to manage problems, and preferred avenues of outside help. In addition, the family may have unique psychological insights into the conditions of life or limitations that the patient may be able to accept, as well as those that may be beyond his ability to endure.

Although this knowledge can be of crucial importance when difficult choices must be made, the family may still be unaware of what options do exist. The nurse may help by encouraging communication with primary physicians and consultants. It is often helpful for questions to be written out and for physicians to be asked to set aside time for a family meeting. Family members may be given literature or references on AIDS and options for treatment.

At Children's Hospital in San Francisco, the clinical sociologist is available to encourage dialogue between patient, staff, physicians, and family. A clinical sociologist uses social-psychological and sociological theory emphasizing the inescapable relationship between the plight of the apparently isolated individual and the social context in which that person lives (symbolic interaction, role theory, and conflict theory) to intervene with individuals and families experiencing social problems. Following a psychosocial assessment with the patient (and with his permission), a family meeting is arranged. The goals of this session include acknowledging the family's distress, providing information about the disease process, encouraging open communication, assessing family resources, and providing information on the availability of hospital and community help. Additional sessions are arranged as needed throughout the illness.

Monitoring comfort. The family can make the patient comfortable by making the hospital surroundings pleasant with music, flowers, cards, foods, or other favorite things from home. The nurse should keep the noise level down and screen visitors and telephone calls. The nurse can further assist the patient and family in recognizing the patient's level of energy, protecting him from stimulation when necessary.

Being an advocate for the patient. Negotiating with medical staff and other personnel in medical institutions is difficult for the healthy person; for the AIDS patient the task may seem insurmountable. If someone can accompany him to tests and take notes during reports, his anxiety will decrease. Helmquist (1984) recommends that significant others establish rapport with physicians and staff and show that they are interested partners in the medical care.

Planning

Developing an intervention plan. In order to intervene most effectively with a family, the nurse should formulate an assessment summary (Wright and Leahey, 1984) and develop a plan of intervention. This plan will evolve from an evaluation of the strengths and weaknesses of the family. If severe dysfunction or pathology exists, the nurse should consider referring the family to a trained family therapist.

The nurse who continues to work with the family should identify problems and priorities. With the family of the AIDS patient, problems may include discussing feelings and beliefs about homosexuality. I have found the following areas of intervention to be crucial in working with these families.

Intervention

Familiarizing the family with the surroundings. The gay patient who lives far from his family of origin many become increasingly dependent on both his lover and the hospital staff, often because he has migrated to a location that accepts an openly gay life-style. In San Francisco, for instance, many young men have left a far more traditional and perhaps rural midwestern setting for a new home in the city.

For the patient and his family, the hospital is an alien environment that demands passivity. The family may need help to find housing, meals, and other necessities to maintain routine living. With a knowledge of local health care delivery systems and community agencies, the nurse can provide the family with consumer information on additional health and welfare services (MacVicar and Archbold, 1976). The nurse can work with discharge planners and family to provide effective aftercare options.

Fortunately, the new urban community may hold excellent resources for the AIDS patient and his significant others. San Francisco has been exemplary in attempting to meet the social, psychological, and medical needs that are emerging. There are presently support and grieving networks (the Shenti Project) and social services (S.F. AIDS Foundation) aimed at the population, as well as a hospice caregiving unit.

In those communities where AIDS is prevalent, there are gay organizations providing support groups, trained counselors, supervised social activities, homemakers, and a buddy system (Perry and Tross, 1984). Often there are special groups designed for the "worried well"—the patient's friends, family, or lovers. In other cities, however, resources specifically for AIDS patients and their significant others are nonexistent. In such cases the caregivers will need to be more diligent in pursuing the meager avenues of help available.

Adjusting to a life-threatening diagnosis. Little progress has been made in the treatment of AIDS. There is currently no treatment known to destroy the AIDS virus or restore the immune system. Significant others may reflect the patient's reactions, such as fear of abandonment, dependency, and separation. The family may be comforted by the knowledge that antiviral drug research is under way and that specific infections may be treated successfully, allowing people with AIDS to lead active lives for long periods of time. As is the case with other patients and families experiencing life-threatening illnesses such as cancer or heart disease, social and emotional support are needed.

Allaying fear of contagion. As a life-threatening disease with no known cure, AIDS is terrifying. The family may need current information about transmission and prevention. At present—despite positive cultures from a variety of body fluids of infected persons—the spread of AIDS from infected persons to others who have no other identifiable risks for infection has not been documented. Nurses can educate significant others regarding the precautions that should be taken to ensure safe contact with an AIDS patient (Price and Scimeca, 1984) by being familiar with current Center for Disease Control regulations. Medical personnel should, of course, be trained systematically in the proper techniques for handling of instruments and similar procedures to decrease occupational exposure to HIV (Martin et al., 1985). By explaining what is known about the transmission of the disease, nurses can reduce the family's fear of contagion. These fears can lead to the use of unreasonable precautions that may alienate the patient from the family.

The AIDS patient's lover may now join the ranks of the "worried well"—those currently without symptoms, fearing that they have or will contract AIDS. Psychological distress may contribute to immune suppression (Coates et al., 1984), therefore placing lovers at greater risk. The preservation of their health becomes an issue deserving immediate attention through information, stress reduction, psychotherapy, and support groups. Topics that may be discussed with the nurse include obsession with AIDS, fear of contagion, sexual issues, loneliness, grieving for friends and lovers, and difficulties with medical aspects of the disease. It may be necessary to remind the AIDS patient's lover to take some time for himself. Therapists must be aware of the network of medical, psychological, social, and political groups that may exist in the community to direct people to appropriate services and activities (Morin, 1984).

Confirming the patient's sexual orientation. For many parents and siblings, the diagnosis will provoke a confrontation about the patient's homosexuality. Many men have not previously revealed their sexual orientation to their families, partially from fear of rejection. To cope with this reality, even if there has been some question, the parents often must grieve for the son they hoped they had and begin to accept him as he is. A case with such concerns is briefly presented below.

CASE STUDY

Although Dan's major concern was his mother's reaction to his being gay, she confided to the therapist that she had "always suspected" as much. Looking back, she could see that she had always hoped that he was "going through a stage," and would "settle down with a nice girl one of these days." She was helped to acknowledge her disappointment, her struggle to make sense of the teachings of an anti-gay fundamentalist preacher she followed, and the dissonance she experienced when she realized "he is still my baby."

Some older AIDS patients may have married in response to ambivalence regarding their sexuality. These patients may have among their significant others children, as well as former spouses. If the children are adolescents, they need help in their struggle to differentiate among their several age-appropriate tasks of achieving autonomy and dealing with their own emerging sexual identity and with their ambivalence regarding their appropriate role and relationship with a sick and dying parent. A woman currently or previously married to a man with AIDS will wonder about the extent of her husband's bisexual activity during their marriage; his infidelity may threaten her self-image and her health.

The nurse can help the family by directing them to accurate information about sexuality and gay life-styles; making referrals to community resources; and facilitating a positive, open relationship with the patient. Questions should be encouraged and answered directly. Individual or family therapy may be appropriate for resolution in some cases.

Dealing with the stigma. A person with a stigma must adjust to a new and painful identity, having been marked with shame or discredit. Time is needed to cope with going "public" in the face of potential social stigma. Parents and siblings may not know what to tell their friends, neighbors, or other relatives. The family members may try to hide the patient's sexual orientation or his illness, mirroring the struggles of "coming out" experienced by the patient. They, too, must decide who they can confide in and how to cope with others' reactions, such as questioning their roles as parents. It may be helpful for the family to talk to a trusted friend or professional to sort out members' feelings.

"Coming out of the closet," or "coming out," the identification or labeling of oneself as gay, is one of the most difficult and potentially traumatic experiences a gay person undertakes. J.A. Lee (1977) has identified four stages involved: coming out to oneself (signification), identifying oneself to others who are gay, identifying oneself to someone who is not gay, and going public. The decision about whether to tell one's parents, worry over their reaction, and efforts to keep them from knowing can be agonizing. The family's adoption of this identity may take a similar course.

Dealing with homophobia. Homophobia is defined as the irrational dread and loathing of homosexuality and homosexual people (Weinberg, 1972), and it is experienced by gays as well as nongays. Homophobic beliefs are a ubiquitous aspect of social mores and cultural attitudes. AIDS represents two taboos: homosexuality and the confrontation of death. Persecution and religious retribution may be seen as just punishment by those who believe in "the wages of sin." It is difficult for the family to remain unaffected by the mass hysteria that is characteristic of the public's response to an epidemic (Rubinow, 1984, p. 28). "Blaming the victim" may result, and patients commonly internalize homophobic attitudes, blaming themselves and/or their life-styles, as does the dominant culture.

Dealing with conflict between the patient's significant others. At this time of increased stress, any latent family conflict may emerge. Family members may bring up old issues, including problems with communication and roles. The nurse can help resolve difficulties arising among family members and deal with the potential withdrawal of social support systems (Morin and Batchelor, 1984).

Many gay people have developed an "extended family" of men and women friends. These close relationships offer an alternative family form that often provides support, reassurance, and devotion during times of crisis. The nurse should include those persons in her definition of "family" so that she can establish visitation rules and provide psychosocial assessment and support; the patient's emotional ties to this "extended family" may be stronger than those to his family of origin.

The patient may live in two different worlds—one with his family of origin, another within his social network. He may, for example, consider a long-term lover his next of kin, but this status may be disputed by his biological family. The nurse may need to help mediate between the patient and the two kin networks, and between the family of origin and others of significance. She can help those who care—but are in conflict—to move beyond their differences and attend to the patient's needs, divide tasks, provide resources, and work together (Furstenberg and Olson, 1984).

Realizing that time for reconciliation is limited. An important task for any patient or family facing life-threatening illness is the resolution of a number of emotional issues. In any relationship, there may be matters that have caused pain and separation. The family coping with AIDS may have intensified struggles, perhaps with some of the issues mentioned above, and the time available for reconciliation is short. Families who have difficulty with this task may require referral to a caregiver with expert therapeutic skills.

Completing unfinished business. One of the most difficult matters for many significant others is helping the patient "get his personal affairs in order." While it is considered rational for all healthy people to have such things settled, many family members are either too eager to approach the issue before the patient has actually come to terms with his impending death, or they are reluctant to discuss such issues as wills, bank accounts, or other financial planning. The nurse might remind significant others to take their cues from the patient and to also avoid "reassurances" to the patient that such arrangements will not be needed and that surely he will recover. Encourage the patient to decide about putting his affairs in order in his own time. Considering that the patient has responsibility for his affairs, discuss the following with him:
- a current will
- the will's location
- a list of bank accounts, charges, and loans
- the giving to a significant other of the legal right to make medical decisions on the patient's behalf in the event that he cannot do so because of disability.

Preparing for the loss of the patient. When death appears certain, anticipatory grief may be observed in family members. In this syndrome, one may go through all of the phases of grief. The emotional stress involved in this serious illness is intense. Often it can be shared with a family member or close friend; however, some feelings may be too personal to share. The nurse can reassure the family that this is a natural response. One patient wrote that because he regarded his diagnosis as a death sentence, he asked his lover, Michael, to leave. His lover refused. "Initially, Michael took the news worse than I. As I look back on those days now, I realize that I didn't have time to think of myself; I was too busy taking care of him..." (Ferrara, 1984, p. 1285).

Many AIDS patients develop both primary (organic) and secondary (related to the disease process) mental symptoms. The nurse can intervene by preparing the family for the patient's possible change in behavior and by making referrals to preventive interventions for reducing stress, emotional disturbance, and psychological dysfunction (Pincus, 1984).

Shifting family roles. When a family member is seriously ill, shifts occur in many family roles, including new patterns of dependency and household and financial responsibility, and new roles within the hospital setting. The feelings aroused within those shifting roles need to be recognized. Sometimes help in the negotiation of these role changes and with the engendered feelings is best provided by health care personnel.

CONCLUSIONS

By assessing and intervening with the AIDS patient's family, the nurse can effectively expand the family's internal and external resource potential (MacVicar and Archbold, 1976).

If necessary, the nurse will need to neutralize her own bias toward gay people, drug abusers, and the disadvantaged and, instead, explore a bias "...more subtle and less conscious...that slight discomfort, awkwardness, or uncertainty that might indicate a concern for our own feelings rather than those of the patient. All patients, but especially those facing so huge a burden, deserve to be treated with full compassion and without bias" (Nichols, 1983, pp. 1085–89).

Caregivers must meet their own psychosocial needs. Nurses must be provided with resources if they are to work with AIDS patients and their families. Liaison services such as clinical sociology or psychiatry can address the salient issues of grief, loss, death, and dying; defuse the emotionalism and restore balance; and provide mutual support (Clark, 1984; Rubinow, 1984; Simmons-Alling, 1984). Psychosocial rounds are useful to stimulate mutual problem solving and teamwork.

Sharing the emotional ordeal of AIDS with the patient and his family is a frustrating and sad experience, but it assists the nurse in becoming a more effective caregiver. The task is one of extraordinary difficulty and immense reward.

REFERENCES

Batchelor, W.F. "AIDS," *American Psychologist* 39(11):1277–84, 1984.

Bell, A.T., and Weinberg, M.S. *Homosexualities: A Study of Diversity among Men and Women.* New York: Simon & Schuster, 1978.

Bowers, M.K., et al. *Counseling the Dying.* New York: Jason Aronson, 1975.

Calliari, D. "Administrative Perspective on Care of Patients with AIDS," *Topics in Clinical Nursing* 6:72–75, 1984.

Clark, E.J. "Intervention for Cancer Patients: A Clinical Sociology Approach to Program Planning," *Journal of Applied Sociology* 1(1):83–96, 1984.

Coates, T.J., et al. "Psychosocial Research Is Essential to Understanding and Treating AIDS," *American Psychologist* 39(11):1309–14, 1984.

Dilley, J.W., et al. "Findings in Psychiatric Consultations with Patients with Acquired Immune Deficiency Syndrome," *American Journal of Psychiatry* 142(1):82–86, 1985.

Durham, J.D., and Hatcher, B. "Reducing Psychological Complications for the Critically Ill AIDS Patient," *Dimensions of Critical Care Nursing* 3(5):300–06, 1984.

Echenberg, D.F. "A New Strategy to Prevent the Spread of AIDS among Heterosexuals," *Journal of the American Medical Association* 254:2129–30, 1985.

Ferrara, A.J. "My Personal Experience with AIDS," *American Psychologist* 39(11):1285–87, 1984.

Furstenberg, A., and Olson, M.M. "Social Work and AIDS," *Social Work in Health Care* 9(4):45–62, 1984.

Goffman, E. *Stigma: Notes on the Management of Spoiled Identity.* London: Penguin Books, 1968.

Goldberg, R.J., and Wool, M.S. "Psychotherapy for the Spouses of Lung Cancer Patients: Assessment of an Intervention," *Psychotherapy Psychosomat* 43:141–50, 1985.

Helmquist, M. *The Family's Guide to AIDS: Responding with Your Heart.* San Francisco: S.F. AIDS Foundation, 1984.

Hill, R., and Hansen, D.A. "Families Under Stress," in *Handbook of Marriage and the Family.* Edited by Christensen, H.T. Chicago: Rand McNally, 1964.

Holmes, P. "Abolishing the Myths about AIDS," *Nursing Times* 19:December 1984.

Holtz, H., et al. "Psychosocial Impact of Acquired Immune Deficiency Syndrome," *Journal of the American Medical Association* 250(2):167, 1983.

Jaffe, H.W., et al. "The Acquired Immunodeficiency Syndrome in a Cohort of Homosexual Men: A Six-Year Follow-up Study," *Annals of Internal Medicine* 103(2):210–14, 1985.

Jay, K., and Young, A. *The Gay Report.* New York: Summit Books, 1979.

Joseph, J.G., et al. "Coping with the Threat of AIDS: An Approach to Psychosocial Assessment," *American Psychologist* 39(11):1297–1302, 1984.

Kosten, T.R., et al. "Terminal Illness, Bereavement, and the Family," in *Health, Illness, and Families: A Life-Span Perspective.* Edited by Turk, D.C., and Kerns, R.D. New York: John Wiley & Sons, 1985.

Landesman, S.H., et al. "The AIDS Epidemic," *New England Journal of Medicine* 312(8):521–25, 1985.

Lee, J.A. "Going Public: A Study in the Sociology of Homosexual Liberation," *Journal of Homosexuality* 3(1):49-78, 1977.

Lopez, D.J., and Getzel, G.S. "Helping Gay AIDS Patients in Crisis," *Social Casework* 387–94, September 1984.

Lusby, G.I. "AIDS: The Impact on the Health Care Worker," *Frontiers of Radiation Therapy and Oncology* 19:164–67, 1985.

MacVicar, M.G., and Archbold, P. "A Framework for Family Assessment in Chronic Illness," *Nursing Forum* 15(2):180–94, 1976.

Mailick, M. "The Impact of Severe Illness on the Individual and Family," *Social Work in Health Care* 5(2):117–28, 1979.

Malyon, A.K. "Psychotherapeutic Implications of Internalized Homophobia in Gay Men," in *Homosexuality and Psychotherapy: A Practitioner's Handbook of Affirmative Models.* Edited by Gonsiorek, J.C. New York: Haworth Press, 1982.

Martin, J.L., and Vance, C.S. "Behavioral and Psychosocial Factors in AIDS: Methodological and Substantive Issues," *American Psychologist* 39(11):1303–08, 1984.

Martin, L.S., et al. "Disinfection and Inactivation of the Human T-Lymphotropic Virus Type III/Lymphadenopathy-Associated Virus," *Journal of Infectious Disease* 152:400–03, 1985.

Morin, S.F. "AIDS in One City," *American Psychologist* 39(11):1294–96, 1984.

Morin, S.F., and Batchelor, W.F. "Responding to the Psychological Crisis of AIDS," *Public Health Reports* 99:4–9, 1984.

Newmark, D.A. "Review of a Support Group for Patients with AIDS," *Topics in Clinical Nursing* 7:38–44, 1984.

Nichols, S.E. "Psychiatric Aspects of AIDS," *Psychosomatics* 24(12):1083–89, 1983.

Nurnberg, H.G., et al. "Psychopathology Complicating Acquired Immune Deficiency Syndrome (AIDS)," *American Journal of Psychiatry* 141(1):95–96, 1984.

Perry, S.W., and Tross, S. "Psychiatric Problems of AIDS Inpatients at the New York Hospital: Preliminary Report," *Public Health Reports* 99(2):200–05, 1984.

Pincus, H.A. "AIDS, Drug Abuse, and Mental Health," *Public Health Reports* 99(2):106–08, 1984.

Price, D.M., and Scimeca, A.M. "The Epidemic of the 80's: AIDS," *Cancer Nursing* 10:283–90, 1984.

Rafferty, C. "Love and Dying," *San Francisco Focus* 6:91–95, 1985.

Rubinow, D.R. "The Psychosocial Impact of AIDS," *Topics in Clinical Nursing* 7:26–30, 1984.

Ryan, L.J. "AIDS: A Threat to Physical and Psychological Integrity," *Topics in Clinical Nursing* 7:19–25, 1984.

Simkins, L., and Eberhage, M.G. "Attitudes Toward AIDS, Herpes II, and Toxic Shock Syndrome," *Psychological Reports* 55:779–86, 1984.

Simmons-Alling, S. "AIDS: Psychosocial Needs of the Health Care Worker," *Topics in Clinical Nursing* 7:31–37, 1984.

Strauss, A., et al. *Chronic Illness and the Quality of Life.* St. Louis: C.V. Mosby Co., 1984.

Strauss, A., et al. "Sentimental Work in the Technologized Hospital," *Sociology of Health and Illness* 4:254–78, 1982.

Viney, L. "Loss of Life and Loss of Bodily Integrity: Two Different Sources of Threat for People Who Are Ill," *Omega* 15(3):207–22, 1984.

Wallis, C. "AIDS: A Growing Threat," *Time* 40–47, August 12, 1985.

Weinberg, G. *Society and the Healthy Homosexual.* New York: St. Martin's, 1972.

Witte, R. "The Psychosocial Impact of a Progressive Physical Handicap and Terminal Illness (Duchenne Muscular Dystrophy) on Adolescents and Their Families," *British Journal of Medical Psychology* 58:179–87, 1985.

Wright, L.M., and Leahey, M. *Nurses and Families: A Guide to Family Assessment and Intervention.* Philadelphia: F.A. Davis Co., 1984.

Zisook, S., and Schuchter, S.R. "Time Course of Spousal Bereavement," *General Hospital Psychiatry* 7:95–100, 1985.

18 Intervening with families at the launching stage and myocardial infarction

J. Howard Brunt, RN, MSN
Assistant Professor
Faculty of Nursing
University of Calgary
Calgary, Alberta, Canada

OVERVIEW

Coronary artery disease (CAD) is the leading cause of death and disability in North America; as such, it affects the functioning of millions of families. This chapter pays particular attention to the nurse's role in helping families cope with an acute myocardial infarction (AMI) in its early phase. Utilizing a crisis intervention approach, three major nursing diagnoses are discussed as they relate to the family with a member in the coronary care unit (CCU). Assessments and interventions for each diagnosis are outlined and alternate approaches described for delivering care to the family through hospital resources.

CASE STUDY

Mr. Stoneguard, a 57-year-old clothing salesman, was admitted to the CCU with the presumptive diagnosis of AMI after experiencing crushing substernal pain while at work. He has a medical history of hypertension, diabetes mellitus, and gout. His father and younger brother both died from massive AMIs. While Mr. Stoneguard's pain is now under control with morphine, he has been having ventricular ectopy and is being treated with a lidocaine drip.

The Stoneguards have two children. Jason is age 27 and works as a lawyer in a large firm; June is age 20 and a student at an out-of-state university.

Mrs. Stoneguard received a call at home from the family's physician informing her that her husband was ill and had been admitted to the hospital with a suspected heart attack; her initial reaction was shock. She immediately called her son and left a message for her daughter to come home as soon as possible.

NURSING PROCESS

Assessment

The health problem: CAD and AMI. Despite ongoing advances in cardiac assessment and treatment, CAD remains a major health concern in North America (Block et al., 1984). Its physical, financial, and emotional impact on individuals, families, and society is staggering. The National Heart, Lung and Blood Institute reports that:

• CAD is the number one killer in America, accounting for one third of all deaths (650,000 annually).

• More than five million Americans are disabled by heart disease, accounting for 22% of all Social Security disability allowances.

• Acute heart diseases account for 18 million lost workdays annually; another 184 million workdays are lost due to heart-related disability.

• Heart disease costs more than $60 billion every year (National Institutes of Health, 1981).

While CAD's individual and family costs—in suffering, pain, depression, and loss—cannot be estimated accurately, they are certainly enormous. The sudden and often unexpected occurrence of an AMI creates an atmosphere of crisis and severely upsets a family's normal equilibrium. Both intrafamily dynamics and relationships with professional health care providers influence the ultimate crisis resolution.

CAD is an insidious disorder marked by gradual atherosclerotic occlusion of the coronary arteries leading to a variety of clinical and functional symptoms. The impact on individual health can be mild to severe. Early stages are typically characterized by short periods of ischemic pain called angina, resulting from an imbalance in the myocardial oxygen supply. This symptom may occur relatively infrequently, during periods of moderate-to-extreme physical activity or emotional stress. As CAD progresses, however, angina may occur with minimal exertion, thus greatly affecting the individual's ability to perform even routine self-care tasks. Worsening angina commonly portends AMI.

AMI results from complete blockage of blood flow to a portion of the myocardium; irreversible damage to the heart's pumping mechanism results. As with angina, the subsequent effects of AMI on the individual range from mild to severe, depending on the area and amount of damaged myocardium. Almost half of all victims die immediately or within 10 days of an AMI. Of those surviving, another 20% will be significantly disabled (Cowan, 1982).

The launching-stage family and CAD. Death and illness are more common among elderly CAD sufferers, but the occurrence of AMIs in those in the prime of life can severely disrupt family functioning (Herz, 1980). There is currently no research into the effects of changing family demographics (for example, the increasing numbers of single-parent and common-law families and the higher incidence of divorce) on the functional impact of CAD. Reports on AMI's implications for families are similarly limited. Both theoretical and research literature deal almost exclusively with the traditional marital dyad.

Developmental tasks of the launching stage. Duvall (1977) has subdivided the fourth through sixth decades of life into two periods, each with relatively distinct developmental tasks. The first phase is marked by the launching of young adult children into the world. Financial demands on parents are higher during this period than at any other time; helping children pay for weddings, advanced education, and the establishment of independent households requires considerable financial outlay.

Another and perhaps more demanding task for the launching-stage family is emotional adjustment; both parent-child and spousal relationships undergo major change. From the childrens' perspective, tension arises from lingering dependence on parents in the face of a need to establish independent adult lives. The launching of the children also removes a major influence on the marital dyad. Whether that influence was positive or disruptive, its loss means that parents must reframe their relationship as husband and wife.

The second half of the launching phase is marked by the numerous developmental tasks associated with middle age. Preparation for a secure retirement is a major undertaking during these years; therefore social and leisure time activities become more important. The children have by now established their financial independence and begun to bring new members—grandchildren and in-laws—into the family. During this period, the wife's influence in major family decisions tends to increase (Duvall, 1977).

Effects of AMI during the launching stage. An AMI during either the child-launching or the middle-aged phase of the family life cycle can significantly hinder the performance of necessary financial, marital, and parent-child tasks. If the earning capacity of the single- or dual-income family is suddenly altered, plans for retirement, weddings, and education can be drastically affected. Emotional ties between parents and children are suddenly heightened, increasing the possibility of guilt on the part of a parent no longer able to adequately support the children. Children might also feel guilty over preexisting strains in the parent-child relationship. Plans for postretirement travel and leisure activities may suddenly be dashed due either to the financial strain of the AMI or its physical effects, compounding the emotional strain on both parents.

The impact of AMI on the marital dyad varies but usually leaves the premorbid relationship largely unchanged. Spouses with marital problems prior to the AMI may suddenly drop their complaints and become close again. At the other extreme, the added stress of the illness or its effects on financial or social plans for retirement may cause dissolution of the relationship. Brown et al. (1982), however, contend that acute illness in the postparental period often has little effect on family functioning, since weaker family units have already dissolved, leaving well-established relationships better able to weather the crisis.

The CCU experience. The CCU is fraught with anxiety-provoking sights and sounds for both patient and family. Indeed, the primary tasks confronting the family in the initial stage of AMI center around adaptation to this foreign, and apparently hostile, environment. Family members must control their fears and anxieties, establish relationships with hospital staff, maintain their own health, and adjust to constant uncertainty about the immediate future (Perlmutter et al., 1984). The typical emergency reaction pattern is characterized by constriction of all nonessential activities, mobilization of all available coping mechanisms, constant readiness for action, and a centralized focus on the crisis (Carter, 1984).

Planning

Because each family member will react differently to the crisis of AMI, the nurse planning care must pay close attention to family interactions. The ill individual's importance within the family structure must be determined (Carter, 1984), especially in a nontraditional family. For example, the father who is unemployed and estranged from his family may have relatively little financial *or* emotional influence on his wife and children. On the other hand, a single parent's AMI could cripple a family's ability to function.

The personality of each member must also be considered in planning nursing care; the strain of the crisis may lead to exaggerated coping behaviors and personality traits that only decrease the family's ability to adapt to its difficult situation. The family's ability to process information, meet self-care needs, and express feelings must be continually assessed (Perlmutter et al., 1984). In addition, it is important to assess the family's understanding of what an AMI is, including its causes, treatments, and usual course.

The nurse who had admitted Mr. Stoneguard met with Jason and his mother in the waiting room. June would not arrive until later that evening. Both were clearly upset, but in control of their emotions. After first assessing Mrs. Stoneguard's and Jason's anxiety levels, the nurse assured them that Mr. Stoneguard was resting comfortably at the moment and gave them a brief explanation of what had happened in the last hour. The CCU's physical layout was described and visitation policies explained. The nurse described exactly what the family would see and hear in the CCU, paying particular attention to the various pieces of equipment in Mr. Stoneguard's room. She then brought Mrs. Stoneguard into the CCU for a short visit with her husband.

Nursing Diagnoses and Interventions

There are many potential nursing diagnoses for a family experiencing AMI (Kim et al., 1984); three of the most common in the CCU are alteration in family process, fear/anxiety, and potential for self-care deficits. The care plan for each is based upon crisis intervention principles and aims to alleviate stress and mobilize the coping mechanisms needed to deal with the crisis effectively. The nurse must make the most of the family's considerable therapeutic influence while providing necessary support for members.

Alteration in family process. Alteration in family process, in this case related to a situational crisis (AMI), is an important potential diagnosis in the CCU setting. Family members of CCU patients feel helpless and unable to meet their loved one's physical and emotional needs. Indeed, Breu and Dracup (1978) report that two of the greatest needs of families in critical care settings are the need to be with and support the patient. The paternalistic attitude that only professional health care workers should help the patient is antiquated and false; the nurse must balance the family's need for patient contact with the patient's need for rest.

The goals of interventions for this diagnosis are twofold: reducing family anxiety and maximizing members' abilities to cope with the crisis. Both decreased anxiety and increased family involvement have been associated with more positive patient outcomes (Chatham, 1978). Nursing interventions that help family members relate honestly and openly with one another are also necessary if these goals are to be met.

As early as 1963, Ujhely proposed that family members be allowed to provide some physical care for acutely ill patients. Nurses need to be sensitive to the relatives' need to help the patient, as well as to the patient's condition and wishes. Hygienic care such as bathing assistance is one area in which the family can be encouraged to interact with the ill member. Reading aloud and other nonphysical interactions should also be promoted during the early post-AMI period. By thus helping relatives meet the needs of the AMI patient, the nurse can take an active role in enhancing family function.

To maximize the family members' ability to interact with the patient during visits, many CCUs have moved away from rigid visitation schedules and restrictions; nevertheless, a few guidelines should be followed. Before the first visit the nurse must prepare family members for what they may see or hear in the CCU. If visits must be restricted, the family must understand the rationale behind that decision. During the visit the nurse should ensure that visitors are as comfortable as possible—providing a chair, for instance, is a common courtesy all too often overlooked. The nurse should be close at hand during the visitation period in order to assess patient-family and interfamily interactions and to answer any questions that arise. Care should be taken to note any particularly stressful and negative interactions. Debriefing sessions after each visit help alleviate unwarranted fears and provide the nurse with additional information about the family's coping abilities.

Over the next few days Mrs. Stoneguard and her children remained at the hospital from early morning until late evening. Mr. Stoneguard had fortunately not experienced any major complications in the first 24 hours, so family members were allowed frequent visits. They were instructed to be sensitive to signs that Mr. Stoneguard was tiring; the nurse frequently assessed family interaction. The next morning Mrs. Stoneguard was encouraged to assist her husband with his bedbath and did so, initially under the nurse's supervision. Because June was tearful and extremely upset when she arrived at the hospital, nursing staff spent extra time with her, explaining what had happened to her father and preparing her for the CCU sights and sounds. Once she had calmed down, June, accompanied by the nurse, visited her father briefly.

Fear/anxiety. A second nursing diagnosis for the AMI family, one closely related to the first, is fear and anxiety. Dread of suddenly losing a family member through death or disability, negative experiences with other AMI or CAD patients, and the frightening CCU environment can all produce anxiety and fear, which can inhibit family members' ability to help care for the patient. The nurse's goal, therefore, is to help them cope with the emotional turmoil associated with the crisis.

Two of the most powerful interventions the nurse can employ at this time are providing information about the CCU routine and the patient's condition/prognosis, and allowing family members to express their fears and concerns.

Despite the nursing curriculum's emphasis on providing information in the CCU setting, Zawatski et al. (1979) found that nurses were not perceived as providing enough education to family members in the CCU. Simple, clear explanations are essential. Irwin and Meier (1973) and Molter (1979) report that three of the supportive behaviors most sought by the families of acutely ill patients are:
• honest explanations of the patient's condition by health care providers
• clear explanations of what is being done and why
• information concerning any changes in the patient's condition.

Gillis (1981) offers a few practical suggestions for keeping families aware of patient status. Prearranged phone calls can keep the family informed, even when relatives cannot be in the hospital. The nurse should set aside at least 15 minutes each shift to talk to the visiting family away from the bedside; such family conferences not only help provide information, but also allow further assessment of coping behaviors and allow relatives to voice their concerns.

The nurse should ask directed questions about how the family is coping with the patient's illness. While CCU nurses must play an active role in alleviating family fear and anxiety, consultation may also be necessary. In some instances, if the family members' anxiety is extreme, the nurse may discuss the need for antianxiety agents with the family's physician.

Perlmutter et al. (1984) describe the use of formal family support groups to help relatives of acutely ill patients acquire information, bring family members closer together, and support less anxious coping behaviors. They outlined five strategies useful to such groups:

- Use language understood by the family members.
- Understand and respect usual family roles.
- Define appropriate and inappropriate behavior.
- Clarify each member's expectations regarding patient care.
- Involve the family in the care plan.

Family support groups may be led by a variety of health care providers including nurses, clinical nurse specialists, psychologists, psychiatrists, social workers, and physicians.

During the first few days of Mr. Stoneguard's hospitalization, the family's anxiety level was extremely high. John and June demonstrated a textbook emergency reaction strategy by "dropping everything" to join their parents despite their own hectic life-styles and obligations. The nurse spent as much time with the family members as possible, informing them of Mr. Stoneguard's condition and answering all their questions. It was decided at once that the family would receive phone calls from the nurse at 11 p.m. and 8 a.m. each day. In addition, Jason was chosen to serve as family spokesperson, keeping other family members and close friends informed of his father's condition. At the family members' request, their pastor was contacted and he met them at the hospital each day at a prearranged time. The family declined an invitation by the CCU's social worker to attend a family support group held each afternoon. When it became apparent that June had difficulty controlling her anxiety, the nurse spoke with the Stoneguard family physician about prescribing a mild antianxiety agent.

During the nurse's daily meeting with the family, fears and concerns were discussed. Family members were encouraged to describe how they were feeling, what coping mechanisms seemed useful, and how they perceived the patient's treatment. Because of the positive family history of heart disease, Jason was worried about his own risk of heart attack. The nurse gave him information on coronary risk factors and encouraged him to enroll in the hospital's public education course on preventing heart disease.

Potential for self-care deficits. A final nursing diagnosis applicable to families in the CCU regards the potential for self-care deficits as a result of the patient's acute illness. Because severe illness is a major family stressor, otherwise healthy relatives often become ill or neglect their own needs. In a study of the perceived self-care needs of spouses of patients in critical care areas, Gillis (1981) found self-care deficits in three major areas: physical health, activity and rest, and nutrition. The nurse must set goals for family members to ensure that they will meet self-care needs and remain in optimal health.

The primary anxiety-related physical complaints include headache, nausea, tremor, hyperventilation, and palpitations. Once again, by offering information and an opportunity to vent negative emotions, the nurse can help lessen family members' anxiety and thereby decrease their symptoms. The nurse must also determine if a family member is in danger of exacerbating a preexisting medical or psychological condition, such as an antoimmune disease sensitive to stress, CAD, or depression. A patient's family members often forget to take prescribed medication, follow special diets, or perform other health-promoting activities required by their conditions; special monitoring may be required.

Problems with activity and rest center around the disruption of the daily routine. Insomnia, nightmares, and fatigue are usually self-limiting, but the nurse should assess the family members for signs of exhaustion and any resulting alteration in their ability to care for themselves. Standard relaxation techniques may be tried during this period, but pharmacologic aids such as mild sedatives may be more effective in helping family members get adequate rest.

Anorexia is another common finding within families of CCU patients; it is due in part to the normal stress reaction, and rarely results in major health problems unless a preexisting condition such as diabetes can be aggravated by deviation from a special dietary regimen. Dependence upon hospital vending machines for nourishment may further reduce the family's appetites. The nurse should make sure that, if possible, the family has access to a cafeteria. Persons with diabetes and other conditions requiring special dietary care should be encouraged to continue their usual diets.

Family members' major self-care problems were related to their anxiety about Mr. Stoneguard's condition. All three suffered from insomnia and by the third day were irritable and near exhaustion. It was suggested that only one family member come to the hospital at a time, and that they schedule visits in 4-hour shifts. The family physician prescribed Dalmane to help them sleep at night. Jason also suffered a flare-up of his duodenal ulcer and was placed on an oral antacid suspension by his physician.

Because Mr. Stoneguard's CCU course was uncomplicated, he was transferred to the step-down unit on the fourth day.

Evaluation

The success or failure of family nursing interventions in AMI can be determined by comparing outcomes with goals. Measuring such outcomes, however, is often difficult in the clinical setting. How, for example, can nurses know if they have maximized the family's ability to cope with the AMI crisis?

Strain (1978) outlined five areas in which the family must adapt during the recovery period (Table 18.1). Together, they form an evaluation framework for the CCU stay.

Table 18.1 Strain's (1978) Framework for Evaluating Family Adaptation to the CCU Experience

Question	Assessment
Has the family accepted the physical/mental regression accompanying illness?	● Observe for signs of intolerance of the patient's condition (argumentativeness, impatience).
Is the family helping the patient reduce illness-related stresses?	● Observe family interactions—does the family discuss its own problems (particularly those arising from the patient's incapacity) in the patient's presence or provide support and reassurance to the ill member?
Can the family tolerate the patient's expressions of fear?	● Assess the family members' ability to conduct serious discussions with the patient—are their comments superficial or do they listen with a willing ear?
Does the family encourage patient autonomy?	● Assess the family's willingness to let the patient perform self-care tasks; work to modify overprotective behavior observed in the CCU.
Is the family able to seek and/or willing to accept support from every available source (friends, relatives, clergy, professional care providers)?	● Evaluate whether the family members are able to articulate *their* needs to those able to provide assistance. Or do they focus only on the patient's needs?

Nurses reviewing the Stoneguards' CCU stay felt that their interventions had met the family's needs. Mr. Stoneguard and his wife were attending the post-MI classes provided in the step-down unit; the aims of these classes were to help the family members integrate the MI experience into their lives and to prepare them for hospital discharge. Questions about sex, diet, physical activity, medications, and coronary risk factor modification were covered in detail during the sessions. Overall, the Stoneguards handled their CCU experience well. They sought advice appropriately and relied on a number of sources for emotional support. While some physical complaints surfaced for each family member, all responded well to nursing and medical interventions.

CONCLUSIONS

The decision to include the family in CCU patient care is an important step toward a positive clinical outcome. If families are treated as nuisances, nurses will lose one of their major therapeutic resources. At the same time, nurses must also see family units themselves as patients, who also suffer the effects of an AMI. Both families and individual patients experience pain, stress responses and grief, loss, and disruption of usual routines. Family members' futures are uncertain and they feel just as helpless and scared as the loved one lying in the CCU bed.

The actions of the CCU nurse during the early stage of AMI care will lay the foundation for effective or ineffective family resolution of the health crisis. By including family members in the care plan, nurses reaffirm their belief in the value of maintaining human dignity through family-centered patient care.

REFERENCES

Block, A.R., et al. "Personal Impact of Myocardial Infarction: A Model for Coping with Physical Disability in Middle Age," *Chronic Illness and Disability Through the Lifespan.* Edited by Eisenger, M.G., et al. New York: Springer Publishing Co., 1984.

Breu, C., and Dracup, K. "Helping the Spouses of Critically Ill Patients," *American Journal of Nursing* 78(1):50–53, 1978.

Brown, J.S., et al. "Family Functioning and Health Status," *Journal of Family Issues* 3(1): 91–110, 1982.

Carter, R.E. "Family Reactions in Reorganization Patterns in Myocardial Infarction," *Family Systems Medicine* 2(1):55–65, 1984.

Chatham, M.A. "The Effect of Family Involvement on Patients' Manifestations of Post-Cardiotomy Psychosis," *Heart & Lung* 7:995–99, 1978.

Cowan, M.J. "Sudden Cardiac Death," in *Cardiac Nursing.* Edited by Underhill, S.L., et al. Philadelphia: J.B. Lippincott Co., 1982.

Dunkel, J., and Eisendrath, S. "Families in the Intensive Care Unit: Their Effect on Staff," *Heart & Lung,* 12(3):258–60, 1983.

Duvall, E.M. *Marriage and Family Development,* 5th ed. Philadelphia: J.B. Lippincott Co., 1977.

Gillis, A.R. "The Expressed Needs and Their Importance as Perceived by Family Members of Patients in Intensive Care Units," Unpublished master's thesis. Toronto: University of Toronto, 1981.

Herz, F. "The Impact of Death and Serious Illness on the Family Life Cycle," in *The Family Life Cycle: A Framework for Family Therapy.* Edited by Carter, E.A., and McColdrick, M. New York: Gardner Press, 1980.

Irwin, B., and Meier, J. "Supportive Measures for Relatives of the Fatally Ill," in *Communicating Nursing Research.* Edited by Batey, M. Boulder, Colo.: WICHE, 1973.

Kim, M.A., et al., eds. *Pocket Guide to Nursing Diagnosis.* St. Louis: C.V. Mosby Co., 1984.

McCullough, P. "Launching Children and Moving On," in *The Family Life Cycle: A Framework for Family Therapy.* Edited by Carter, E.A., and McGoldrick, M. New York: Gardner Press, 1980.

Molter, N.C. "Needs of Relatives of Critically Ill Patients: A Descriptive Study," *Heart & Lung* 8(2):332–39, 1979.

National Institutes of Health. *Eighth Report of the Director: National Heart, Lung and Blood Institute.* Washington, D.C.: National Institutes of Health, 1981.

Perlmutter, D.R., et al. "Models of Family-Centered Care in One Acute Care Institution," *Nursing Clinics of North America* 19(1):173–88, 1984.

Strain, J.J. *Psychological Interventions in Medical Practice.* East Norwalk, Conn.: Appleton-Century-Crofts, 1978.

Ujhely, G. *The Nurse and Her Problem Patient.* New York: Springer Publishing Co., 1963.

Zawatski, E., et al. "Perceived Needs and Satisfaction with Nursing Care by Spouses of Patients in the Coronary Care Unit," *Perceptual and Motor Skills* 49:170, 1979.

19 Intervening with families at the launching stage and heart attack recovery

Ann W. Burgess, RN, DNSc
Professor of Psychiatric Mental Health Nursing
University of Pennsylvania
Philadelphia, Pennsylvania

Carol R. Hartman, RN, DNSc
Associate Professor and Coordinator
    Graduate Program in Psychiatric Mental Health
    Nursing
Boston College
Chestnut Hill, Massachusetts

Debra J. Lerner, PhD
Boston University
Boston, Massachusetts

OVERVIEW

This chapter presents the nursing intervention framework used in a randomized clinical trial studying a patient's return to work after myocardial infarction. The model of nursing intervention developed for this cardiac rehabilitation project is meant to complement existing nursing interventions, during both the cardiac crisis and the recovery period.

The model assumes that issues must be confronted by not only the patient, but also his family and work/social networks. Further assumptions in the model convincingly support the hypothesis that attributional processes (beliefs about what caused the heart attack, what is expected of one and others, and expectations for recovery) influence the patient's stress levels and shape his motivation to participate in recovery planning. Further, these expectations influence the emergent pattern of postillness interpersonal relationships among the patient, family, and work-social network.

This chapter considers the case of Mr. Byrd. The critical phases of the heart attack and recovery are described. The tasks required during these phases become the crucial areas of nursing assessment. Next, there is a section on planning; the purpose of planning is to make accurate, dynamic formulations that structure strategic intervention efforts aimed at specific outcomes. The next section illustrates the use of intervention strategies, and the final section deals with the evaluation of the response to the efforts.

CASE STUDY

There are five members of the Byrd family: Don Byrd, 53, the director of the Career Counseling Center at a university; his wife, Marion, 51, a public relations specialist for a large investment firm; the oldest son, Mike, 28, who is married, works for an engineering firm, and lives with his wife, Laura, and their new-born baby 2,000 miles from his parents; a second son, Bob, 25, who recently moved to the same distant area and is an economist for an oil company; and a daughter, Ellen, 23, a secretary who recently moved back into the family home after terminating a relationship with a male partner.

With both husband and wife working, the family could be called middle class. The extended family includes the husband's elderly parents, who are visited at least weekly. The identified patient is the father, Don Byrd.

Mr. Byrd suffered a heart attack 6 weeks into the university semester. This was his second myocardial infarction; he had experienced his first attack 6 years earlier. This infarction was nontransmural, and the physicians told him they believed it was a reblockage.

Family health care was initiated on Don's fourth day in the hospital, during the cardiac crisis. He had just been transferred from the coronary intensive care unit to the cardiac general care floor. Don and Marion Byrd were inter-viewed separately regarding their memories of the cardiac event; they were re-interviewed together several days before discharge in order to plan for it. Altogether, Don was interviewed six times—twice alone, twice with his wife present, once with his wife and daughter, and once in the work place, with his supervisor and a co-worker. Following discharge, the nurse clinician continued the family health care, using a community model of home visit for three ses-sions and for one meeting at the work place.

Each family member was assessed at critical phases of the recovery contin-uum. The rationale for doing so was that the patient and family members assimilate the information necessary for understanding and coping with the heart attack phase by phase; such assimilation is necessary for full recovery. The phases of assimilation have been broadly defined in a time and activity context (Burgess et al., 1983).

Critical Phases

Crisis. Begins with the heart attack and the emergency measures taken. A survival level of functioning is the aim of hospitalization; ultimate cardiac stabilization and discharge are also included.

Immediate post crisis. Involves the hospital/home transition and imme-diate return to family activities. The objective is an expanded mainte-nance level of functioning.

Transition to optimal level of functioning. Includes maximizing functional levels within the home and first days back in the work place.

Total integration. Integration within home and work. The aim is to obtain and maintain optimum health functioning and to return to the pre-cardiac crisis state.

Family Functioning

A family functions as a subsystem within the larger community and is the basic building block of human society. The family ensures physical survival and is organized around member regulation, support, nurturance, and socialization. The family must also provide a foundation for one of the most basic human survival requirements: adaptation to change. When crisis disrupts a family routine, assessment of coping and adaptation skills is necessary. When assessing the Byrd family's functioning during the crisis phase, the nurse used the following guideline questions (Shapiro, 1985) and obtained the accompanying findings:

• Is the family maintaining adequate nutrition, health, and shelter? *Yes.*
• Is the family able to generate adequate economic resources to meet its material needs? *Yes.*
• Are there appropriate rules for guiding behavior within the family and outside? *Yes.*
• Are all family members at the appropriate stages of growth and development for their place in the life cycle? *Yes, the family is in the launching phase of the family cycle.*
• Have the children mastered skills of daily living? *Yes; the results of that learning are confirmed by the two older children's independence.*
• Do family members have workable decision-making and problem-solving skills? *Yes.*
• Are members able to look to one another for support and love? *Yes (directly observed).*
• Does the family have a viable method of resolving conflicts? Does it allow airing of differences? *Yes (directly observed).*
• Can family members work together to meet their goals? *Yes; this was demonstrated early in the crisis phase.*
• Do family members have a peer group outside of the family? *Yes (observed from visiting patterns in the hospital and the home).*
• Do family members have a healthy balance of time with the family and time with others? *Yes (directly observed during home visits).*

In summary, the Byrd family demonstrated major strengths in coping and crisis adaptation. General problems identified through the family assessment included presence of a life-threatening illness, accumulation of family- and work-related stressors, and ambivalence over work.

A focused assessment of husband and wife identified Don as a stoic, responsible, future-oriented man with marginal denial of life stressors. Marion was found to maintain a loyal, traditional, stoic role towards her husband. She admitted multiple stress-causing concerns, including the dependence of Mr. Byrd's elderly parents on her husband and her daughter's distress over the disruption of her partner relationship and her return home. Mrs. Byrd denies the impact of stress on herself, refusing to openly discuss it. Rather, she views herself as a bearer of consequences.

Planning

Planning for the Byrd family was based on the rationale that, following the diagnosis of life-threatening illness, it is essential to reestablish the links between patient, family, and eventually the work place. The Byrds' nurse laid the groundwork for working not only with individual family members but also with husband and wife; husband, wife, and daughter; and Don's supervisor and co-worker. It was also important to deal with the patient's work stressors—his difficulty delegating tasks to department members and setting limits on student requests for career counseling.

Plans to help the Byrds through the crisis phase included educating patient and family about positive health behaviors related to heart attack recovery, sorting out specific stress items, facilitating husband-wife communication, and exploring a possible career change for Don.

Intervention

Major interventions in any family health care program include managing stress through individual cognitive-behavioral reframing and relaxation; defining family stressors and altering expectations accordingly; and decreasing stress in the work setting.

For the Byrds, as in most cardiac cases, intervention was designed to limit strain on the patient's intra- and interpersonal social networks and to attend to potential problems concerning reintegration into family life and, later, into the work place.

Because of the variety of possible conflicts that could arise during crisis and convalescence, the nurse clinician tried to guide all participants toward identifying and anticipating each other's needs and toward developing strategies for their adequate fulfillment. Specific interventions were primarily cognitive/behavioral: reframing attitudes toward the self and others; evaluating expectations and methods of expression; setting goals; renegotiating changes; and teaching relaxation techniques. Structured family "talks" were also instituted.

Evaluation

The Byrd family achieved several key goals. First, by fully exploring both individual and family expectations, family members resolved their anxieties about the life-threatening nature of Mr. Byrd's heart attack.

Second, new communication lines were opened. Third, all family members were able to apply the health crisis to a positive review of their own life goals, in light of the family's goals and their own newly recognized mortality. Don decided to stay at his job and learn to delegate some of the stressful tasks; Marion learned to be more open regarding her desires, in particular, special experiences she wished to have with her husband. This took on more meaning now that the children were grown. The daughter was able to seek out a new group of friends and began exploring a living arrangement with several young women from work.

NURSING PROCESS

Assessment

The health problem: Myocardial infarction. The terms "heart attack" and "myocardial infarction" terrify and bewilder most people. Normal anxiety and confusion can easily become fixated, making the illness a primary and crucial element in individual self-identification. In one instance, a man coming to a family evaluation because of his adult daughter's deep depression identified himself as follows, "I am Mr. Chase. I am a cardiac."

Primary preventive efforts as well as early medical crisis intervention with heart attack victims are shifting the focus from the immediate probability of recovery to the more complex long-term quality-of-life issues. Despite reduced hospitalization and earlier return to more vigorous physical activities, it is important to remember that damaged hearts take time to heal. The residual structural and functional recovery tax a client's understanding of and adaptation to altered physiological and physical processes. Every sharp pain in the chest area can be interpreted as a signal of impending heart attack unless the client learns to differentiate sensations. Time, testing, and acclimatization are needed to define tolerance limits.

The assessment process must encompass such physiological factors as infarction type and extent, as well as psychological factors, such as belief patterns, coping style, and levels of anxiety and distress. Social assessment should include relationships with family members, friends, co-workers, and colleagues.

Family development and crisis management. Clinicians identify two main types of crises: internal, or developmental, life cycle crises and external, or situational, crises. With heart attack victims, age clearly influences how the victim handles the crisis and what the priority issues are.

According to Erikson (1963), adult members of launching-stage families are generally in the second stage of adulthood, or middle years, between the ages of 30 and 60. During this period, a sense of generativity leads to productivity and creative work. Discussing midlife research on men, Levinson (1978) proposes a universal human life cycle consisting of specific eras and periods in a set sequence from birth to old age: preadulthood, 0 to 20 years; early adulthood (20 to 40); middle adulthood (40 to 60); late adulthood (60 to 80); and late, late adulthood (80 to death). Each era has its own distinctive character; change between eras is profound and requires a transitional period of some 4 to 5 years. Within each phase, the concept of work is extremely important. Work is defined by the patient, and that definition depends upon the individual's functional level relative to the developmental phase. It is most important to assess how the patient's definition of work relates to his family's and co-workers'. Many patients define work primarily as doing tasks; anything less is considered a personal failure. Reframing client expectations can be critical; for example, teaching others to carry out a specific work assignment is as important, if not more so, than doing the job itself.

Successful occupational function has both psychological and practical import. Besides helping the individual establish an identity and maintain self-esteem, it carries obvious economic rewards and the social sanction afforded those who hold jobs (Croog et al., 1968).

Time lost by the working population from cardiovascular disease in the United States varies from 20% to 60% (Mitchell, 1975; Stern et al., 1977). While research indicates that the period of time cardiac patients must remain out of the work force is on the decline (Burgess et al., 1983), there is a high-risk group who cannot return to their jobs at all.

Key work-related assessment issues include the meaning of work to individual and family, as well as perceptions of job stress and its relationship to the heart attack. In the Byrd family, both Don and Marion identified work as a stressor related to Mr. Byrd's illness. Part of the intervention strategy was to isolate work-related stresses and identify available controls for the patient, spouse, supervisor, and co-worker. This goal was accomplished by meeting with key supervisors and Mr. Byrd. Besides airing existing tensions, this meeting allowed clarification of changed expectations related to Don's new relationship to the work setting; in short, it allowed more realistic appraisal of possibilities. Unconscious concerns regarding aging and career pursuits were also indirectly approached, thus reducing unconscious stress associated with competence and competition.

Planning

Myocardial infarction is both physically and psychologically life threatening. The severity of heart damage determines short-term survival. After the initial physical peril is past, the question becomes how long will disease-related emotional distress—the acute post-traumatic stress response—continue? The answer to this question is crucial for the nurse planning care.

The first level of dynamic formulation regarding anxiety is to recognize its signs as part of acute post-traumatic stress. This gives the nurse a starting point for patient, family, and colleague education about personal response patterns.

Intrusive thoughts and other disturbing initial personal responses can be approached more directly from a stress framework. Relaxation strategies, for example, imagery or thought stopping, can be aimed at target symptoms.

Many heart attack patients display diminished responsiveness to the environment, or "psychic numbing," usually beginning soon after the trauma, which might be referred to as "emotional anesthesia." The patient may describe feeling estranged or detached from others, without interest in formerly enjoyable activities. He may be unable to experience emotions, especially those associated with tenderness and intimacy; sexuality may be markedly decreased.

Symptoms of excessive autonomic arousal may also develop. Hyper-alertness, a pronounced startle response, and sleep disturbances may arise after the person returns home from the hospital. The person may complain of difficulty concentrating, impaired memory, or difficulty completing tasks. Guilt or self-blame over former behavior patterns or behavior patterns used to survive the traumatic event might arise. Environmental associations triggering a flashback to the event may be consciously avoided.

If initial distress symptoms are not relieved, another planning level becomes necessary. This second level shifts its emphasis from the acute post-traumatic stress response to the emerging belief patterns that maintain high anxiety levels and limit patient functioning. At this point, strategies aim not only at education but also at reframing fixed beliefs. Helping people identify the positive consequences of what they are going through, and increasing communication and verbalization of fears and expectations are the desired outcomes. Second-level planning involves deciding with whom to meet, and in what context.

Research results suggest that most cardiac patients experience post-traumatic stress (measured through Horowitz's [1975] Impact of Events Scale) but recover within 6 months. However, a small group of patients fix on the attack's immobilizing aftereffects and do not return to pre-crisis functioning (Burgess et al., 1983).

Intervention

The Cardiac Return to Work program. The Cardiac Return to Work program was a 3-year randomized clinical study using a nursing intervention strategy designed to modify the psychological, social, and occupational characteristics that, according to prior research, impeded postinfarction employment (Burgess et al., 1983). The study's aim was to determine whether adding a special cardiac rehabilitation program to conventional care would improve the rate at which heart attack patients returned to work. Nurse clinicians began administering the program during the first or second week of hospitalization, continuing it for up to 3 months after discharge. Using both hospital and community models of care, the program's three objectives were:
- decreasing post-traumatic distress during cardiac crisis
- minimizing strain on patients' social support networks
- facilitating job reentry.

This intervention assumes that not only the patient but also the family and co-workers must move through the various phases of post-traumatic response in order to deal with the recent heart attack. These four phases, identified earlier, are crisis, immediate postcrisis, transition to optimal level of functioning, and total integration.

The crisis phase. Mr. Byrd's cardiac crisis interview went as follows: At 2 p.m., Don was alone in his car waiting for Marion to finish shopping when he experienced chest pain suggesting heart attack. His first affective reaction was anger, followed by anxiety and then denial. He waited 8 hours before asking Marion to drive him to the emergency department of the community hospital.

Mr. Byrd believed his heart attack had been caused by stress at work. At the time of the interview he noted that he had had a previous attack, and he continued trying to "put the pieces together" as to what that meant.

The patient's usual coping mode is action ("Let's get with it; it shouldn't have happened; let's fix it") and his emotional style is controlled ("especially on the job and working it out with staff"). Don's social support system is strong and includes family, friends, and co-workers. His primary prior crisis experience was illness (heart); he ranks this heart attack as an 8 (out of 10) on the crisis scale. He feels very vulnerable (a 5 out of 5). He tells the nurse: "On my last heart attack, it was the nurse in the ICU who was the only one who really knew what it was like for me. The doctors didn't understand. She was right on target. She said, 'All your life you've been helping people—your work is counseling. Now you need help. You are in that position.'"

Mrs. Byrd's cardiac crisis interview went as follows: At 10 p.m., Marion was asked to drive her husband to the hospital. He told her that during the afternoon, while she was shopping, he experienced chest pain. He hoped it would dissipate, but when it did not he decided to go to the hospital. Her first thought was of his heart; she was not surprised ("I didn't panic or sense an urgency; I was determined to stay low key; I had to stand by") although her affective reaction was helplessness; she drove him to the hospital.

Mrs. Byrd believed her husband's attack was from stress and smoking ("It's all related; he internalizes his stress and he smokes"). It has happened before and she believes its meaning is a warning. Her usual coping mode is cognitive ("I'm a thinker and a planner; it relieves my anxiety"); her emotional style is controlled. Marion has a strong social support system (daughter, son, husband, close woman friend, friends) and her prior crisis experience has been illness-related (husband, daughter, self). She ranked the husband's heart attack as a 7 ("Lower because it was mild") and her own personal vulnerability is between 3 and 4 ("The decision process will be tough; it depends on his attitude and if he denies things"). She asked the nurse for assistance with what seemed an impossible task ("If you keep the work issue up front you may be able to help. You can be a bridge between my husband and myself. I am less convinced we can work it out alone").

The couple clearly identified the nature of the nurse's task. The husband needed a role reversal—someone to listen and to help him adjust to the second heart attack. The wife was pessimistic, believing that her husband could not change his basic coping style of internalizing stress. The wife challenged the nurse to bridge the chasm of communication.

Immediate postcrisis phase. During a home visit, the nurse found Don and Marion in good spirits, although Mr. Byrd was having difficulty adjusting to the slow pace at home ("It's boring to be confined; sleep is a waste of time"). He explained that he was involved in a total life review. He had stopped smoking, was watching his diet, and had increased his exercise level. However, Don was still uncertain about returning to work. He was experiencing recurrent images and conducting internal dialogues with Marion, his supervisor, and his co-workers concerning his work behavior.

Transition to optimal level of functioning. During this phase the nurse met with Mr. Byrd's co-workers and supervisor. All members of the department confirmed the presence of work-related stress and overload. One co-worker talked of her own stress that year ("My father died, my mother is ill, my father-in-law is having bypass surgery; I have had to double up on the work with Mr. Byrd's illness"). The supervisor also commented on the stress level of work and the methods he used to reduce the pressure on himself. During this phase, Don returned to work on a part-time basis, gradually increasing his work load. He initiated weekly staff meetings to help defuse stress-producing situations.

Total integration. By the nurse's final visit at 6 months, Mr. Byrd was back to work full time. Communication had improved markedly within the family as well as at work.

Cognitive interventions. In each phase of intervention there is a reorganization of the individual's preexisting ideas about the nature of his illness, his existence, his death, his self-worth, and so on. A patient's belief system provides a method of determining how the heart attack experience will be processed and stored by the individual. Also derived from the belief system is the patient's characteristic behavior pattern; therefore, attention to both cognitive and behavioral patterns is necessary for effective monitoring of patient recovery, as well as for determining how best to plan interventions.

Those subject to chronic heart disease often hold belief systems that, while associated with success, are just as clearly associated with stress. Attempts to force such individuals to change their behavior—for instance, their smoking or eating habits—may be short lived despite a strong impetus for change. A cognitive behavioral approach, however, can identify ways in which belief systems can be used to make such changes seem desirable to the individual and under his control. This result is likely to result in long-term adherence to the changed patterns.

The studies of Beck (1976), Ellis and Harper (1975), Rehm (1977), and Seligman (1975) all center upon individual control of cognitive processes. As such, they provide a useful theoretical and empirical basis for an intervention model. The Neurolinguistic Programming Model (Bandler and Grinder, 1976; Bandler-Cameron, 1980; Diltz et al., 1980) provides a technology for examining both cognitive and behavioral patient aspects and tailoring a therapeutic intervention for the individual client.

During Mr. Byrd's hospitalization, for instance, he insisted on having office work brought to him. This, he explained, was because he was working on a particular program that no one else in the department could manage. Mr. Byrd's supervisor was contacted and expressed surprise that Don had requested the work, but appreciated Mr. Byrd's attention to the program since it was a complicated one. Marion was distressed by what her husband was doing but commented that he was a determined man and that she, rather than upset Don, had gone along with the request.

Why did Mr. Byrd behave this way? And what should the nurse have done about his behavior and concern for his work? There are theories that would assume a psychological etiology for his response. Psychoanalytic models, for example, suggest unconscious conflict and the threat of helplessness as a possible basis for such behavior and claim that these patient responses originate in early childhood. Therapeutic interventions attempt to illuminate unconscious fears concerning death, retaliation, and guilt based on childhood relationships. A crisis model, on the other hand, might see Mr. Byrd's behavior as an attempt to regain control; therapy would be directed not only towards Mr. Byrd but also towards his social network. Behaviorists might see Don's actions as a means of reducing tension and would therefore attempt to substitute relaxation measures for work as a means to the same end.

The differences in these models lie primarily in the assumed role of mentation in motivating behavior. Behaviorism places the least emphasis on the personal meaning of behavior and emphasizes drive or tension reduction. The other models speculate on the meanings of the behavior and address efforts to the hypothesized etiological foundations of the meaning in the hope that thinking and thus behavior will change.

The nurse had no doubt that Mr. Byrd's thinking patterns and beliefs influenced his behavior; she concluded that the cognitive and behavioral responses of his wife and co-workers inadvertently influenced and supported his beliefs about himself and his work—beliefs that placed him at risk for undue stress and repeated heart attack. Cognitive models for intervention were adopted. Activities addressing the patient's belief structure, the behavior patterns that logically derived from them, and the beliefs and behaviors of his wife and employer were all initiated.

Mr. Byrd believed that no one else could handle his special work program. The nurse, seeking to persuade him otherwise, needed to challenge some of his presuppositions: that the program was beyond the comprehension of other qualified department members; that he was the only counselor who could organize the program; and that it was absolutely necessary that the work be done immediately, by him. Each of these presuppositions defied reality. There were other counselors in the department qualified to handle the program, she said, and even if there were not, the work could have been delayed. However, the challenging nurse also had to overcome the unconscious reinforcement offered by Mr. Byrd's wife and co-workers. How could the patient's position be challenged? What would be the consequences of challenge? What was the desired outcome? How would the nurse know the outcome had been achieved?

Mr. Byrd's thinking exemplified cognition as the mediator of behavior; an event experienced at point A does not determine how a person reacts at C; rather, it is the thoughts experienced at B that do so. People, it follows, are predisposed to certain emotional reactions and behaviors. Don, for example, believed that the program he was working on could only be handled by himself and looked only for information to confirm this. Second, Mr. Byrd supported his experiences through self-evaluation: "I am a good person if I do this work, a terrible one if I don't." Third, he preserved past negative emotional events and dwelt upon future ones, imagining his students' disappointment and complaints and saying to himself, "I will let people down if I don't do the work." Fourth, Don indirectly created a situation where behavior consistent with his emotional state could be enacted. By having the work sent to him, he consciously and unconsciously reinforced his beliefs.

From this it can be seen that Mr. Byrd's selective perceptions and the attendant emotional arousal served to further ingrain beliefs and to make their activation more likely in the future. When Don returned to work, and if his supervisor asked him to do extra work, he would in all likelihood agree, even if he was tired. Similarly, by labeling the uncompleted work as a negative event, he created the possibility of a negative or unbearable emotional state: "I will feel bad if the work is not done." Belief systems may reflect a presupposition that the failure to complete work must not happen.

Behavioral interventions and neurolinguistic programming (NLP). A critical assumption of cognitive-behavioral nursing intervention is, then, that an individual may control his behavior and thereby his emotional state. It was necessary that the nurse convince Mr. Byrd of this presupposition and make him view the process of behavior change as resulting from his own efforts. This provided the basis for NLP—examining the structures, rather than the content, of communication.

Of particular importance to intervention efforts are the systems of meta programs and patterned operations. NLP facilitates structural mapping of meta programs and pattern assessment for verbal and nonverbal behavior, all based upon time, activity, person, and criteria for closely held beliefs (Bandler-Cameron, 1980). Mr. Byrd's case illustrates how these concepts are used.

Before intervening in any way, Mr. Byrd's nurse needed to answer some fundamental questions. Did Mr. Byrd prefer to categorize his world by person, place, information, activity, or thing? If one were to ask him how he spent his vacation, would he probably reply that he had been too busy with work but had managed to get away for a little fishing? Thus, Mr. Byrd defined personal experience by activity rather than people, places, or things.

Did Don focus primarily on past, present, or future? Obviously, from his work-oriented behavior in the hospital, he looked to the past and predicted—thus revealing an orientation towards—the future. Rather than agreeing with others, Mr. Byrd offered counterexamples to their suggestions, but his behavior was primarily initiated by what he perceived others to be thinking or feeling. These perceptions, however, were based upon his own internal processes. He ignored behavior in others that indicated they did not want or expect him to work; he was selectively attentive only to those behaviors that confirmed his beliefs.

Mr. Byrd felt that others would consider him "wrong" if he did not do his work, thus revealing that, where right and wrong were concerned, he relied upon others' beliefs. For him, others were a relevant referent for "correct" behavior.

NLP was a valuable tool for the nurse in assessing Mr. Byrd's personal parameters of time, activity, person, and criteria from his linguistic patterns. It also helped identify what was most valued by and familiar to the patient, thus revealing the structure of his belief system. With this information, the nurse could design an intervention specific to Mr. Byrd, one that respected and was sensitive to his belief system and allowed him to detail his own changes.

Structures can potentially limit choice, but therapeutic interventions are designed to increase flexibility and expand choice. Behavior may be changed by engaging the patient in one or more of the following activities: combining, sorting, separating, or adjusting criteria, and rehearsing new behavior. Mr. Byrd, for example, by altering the criteria of what he valued, could achieve more flexible dealings in work situations. The nurse could challenge his premises by inducing him to look for information contradicting the opinion that only he could manage the program in question. He could be guided to a separate sense of himself by asking, for example, how he might react in a situation where a young and talented basketball player, recovering from knee surgery, insists on playing in an important game because there is no adequate replacement—in other words, by forcing him to use varied criteria in a situation analogous to his own.

Memory is stored through the sensory system; that is, auditorially, visually, and kinesthetically. Eye movement is a useful indicator of what sensory system a person uses to store events. Movement above a median line indicates that the person draws upon visual representations, while lateral eye movements indicate internal, auditory experience. Looking down to the right or left, respectively, indicates kinesthetic experience or attention to internal dialogue. Consider the following dialogue between Don and the nurse:

Don: I don't know... (looking down to his left).
Nurse: What is on your mind?
Don: I keep saying to myself, "Why me?"

Nurse: (moves patient out of a conscious representational system by asking) When you say that to yourself, what do you see?

Don: (looking up to the right, then to the left) I see myself painting the house last year and now I picture myself too weak to climb a ladder.

Nurse: That is quite a picture you have of the future. Are you wearing a hospital gown?

Don: (laughing) No. I guess I could talk myself into a bleak future. It's just not knowing.

The nurse, by attending to Mr. Byrd's patterns, could alter his mood and allow him to express concerns. Before his attention was drawn to it, Don probably had only a negative view of the future; it is the nurse's task to help the patient think resourcefully and resolve crises.

The combination of cognitive-behavioral intervention and NLP provides a comprehensive assessment and intervention strategy when applied to post-traumatic response as experienced by post–heart attack patients, their spouses, and fellow workers.

Evaluation

Evaluation of nursing assessment, planning, and intervention in cardiac care is multidetermined. Both nurse and family must look back upon the work that has been done. Were the goals accomplished? In this case, Mr. Byrd returned to work and communication between the wife and daughter improved.

Other questions to explore in the final family meeting include the following: What did each family member learn in the process? What has changed? What was helpful? What was not helpful? New issues or problems should not be explored at this time, but a mechanism for additional work in the future may be set up.

CONCLUSIONS

Nurses can implement a variety of interventions in families where children are beginning to leave the home and be independent. This chapter has focused on a family in which one member suffers a heart attack. The nurse can help families identify the nature of the particular crisis they are experiencing, can facilitate communication about stressful issues, and can support family members in problem solving. In some families, the nurse may help the members strengthen diffuse boundaries by changing stressful behaviors. In other families, the nurse may support the relaxation of overly rigid boundaries by fostering communication between isolated members. In all families, the nurse can facilitate relationships by helping members to talk directly with each other.

REFERENCES

Bandler, R., and Grinder, J. *The Structure of Magic,* vol. 1. Palo Alto, Calif.: Science and Behavior Books, 1976.

Bandler-Cameron, L. *They Lived Happily Ever After.* Cupertino, Calif.: Meta Publications, 1980.

Beck, A.T. *Cognitive Therapy and the Emotional Disorders.* New York: International University Press, 1976.

Burgess, A.W., et al. "Policy Issues for Cardiac Rehabilitation Programs," *Image: The Journal of Nursing Scholarship* 15(3): 75–79, 1983.

Croog, S.H., et al. "The Heart Patient and the Recovery Process: A Review of the Directors of Research on Social and Psychological Factors," *Social Science and Medicine* 2:111–64, 1968.

Diltz, R., et al. *Linguistic Programming: The Study of Subjective Experience,* vol. 1. Cupertino, Calif.: Meta Publications, 1980.

Ellis, A. *Reason and Emotion in Psychotherapy.* New York: Lyle Stuart, 1962.

Ellis, A., and Harper, R.A. *A New Guide to Rational Living.* Englewood Cliffs, N.J.: Prentice-Hall, 1975.

Erikson, E.H. *Childhood and Society,* 2nd ed. New York: W.W. Norton & Co., 1963.

Levinson, D.J. *The Seasons of a Man's Life.* New York: Alfred A. Knopf, 1978.

Mitchell, K. "Motivational Factors of a Successful Return to Work after a Myocardial Infarction," Unpublished doctoral dissertation. University Park, Pa.: Pennsylvania State University, 1975.

Rehm, L.P. "A Self-Control Model of Depression," *Behavior Therapy* 8:787–804, 1977.

Seligman, M. *Helplessness: On Depression, Development and Death.* San Francisco: W.H. Freeman, 1975.

Shapiro, G.E. "Family Assessment and Intervention," in *Psychiatric Nursing in the Hospital and the Community,* 4th ed. Englewood Cliffs, N.J.: Prentice-Hall, 1985.

Stern, M., et al. "Life Adjustment Post Myocardial Infarction," *Archives of Internal Medicine* 137:1680–85, 1977.

20 Intervening with middle-aged families and terminal cancer

Jane Marie Kirschling, RN, DNS
Assistant Professor
Department of Aging Family Nursing
The Oregon Health Sciences University
Portland, Oregon

OVERVIEW

This chapter applies the nursing process to the case of a middle-aged family experiencing terminal illness. Assessment, planning, intervention, and evaluation are discussed in relation to the case, and overall recommendations are made.

Middle-aged families with a terminally ill adult member develop a variety of needs both prior to and following the death. Today's trend toward home care means that more families are assuming the caregiving role, one that is often emotionally and physically exhausting. Health care professionals must strive to provide constant, comprehensive care as the terminally ill person moves between hospital and home. This includes providing the family with instructions for home care, developing treatment regimens for controlling the patient's symptoms, offering respite for the caregiver, and exploring sources of support during the grief process.

CASE STUDY

At age 52, Paul Jarvis was told he had lung cancer. The father of three grown sons, Paul had been a traveling salesman most of his life. His wife, Susan, was 3 years younger and had worked as a secretary during the early years of their marriage. The Jarvises had sent their last child to college 2 years previously and, before the diagnosis, Paul and Susan had looked forward to playing tennis and spending time together without interruption.

Aggressive chemo- and radiation therapy left Paul increasingly weak during the final year of his life. As the cancer metastasized, he was forced to quit his job; Susan provided for his physical needs at home. Paul died in an inpatient hospice unit 10 months after diagnosis, in the presence of Susan and a son. As a hospice team member, the author cared for Paul and his family during inpatient hospice admissions and worked with Susan and her sons following Paul's death.

Impact on the Family

Cancer has been labeled a family disease (Cohen and Wellisch, 1978; Johnson and Norby, 1981; Lewis, 1983; Welch, 1981). For Susan and Paul, the cancer diagnosis seriously altered their plans for the future. Paul's physician referred him for hospice care 8 months after the initial diagnosis. Although reluctant, the Jarvises agreed, and the hospice staff began working with the family in its home. Susan displayed a high degree of denial toward Paul's illness, despite his increasing fatigue, appetite loss, nausea, vomiting, and pain.

NURSING PROCESS

Assessment

The health problem: Terminal cancer. Terminal cancer is not often thought of as a middle-aged phenomenon. However, in 1980, malignant neoplasms accounted for 31.5% of all deaths in the 45 to 64 age group in the United States (Fruehling, 1982); only heart disease claimed more lives among that population. To accurately assess the effects of terminal illness on a middle-aged client family, the nurse must be aware of certain facts:
- definition of the middle-aged family
- developmental tasks in family middle age
- a theory for family assessment during terminal illness.

Comprehensive nursing assessments, although time- and energy-consuming, are crucial to successful intervention with the middle-aged family facing terminal illness. The healthy spouse commonly serves as family spokesperson, but all members should be assessed both individually and collectively.

Defining the middle-aged family. Middle age, in the family sense, begins when the last child leaves home and ends with retirement; individuals are said to be middle aged at 45 to 64 years (Feldman and Lopez, 1982). The typical middle-aged family is multigenerational (including the middle-aged parent(s), their parents and siblings, and adult children and their mates) and may be spread over a wide geographic area. These facts may be important to the nurse in helping her plan or coordinate care of a terminally ill patient. In addition, the family can include members who are not blood relatives but are identified as a part of the family for one reason or another.

Paul and Susan Jarvis were 52 and 49 years old, respectively, and had sent their last child to college 2 years earlier, therefore meeting the criteria for middle age.

Developmental tasks. Wright and Leahey (1984) and Friedman (1981) have identified developmental tasks for the middle-aged family. While pursuing independent interests in the absence of their children, middle-aged parents need to reinvest in their identity as a couple. Ideally, this reinvestment strengthens the marital relationship. The couple should also realign relationships with other family members. As their children marry, parents need to develop roles as in-laws and, eventually, as grandparents. The middle-aged couple must also deal with the physical limitations accompanying age and with the reality of eventual death. A final task identified by Friedman is the pursuit of a healthier life-style.

Family assessment models. The numerous theories and models designed to assess middle-aged families experiencing a terminal illness include Aguilera and Messick's (1982) theory of crisis intervention; Kahn and Antonucci's (1980) model of attachment, roles, and social support; and Lazarus' theory of stress and coping (Lazarus, 1981). The theory of stress and coping provided the foundation for assessing Paul and Susan.

Lazarus's theory is grounded in the transaction between environment and person. During each exchange, the person cognitively appraises the situation in order to determine its impact on personal well-being. The person considers the environmental demands and constraints, available resources, and existing options. Stress is experienced when the person perceives the demands as too great and/or the resources as too few.

When a person cognitively classifies a transaction as stressful, coping behaviors are initiated. According to Lazarus (1981), coping has two major functions:
• to change the situation for the better (includes altering individual action and/or the environment)
• to manage the emotions associated with the transaction so that "they do not get out of hand and do not damage or destroy morale and social functioning" (Lazarus, 1981, p. 197).

Case analysis. Paul and Susan Jarvis had made noticeable progress toward accomplishing the developmental tasks of middle age. With their children gone, the couple talked about the activities they enjoyed together and the hobbies they pursued independently (Paul golfed while Susan worked on ceramics). They had assumed the roles of in-laws and grandparents and had faced the responsibility of coping with disabilities in aging parents (Susan's mother had moved across the country in order to be near her daughter in case of emergency).

The developmental tasks associated with establishing a healthy environment assumed priority when Paul's cancer was diagnosed. Put into the framework of Lazarus's theory, the demands of Paul's environment and his own available resources changed daily. Initially, the prognosis was good and Paul felt in control of his disease. This feeling of control eroded, however, as the cancer metastasized and aggressive radio- and chemotherapy left him drained both physically and psychologically.

Paul continually perceived transactions with his environment as stressful, but the terminal diagnosis left him with very few avenues for coping. He could not change the course of the disease and therefore had to deal with a broad range of negative emotions including anger, denial, indifference, and sadness.

Susan's environment interactions placed additional demands on her physical and psychological well-being. As Paul's disease advanced, he required assistance with activities of daily living (ADL); frequent trips to the hospital for therapy and Paul's pain, nausea, and vomiting required 24-hour attention. Susan gave up her ceramic work to devote her time to his care.

The resources available to Susan for Paul's care were limited by a number of factors. Susan considered herself a private person and did not like to ask for help from her children or friends. Consequently the demands of Paul's care fell largely on her shoulders. Although she could have changed her situation by requesting help, she chose not to do so. Susan also limited her own coping resources by presenting a strong front to health care professionals. The radiology staff and primary physician caring for Paul were known to be sensitive to family needs, and a referral for home health care would not have been unusual. However, none was ever initiated.

Every family member was forced to cope with difficult emotions. Early in the disease trajectory, Susan expressed hope that they would "beat the cancer." However, as the illness metastasized, family members vacillated between such signs of anticipatory grieving as depression, heightened concern for the patient's well-being, rehearsal of the actual death, and attempts to adjust to the death's consequences (Fulton and Fulton, 1971).

Lazarus' theory of stress and coping is but one framework for family assessment. Members' appraisals of their interactions with the ill member, with other family members, and with the world in general provide valuable insight into what the family unit perceives as stressful. The nurse may also utilize any of the following methods for gathering necessary information:
• observation of family interaction patterns

- one-on-one contact with individual family members
- a family meeting with the nurse serving as facilitator
- a written questionnaire.

Whatever method(s) the nurse uses, one question must be answered: How does this person view the present situation? With this information the nurse can work with other health professionals to develop a plan for meeting the needs of the middle-aged family facing terminal illness.

Planning

The middle-aged family with a terminally ill adult member faces a wide range of issues that its members have probably never encountered before. These issues include the need for the family to assume the care-giving role for one of its members, the financial demands of the illness itself and the loss of a wage earner, the trauma of an adult dying in the prime of life, and the social implications of being a middle-aged widow or widower.

As the nurse plans family intervention, it is essential that family members identify their immediate and projected needs. Even then, the nurse must anticipate needs the family may not have identified but is likely to experience, and plan accordingly.

Though the availability of a hospice program can facilitate family care planning, such care is not essential. In every case, planning must allow continuity of care between inpatient facilities and home. Nurses working with the family in the inpatient setting, physician's office, and home must communicate with each other, as well as with the other health care providers, to ensure quality health care. As hospitalizations grow shorter and less frequent, the planning emphasis will shift toward providing home health care during the initial and recurrent phases of the disease.

Case analysis. Plans for Paul's care were fragmented prior to his hospice referral, 8 months after the initial diagnosis; he remained home and Susan assumed the role of primary caregiver. Ideally, hospice referrals are made 6 to 12 months before death. In reality, most come later in the disease trajectory and force rapid care plan implementation.

Paul's hospice program included home care, an inpatient facility, and bereavement counseling. Upon referral, the hospice nurse coordinator contacted Paul's attending physician to validate the prognosis, obtain a medical history, elicit the physician's perception of the family response to Paul's illness, and secure orders for hospice care.

A hospice nurse then contacted the family to schedule an initial home assessment. Besides obtaining baseline data on Paul's physical and psychological well-being, the nurse questioned Susan about Paul's condition, her ability to care for Paul at home, and the children's involvement in their father's care. The hospice philosophy was also discussed, and Paul and Susan signed a consent form.

Based upon feedback from the family, the attending physician and the nurse who made the initial home visit met with the interdisciplinary hospice team to develop Paul's care plan. The identified problems included:
• caregiver fatigue due to the client's increasing dependence and the caregiver's reluctance to request assistance
• potentially unsafe home environment due to caregiver fatigue and knowledge deficit
• deteriorating (patient) physical status with pain, nausea, and vomiting, due to disease process
• potential psychological, physical, and financial distress for surviving family members due to client's impending death.

Having identified the problems, the hospice team identified family intervention strategies.

Intervention

Strategies. Because the middle-aged family can face such a wide array of problems, interdisciplinary intervention is recommended. For example, the social worker may need to assist the family with financial problems; the physical therapist may need to evaluate the terminally ill person's ability to ambulate safely; the nurse may need to evaluate symptom control. Additional hospice team members can include physicians, an occupational therapist, a speech pathologist, clergy, pharmacists, and volunteers. Each team member brings a repertoire of skills for helping the middle-aged family manage terminal illness, and, hopefully, help itself.

Intervention strategies must be tailored to meet the family's collective needs, as well as those of individual members (see Table 20.1). The health care professional should listen carefully to each member, as well as to the family as a whole, in order to grasp the larger family situation.

The caregiver must also remember that family members will cope with terminal illness relative to their years of experience with each other. If the family has traditionally worked to resolve its problems, members will probably attempt to do so again. Conversely, if the family has avoided resolving its problems, then the members will probably avoid dealing with those associated with terminal illness (Haley, 1973).

Therefore, health care professionals need to be particularly cognizant of the impact of the caregiving role on the family. Most family caregivers accept the role without question (Abrams, 1974) and generally perceive shouldering the burden as the only way to manage the situation (Calkins, 1972). Intervention strategies must be designed to help the caregiver provide needed care.

Table 20.1 Family-Focused Intervention Strategies for Terminal Illness

- Keep the family informed of the ill member's condition (Hampe, 1975); avoid delivering upsetting news without preparing the family.
- Answer questions openly, willingly, and honestly (Skorupka and Bohnet, 1982).
- Facilitate intrafamily communication and encourage expression of feelings (Rogers and Mengel, 1979; Northouse, 1981).
- Reassure the family about the dying member's comfort (Hampe, 1975).
- Elicit family input into the treatment plan.
- Inform the family of available support resources.
- Ensure that health care professionals are available in case of emergency and that the family knows how to contact them (Skorupka and Bohnet, 1982).
- Make sure the caregiver has periods of respite.
- Help the caregiver obtain proper home care equipment.

The health care professional should be aware of appropriate community support providers and should initiate contact in order to facilitate the family's entry.

Golan (1981) identified community-based resources that might be considered when designing intervention strategies. The family's natural helping system—friends, neighbors, relatives, for example—can be called upon, as can informal and formal support groups. Finally, non-professional support services should be considered.

The caregiver(s) must be taught how to keep the terminally ill person comfortable (Skorupka and Bohnet, 1982). The health care professional will have to develop a treatment regimen for controlling the patient's symptoms, a process that involves not only ongoing assessment, but also patient and family compliance with the regimen and a willingness on everyone's part to explore various intervention strategies.

Groebe et al. (1981) interviewed terminally ill persons and their families regarding their need for education before providing care. Most (64%) of the active family caregivers expressed at least one learning need (for example, ambulation, bowel management, comfort, dietary control, pain management, or wound and skin care). The researchers also found that many family members acquired skills by trial and error and rarely received professional follow-up.

Grief assistance. Finally, intervention must persist through the grief process. The death of a terminally ill family member is a particularly stressful life event. When death comes during middle age, it will be perceived as untimely; the surviving spouse faces widowhood prematurely, parents must assimilate the painful loss of an adult child, and children experience the deprivation of a leader and guide.

The use of multiple intervention resources helps buffer the "double loss" experienced by numerous families. Health care professionals involved in a case prior to death often reduce or discontinue family contact soon after the patient's death. Often, the family perceives this as a second loss, in addition to the death of the terminally ill relative. The use of resources from outside the health care arena, however, can mitigate this loss.

Health care professionals must understand the grief process in order to assist families during this phase. Rando (1984) proposed strategies for intervening with grieving individuals, emphasizing those designed to help the bereaved complete the grief process. The choice of strategies will require consultation with the family and a careful assessment of the situation.

Family members should be encouraged to verbalize their feelings and recall positive memories of the deceased. Helping the family identify and resolve secondary losses and unfinished business is part of the health professionals' role. Finally, the bereaved family needs support in order to adjust to the loss and reinvest in a new life.

Not all health care professionals have the opportunity—even when they do have the necessary skills—to intervene with families following a death. However, every professional must be aware of and pass along to the family as much information as possible on available bereavement services.

Case analysis. The experiences of Paul and his family resembled those of many middle-aged families. Intervention strategies specific to the problems identified by the hospice team follow.

Caregiver fatigue due to the client's increasing ADL dependence and caregiver reluctance to request assistance. The goal of intervention was to provide Susan with regular breaks from the home care routine. Intervention strategies included provision of a home health aide three to five times a week to bathe Paul and assist with light household chores and assignment of volunteer(s) to stay with Paul for 3 hours twice a week. The home care nurse also explored Paul and Susan's feelings about involving other family members in Paul's care.

Potentially unsafe home environment due to caregiver fatigue and knowledge deficit. Intervention strategies were preventive in nature, focusing on education and caregiver relief. The nurse assessed Susan's understanding of medication administration and compliance with the prescribed regimen; she also provided ongoing education and developed a system by which Susan could record medications administered.

The nurse also assessed Susan's skill at helping Paul with ADL. Where her skills were inadequate, the nurse instructed her on correct techniques and efficient assistive skills.

An occupational therapist was invited to evaluate the need for additional equipment in the home; a primary goal was to involve Paul in his own care. Eventually, the home was equipped with a hospital bed, trapeze, and bedside commode.

Paul was admitted to the inpatient hospice unit as his death neared. Though the goal of hospice care is to allow terminally ill persons to die at home, circumstances arise in which the caregiver feels incapable of carrying the burden of care. In this case, for a variety of reasons, Susan preferred that Paul not die at home.

Deteriorating physical status with pain, nausea, and vomiting due to disease process. The hospice team worked closely with Paul's primary physician to control his symptoms. Several pain medications and antiemetics were used with variable success. In addition, efforts were made to inform the family of Paul's condition.

Potential psychological, physical, and financial distress for surviving family members due to client's impending death. The hospice social worker helped Paul and his family resolve their financial concerns, make funeral arrangements, and emotionally prepare for his death. The bereavement follow-up was conducted by volunteers and included both written and verbal correspondence with the family for 1 year following Paul's death. Team members participated in the funeral home visitation and service; Susan participated in a 6-week support group for hospice families.

The hospice team coordinated all of the services Paul and his family received. Though other avenues of intervention might have been explored, these appeared beneficial. The use of trained hospice volunteers in the home prior to and after the death, for example, allowed Susan respite and offered continuity of care following the death.

Evaluation

Evaluation forms an integral part of the nursing process; it is a key component of intervention in cases like the Jarvises'. The health care professional will want to evaluate intervention strategies in light of their impact on the family's overall well-being. On a more global level, evaluation means identifying intervention strategies that might help other families.

Whatever evaluation method is used, the health care professional must strive to be systematic and thorough. Professionals who are closely involved with a family over a period of time may not be able to evaluate an intervention objectively; therefore, a disinterested observer should help evaluate each case.

Because they risk losing their objectivity, terminal care professionals may have difficulty evaluating their own effectiveness. For those who work with middle-aged families experiencing terminal illness, professional self-evaluation should encompass a number of areas (Table 20.2).

The answers to the questions outlined in Table 20.2 do not depend solely upon the work of health care professionals. The family and terminally ill person can, and do, have an impact on the effectiveness of intervention strategies. The health care professional must examine this information and assess what might have been done differently.

Research focused specifically on the family as a unit is essential to the effort to provide comprehensive services in terminal illness. Longitudinal research with families prior to and after the death of an adult member is also needed to more fully understand the impact of various intervention strategies.

Table 20.2 Questions to Ask When Evaluating the Effectiveness of Family Care

- Has the focus been on the family or on the patient?
- Has the family been included in development of the treatment plan?
- Has the caregiver received comprehensive instruction about caring for the terminally ill person at home?
- Has the caregiver had adequate respite time?
- Have the terminally ill person's symptoms been controlled?
- Have family members received support through the grieving process?

CONCLUSIONS

Most families are committed to caring for their terminally ill members, as the case of Paul Jarvis and his family demonstrated. With Paul's death, Susan and her sons were forced to make major adjustments. Although they continued to experience sadness, as time passed the question, "Why did Paul have to die?" was asked less frequently. The work of the hospice team helped shape the last months of Paul's life and supported the surviving family members during the grieving process.

Middle-aged families with a terminally ill adult member should be assessed according to the developmental tasks that they want to accomplish. Lazarus' theory of stress and coping provides one way to perform this assessment. Continuity of care must be reflected in the treatment plan. Hospice care is one form of intervention for middle-aged families facing terminal illness.

REFERENCES

Abrams, R.D. *Not Alone with Cancer.* Chicago: Charles C. Thomas, 1974.

Aguilera, D.C., and Messick, J.M. *Crisis Intervention Theory and Methodology,* 4th ed. St. Louis: C.V. Mosby Co., 1982.

Calkins, K. "Shouldering the Burden," *Omega* 3:23–36, 1972.

Cohen, M.M., and Wellisch, D.K. "Living in Limbo: Psychosocial Intervention in Families with a Cancer Patient," *American Journal of Psychotherapy* 32:561–71, 1978.

Feldman, H.S., and Lopez, M.A. *Developmental Psychology for Health Care Professionals, Part 2: Adulthood and Aging.* Boulder, Colo.: Westview Press, 1982.

Friedman, M.M. *Family Nursing: Theory and Assessment.* East Norwalk, Conn.: Appleton-Century-Crofts, 1981.

Fruehling, J.A., ed. *Sourcebook on Death and Dying.* Chicago: Marquis Professional Pubs., 1982.

Fulton, R., and Fulton, J. "A Psychological Aspect of Terminal Care: Anticipatory Grief," *Omega* 2:91–99, 1971.

Golan, N. *Passing Through Transitions: A Guide to Practitioners.* New York: Free Press, 1981.

Groebe, M.E., et al. "Skills Needed by Family Members to Maintain the Care of an Advanced Cancer Patient," *Cancer Nursing* 4(5):371–75, 1981.

Haley, J. *Uncommon Therapy: The Psychiatric Techniques of Milton Erickson, M.D.* New York: W.W. Norton & Co., 1973.

Hampe, S.O. "Needs of the Grieving Spouse in a Hospital Setting," *Nursing Research* 24(2):113–19, 1975.

Johnson, J.L., and Norby, P.A. "We Can Weekend: A Program for Cancer Families," *Cancer Nursing* 4:23–28, 1981.

Kahn, R.L., and Antonucci, T.C. "Convoys over the Life Course: Attachment, Roles, and Social Support," in *Life-Span Development and Behavior,* vol. 3. Edited by Baltes, P.B., and Brim, O.G. New York: Academic Press, 1980.

Lazarus, R.S. "The Stress and Coping Paradigm," in *Models of Clinical Psychopathology.* Edited by Eisdorfer, C., et al. New York: Springer Publishing Co., 1981.

Lewis, F.M. "Family Level Services for the Cancer Patient: Critical Distinctions, Fallacies, and Assessment," *Cancer Nursing* 6:193–200, 1983.

Northouse, L.L. "Living with Cancer," *American Journal of Nursing* 81:961–62, 1981.

Rando, T.A. *Grief, Dying, and Death: Clinical Interventions for Caregivers.* Champaign, Ill.: Research Press, 1984.

Rogers, B.J., and Mengel, A. "Communicating with Families of Terminal Cancer Patients," *Topics in Clinical Nursing* 1(3):55–61, 1979.

Skorupka, P., and Bohnet, N. "Primary Caregivers' Perceptions of Nursing Behaviors that Best Meet Their Needs in a Home Care Hospice Setting," *Cancer Nursing* 5:371–74, 1982.

Welch, D. "Planning Nursing Interventions for Family Members of Adult Cancer Patients," *Cancer Nursing* 4:365–70, 1981.

Wright, L.M., and Leahey, M. *Nurses and Families: A Guide to Family Assessment and Intervention.* Philadelphia: F.A. Davis Co., 1984.

21 Intervening with aging families and stroke

Naomi R. Ballard, RN, MA, MS
Associate Professor
Department of Adult Health and Illness
School of Nursing
The Oregon Health Sciences University
Portland, Oregon

OVERVIEW

A case study demonstrates the importance of a family-oriented approach to the nursing care of a stroke patient and his aging family. Family stress theory provides a comprehensive framework for intervening with families with a life-threatening illness. The Calgary Family Assessment Model is used to evaluate the family's strengths and weaknesses. Interventions are suggested for the following nursing diagnoses: fear, sensory-perceptual alterations, alterations in family processes, and sexual dysfunction.

CASE STUDY

John Dufour, a 67-year-old dentist, was preparing to examine a patient when his assistant noticed that he seemed to be having difficulty selecting the appropriate tool. She asked if anything was wrong. He dropped the tool and slumped to the floor. He said, "I can't move my arm or leg." The assistant quickly called the rescue squad, and he was transported to the hospital.

When the nurse admitted him, John was lethargic but oriented to time, place, and person. He was able to describe the onset of his illness. When he tried to raise the head of the bed, however, he could not figure out how to operate the controls. Upon physical examination, John's pupils were small, equal, and reactive, but he had a marked left visual field cut. He had no sensation on the left side of his face, his left lower eyelid sagged, his mouth drooped toward the affected side, and the nasolabial fold was flattened. His tongue deviated to the left. He had attenuated gag and swallowing reflexes. When John tried to talk, he had difficulty articulating. Carotid bruits were auscultated on both sides of his neck. He had left hemiplegia and left hemi-anesthesia and the muscles on the affected side were flaccid. Deep-tendon reflexes were hyperactive, and he had a positive Babinski response on the left side. All other findings were within normal limits.

Just as the nurse was completing her admission assessment, John's wife, Diane, his youngest daughter, Susan, and the daughter's two children arrived. They were tearful as they approached the bed. Diane wiped her eyes, smiled, and said, "David (the physician) says that he'll let you out of Saturday's game, but that he will expect you back on the greens by the end of the summer." John smiled wanly and nodded off.

NURSING PROCESS

Assessment

The health problem: Cerebrovascular accident. Cerebrovascular accident (CVA) is the third leading cause of death in the United States today; almost a third of each year's 500,000 stroke victims die (American Heart Association, 1985). For the survivors, living sometimes seems worse than death. They and their families must learn to cope with a variety of deficits, many of which can alter their lives. Dealing with this crisis requires full cooperation from all members of the health care team, as well as patient and family.

The term *stroke* refers to "the acute occurrence of symptoms and signs of neurological deficit resulting from disease of the arteries or veins serving the central nervous system" (Toole, 1979, p. 2). The three most common forms of stroke are thrombosis, embolism, and hemorrhage. From John's symptoms, the nurse inferred that he had an embolism (Rudy, 1984, p. 212) lodged in the right middle cerebral artery. Because John had no history of cardiac problems, his embolus probably originated with atherosclerotic plaques in the carotid arteries, the cause of the bruits. If additional emboli were to break off from these sites, John could have developed multifocal infarctions. However, because the stroke made him a high-risk surgical candidate, John was not considered at the time of admission for carotid endarterectomy. The option was left open for later consideration. Meanwhile, John was expected to improve as the edema surrounding the infarcted area subsided and other parts of the brain were trained to compensate for lost functions (Stonnington, 1980, p. 88).

The incidence of stroke increases with population age and was therefore projected to increase during the latter part of the twentieth century. However, in the past decade, it decreased by almost 30% (Ballard, 1983, p. 1445). This unexpected finding has been attributed to increased emphasis on identifying and treating diabetes and hypertension, two major risk factors, as well as improvements in management, which have allowed a larger percentage of stroke patients to survive. In 1982, an estimated 1,900,000 stroke victims were living in the United States alone (American Heart Association, 1985).

According to McDowell (1976, p. 145), 70% of stroke survivors have a functional disability that interferes with activities of daily living. Of these, 10% require nursing home care and 30% depend upon others. This increase in the number of stroke survivors is concurrent with a shortening of hospital stays secondary to cost containment efforts, meaning that families have to assume much of the burden for stroke care and rehabilitation.

The aging family. CVAs pose a particular challenge for the aging family. Although dealing with illness and the loss of a spouse is anticipated at this life cycle stage, it nevertheless interferes with healthy spouses' abilities to meet their own needs and with families' abilities to complete the following developmental tasks associated with aging (Duvall, 1977, p. 390):

• establishing/maintaining satisfying living arrangements as aging progresses
• adjusting to a retirement income
• establishing comfortable routines
• safeguarding physical and mental health
• maintaining love, sex, and marital relations
• maintaining contact with other family members
• keeping active and involved
• finding meaning in life.

The degree to which developmental tasks are met in old age—or have been met at earlier life stages—influences the family's ability to cope with the stress of stroke or any life-threatening illness.

Theoretical approaches to family assessment. Several theoretical models can help the nurse understand a family's response to a life-threatening illness. By describing how the life cycle stage alters the demands placed upon a family, the developmental perspective (Aldous, 1978; Duvall, 1977; Rodgers, 1973) is useful for predicting how families will cope with the health crisis. Rodgers (1973) attempts to expand the developmental model by accounting for societal-institutional, interactional-associational, and individual-personality variables in family phenomena. Thus, he facilitates both macro- and microanalysis within the developmental perspective. However, other theories—for example, the structural-functionalist and interactionist approaches—seem to cover those relationships more comprehensively.

Family stress theory. None of these theoretical perspectives—developmental, structural-functionalist, or interactionist—adequately explains family responses to one key variable: *stress,* either at various stages of the life cycle or in relation to the individual, family, and community. This is where family stress theory can provide key insight.

The family stress perspective actually integrates the family system (Broderick and Smith, 1979) and developmental approaches; the Double ABCX Model (Table 21.1; McCubbin and Patterson, 1982) seems to be one of its most promising applications. This theoretical perspective is supposed to be predictive; however, it requires additional testing and refinement. Currently, especially when used with information gleaned from a Calgary Family Assessment Model evaluation, it provides a guide for assessing a family's response to the stress of life-threatening illness.

The Calgary Family Assessment Model. If used at the very beginning of the crisis and later, after the family has adapted, the Calgary Family Assessment Model provides most of the information necessary to apply the Double ABCX Model. Therefore, this model, adapted from Wright and Leahey (1984), was used to assess John's family. In addition, data from John's physical assessment (Supra) and data related to the family's perception of and adaptation to the crisis were needed.

Table 21.1 Elements of the Double ABCX Model

Double Factor	Variable(s)
A	**Stressor:** Event Family change secondary to developmental stage and stress response

B	**Resources:**
	Initial
	Developed through dealing with stressor
	    self-reliance/esteem
	    family integration
	    social support
	    social action

C	**Perceptions:** Of the stressor Of the crisis
X	**Interaction between double A, B, and C:** Crisis Adaptation

Source: McCubbin and Patterson, 1982

Structural Assessment

Internal structure. The Dufour family is composed of John, 67, a practicing dentist, his wife, Diane, 65, one son, 45, and two daughters, 42 and 30. The oldest children are married and live in adjacent states. The youngest daughter, a nurse, is a divorced mother of two who lives within a 10-minute drive of her parents. Diane's mother, 87, is in a nearby nursing home; Diane visits her daily. Diane has very close relationships with both her youngest daughter, Susan, and her mother, but is less close to her husband, who spends many of his free hours with his golfing buddies. There is minimal interaction between the major family subsystems, Diane and John, Diane and Susan, and Diane and her mother.

External structure. Both John and Diane are third-generation Americans of Scandinavian descent. They are Lutheran but attend church only on special occasions. John is an active partner in a private dental practice. Both his and Diane's families operated small businesses. Their son is a college professor and the oldest daughter is a pharmacist. The youngest daughter, a nurse, has needed financial assistance to meet house payments since her divorce 6 years ago. John and Diane rarely see their own siblings.

The Dufours live in a four-bedroom, single-level house with eight steps at the entrance. John regularly mows their half-acre lawn with a tractor mower. The bath in the master bedroom, which John usually uses, is very small and cannot be readily adapted for the disabled. The second bathroom can be, but it does not have a shower, which John prefers.

Developmental Assessment

Tasks. Because of their ages, John and Diane are in the last stage of the family life cycle. However, they have barely begun to work on the developmental tasks of the aging family. John has steadfastly refused to retire. He invested his money wisely over the years, so income is no problem, but he has made no arrangements to divest himself of the dental partnership. He, more than Diane, has avoided facing his own mortality. Neither has modified living arrangements or daily routines to adapt to this family life stage.

Attachments. Because each continues to pursue separate interests, John and Diane are only slightly attached to each other. Nevertheless, their relationship is positive. In contrast, John's relationship with his youngest daughter is negative; he blames her for her divorce, the first in his family. Diane's relationships with both her mother and her youngest daughter are very strong.

Functional Assessment

Instrumental. In the past, both John and Diane have proven very competent in managing the family's instrumental tasks. However, they have followed very traditional gender roles. John controlled the finances and took care of the lawn and household repairs. Diane assumed responsibility for housework and social relationships.

Expressive. John has the most decision-making power; his wife is usually supportive. Communication between the two is direct, but both partners tend to avoid emotional extremes. They are affectionate with each other when alone.

Planning

Daily, the nurse met with the Dufour family to discuss John's progress and plan his care. On the 10th day of hospitalization, the family was informed that John would be going home in 4 days.

At discharge, John had regained function in his left side, although it remained weak. He had no difficulty eating but still needed assistance in other activities of daily living (ADLs); his visual field cut had not improved. John displayed severe unilateral neglect, occasionally forgetting to dress the affected side. Lingering spatial-perceptual deficits (at times, he even found it difficult to find his room) made it difficult for him to do any skilled work with his hands, which he found particularly frustrating. These deficits, combined with a quick/impulsive behavioral style, presented a challenge to both family and staff.

All health care team members, including the family, met to plan for John's long-term care. They identified the following goals for the family system:
- to cope effectively with the fear accompanying life-threatening illness
- to resolve the grief associated with object loss
- to facilitate John's ability to perform ADLs
- to provide a safe family environment
- to cope effectively with the role transitions necessitated by John's illness
- to develop a functional social support system
- to strengthen the husband/wife bond
- to maintain Diane's—the primary caregiver's—health status.

The health care team cooperated to accomplish these goals. Prior to John's discharge, the physician placed him on antiplatelet aggregants and scheduled a left carotid endarterectomy in 3 months. He also arranged to see John every 2 weeks prior to surgery. The social worker and nurse helped the family deal with feelings of loss and develop coping mechanisms. With the social worker's assistance, for instance, the family could confront the need to call in its attorney and begin dissolving the dental partnership.

The home health care nurse and physical therapist evaluated the home and arranged for necessary modifications prior to John's return. The nurse, physical therapist, and occupational therapist also developed and implemented a program to help John resume ADLs. During his first 6 weeks at home, John continued to see the physical and occupational therapists on an outpatient basis; the home health care nurse visited weekly.

Interventions

A comprehensive nursing care plan for John and his family is beyond the scope of this chapter. (For more complete information, see Ballard, 1983; Hickey, 1981; O'Brien and Pallett, 1978; Pallett and O'Brien, 1985; Rudy, 1984; Snyder, 1983; and Taylor, 1985; also see Table 21.2 for general guidelines.) This discussion is limited to the four nursing diagnoses (Carpenito, 1983) that contributed most to meeting the family's defined goals:
* fear related to a life-threatening illness
* sensory-perceptual alterations related to the cerebrovascular accident
* alterations in family processes related to an ill family member
* sexual dysfunction related to a change in body image.

These diagnoses are commonly overlooked by those caring for stroke patients and their families.

Fear related to a life-threatening illness. For both patient and family, the onset of a life-threatening illness produces fear, which may be expressed in a variety of ways. In the Dufours' case, Diane joked and John withdrew; however, their physical demeanor revealed their concern. Much has been written about handling patient fears, yet little has been done in relation to their families. In a study of the perceived needs of families of brain-injured patients, Mathis (1984, p. 41) found that the following needs were deemed most important to family members during this critical period:
* to feel that hospital personnel care about the relative
* to know they would be called at home if there were any changes in the relative's condition
* to know exactly what was being done for the ill relative
* to be reassured that the best care possible was being given the relative
* to have questions answered honestly
* to be told about the relative's medical treatment
* to receive information about the relative's condition at least once a day

- to feel accepted by hospital personnel
- to feel there was hope
- to have specific facts concerning the relative's progress.

Table 21.2 Helping Families Adapt to Stroke

The following nursing actions facilitate the adaptation process in families coping with stroke:	
	• Base nursing interventions on *good* patient and family assessments; inaccurate or incomplete data may lead to inappropriate intervention. Examples in which this has occurred include the failure to differentiate between homonymous hemianopsia and blindness and failure to acknowledge the longtime mistress of a priest as a significant other.
	• Begin rehabilitation upon admission. For example, following the initial health assessment, use careful positioning to help the patient maintain function. Also share findings with the family to help maintain family cohesiveness.
	• Develop a long-term rehabilitation plan encompassing diet, exercise, rest, sexual activity, and medical therapy.
	• Include patient and family in planning whenever possible. In the initial stage of the crisis, their participation might not be effective or efficient, but inclusion will promote long-term participation in the health care team.
	• Provide opportunities for both family and patient to express fears related to the life-threatening illness. Usually, all that is required is sitting down with them!
	• Titrate denial (Goodstein, 1983, p. 145). Do not force patients or families to face the extent of the stroke problem until they have gotten over their initial vulnerability, yet try to reduce the denial to the degree that it might be interfering with the treatment plan.
	• Help the family differentiate between behavioral changes resulting from the patient's brain injury and behavioral responses to the disease.
	• Identify and positively reinforce the patient's and family's gains, no matter how small.
	• Provide models for patient and family emulation.
	• Maintain open communication with all members of the health care team, including patient and family.
	• Help the family identify and mobilize resources.
	• Do an environmental assessment and alter the surroundings, if necessary, prior to discharge.
	• Help the family members identify community resources that may facilitate adaptation. These might include anything from craft stores where they can obtain materials for a new hobby to a self-help group.
	• Arrange at-home follow-up visits.
	• Affirm family members' right to attend to their own needs.

In contrast, four needs were ranked as "not important." These were to have visiting hours changed because of special conditions, to talk to someone about such negative feelings as guilt and anger, to be encouraged to cry, and to have another person along when visiting at the relative's bedside (Mathis, 1984, p. 43). Overall, these guidelines proved useful in helping John and his family cope with their fears.

Nevertheless, the Dufours found it difficult to begin long-term planning only 10 days after the stroke. With additional time, they probably could have coped very well, but, because of Medicare's limited hospital coverage, they had to adapt more quickly. The social worker was called in to help them deal with their feelings about the illness before they would proceed with planning.

In many cases, nurses try to reduce families' fears by involving members in the actual physical care of the ill member. However, according to Mathis (1984, p. 41), families are very ambivalent about this intervention. Diane wanted to be involved, so she was taught to help John with range-of-motion exercises. Although the effectiveness of this intervention has recently been questioned (Clough and Maurin, 1983), it does not seem to do any harm and was used, in this case, to bring the marital dyad closer together. At the same time, Diane's offer to feed John was refused. Because of the danger of aspiration, feeding by an unskilled caretaker is potentially dangerous in patients with attenuated gag and swallowing reflexes and should not be attempted. The only family members that need to be involved in feeding the stroke patient are those that are going to have to do it at home. Those relatives should be taught the correct method.

The fear of death from a stroke does not end when the patient leaves the hospital. Family members and the patient often fear a recurrence. Such commonly used expressions as "I got so mad, I thought I'd have a stroke" tend to lend credence to these fears. Consequently, family members are often overprotective of the recovering patient (Stroker, 1983, p. 363).

This was particularly true of John's family prior to the planned surgery. Encouraging Diane and the children to verbalize fears helped alleviate them. It was revealed that, for example, Diane was afraid for John to take a walk, lest he have another stroke and lie on the street for a long time without being found. When she was able to identify this and other fears, she realized that they were unrealistic and was able to give her husband freedom.

Sensory-perceptual alterations related to cerebrovascular accident. One of John's poststroke problems was potentially dangerous. Sensory-perceptual deficits would make it easy for him to get lost while taking walks in the neighborhood. Or he could, for instance, leave a dishcloth on a stove burner. Many times health professionals, patients, and their families do not understand these phenomena, or how to compensate for them. Many stroke patients' difficulties performing ADLs are attributable to just such deficits. Families and health professionals who do not recognize the etiology tend to think that the patient is just being difficult. For families, Fowler and Fordyce's booklet, *Stroke: Why Do They Behave That Way?*, available through the American Heart Association, is very helpful.

One-sided neglect. John did not eat the food on the left side of his tray; he forgot to shave the left side of his face; he tended to bump into things on his left side; and, on occasion, he forgot to put his left arm in his sleeve. This one-sided neglect was partially a product of John's reduced visual field, or homonymous hemianopsia. However, it also involved proprioception, or the ability to locate oneself in space. Spatial orientation requires the acquisition, interpretation, and integration of information to establish an awareness of self. It is believed to be a function of the nondominant parietal lobe (Pallett and O'Brien, 1985, p. 306), which is supplied by the middle cerebral artery. In the acute stage of stroke, when proprioception is often impaired, staff and family need to compensate for such deficits as John's. However, during the rehabilitation phase, the patient must learn to attend to the affected side.

John's family was taught to place equipment that he needed to use on his left, or affected, side. The television, for instance, was moved to his left. John was also encouraged to play checkers, which required him to attend to the entire board. His clothing was marked on the left side to remind him to put on that side first. Gradually, the necessary skills became habitual.

Spatial orientation. However, when confronted by more complex tasks—for instance, finding the men's department in a store—John was overwhelmed. Diane learned to give him simple verbal directions; sometimes, she even wrote them down. If not distracted, he was able to accomplish complex tasks such as putting a bike together for his granddaughter by following written directions. Nevertheless, the family members had to continuously remind themselves not to overestimate his abilities; for example, one morning Diane discovered John combing his hair with his toothbrush.

Alterations in family process related to an ill family member. John's stroke rendered long-standing family processes ineffective. Suddenly, John and Diane were compelled to adapt to their chronological stage of family life—the aging family. In the past, John in particular had avoided dealing with age and mortality, and because of the couple's adherence to traditional gender roles, neither had the skills to perform multiple family functions. These problems were accentuated by the emotional changes associated with right-hemisphere brain damage (Binder, 1984, p. 175). John tended to ignore or deny his limitations and was inclined to act impulsively. Furthermore, he found it difficult to pick up emotional intonation in conversations. These deficits frequently caused friction in family interaction and, in turn, potentiated the depression associated with object loss.

Roles. John's first few weeks at home were very frustrating for both him and Diane. In addition to the increased demands of home care, there were outpatient appointments almost every day. Both were very fatigued, yet John kept trying to perform his usual home activities and had to be watched constantly. He had three wrecks on his tractor mower before he agreed to let someone else care for the lawn. He became so frustrated when he tried to balance a checkbook that he threw it across the room. His depression increased with failure after failure. Diane, too, felt frustrated because she could not meet all the demands being placed on her. She experienced role overload. Additional stress arose from John's continual presence in the household, which altered Diane's daily routine. Each week, the nurse discussed with them the role modifications they were making and helped them use problem-solving techniques to identify and alleviate sources of strain. John hired a neighbor boy to mow the lawn; Diane hired a housekeeper to come in once a week and do the heavy cleaning. John's attorney and his business partner helped Diane figure out the finances so that she could take over their actual management, although all decisions were discussed with John.

The intervention that proved most effective was the substitution of other roles for those John had had to relinquish. This solution occurred almost by accident; the nurse had encouraged John and Diane to join a support group to learn how others dealt with role transitions. Not only did this help them accept what was happening between them, but John quickly became a leader of the group. The satisfaction that he derived in this capacity helped compensate for some of his losses.

To counteract the Dufours' frustration, the nurse encouraged John and Diane to begin doing at least one activity each day that they could enjoy together. After much discussion, they decided that Diane would read to John each night before going to bed. Diane had always enjoyed reading aloud, and John enjoyed reading but had been frustrated in poststroke attempts because of his reduced visual field. So, each evening, Diane read to John for almost an hour. They both enjoyed it and frequently spent time afterwards discussing ideas that the reading stimulated.

Social support. The family's primary sources of social support during the recovery period were the stroke club and each other. They interacted with others more as a couple, since John was dependent upon Diane to offset some of his limitations. In addition, Diane's mother and Susan continued to make demands upon Diane's time. She and Susan were able to work out a satisfactory arrangement. Susan stayed with John one evening a week, while Diane and John watched the grandchildren on Sunday afternoons. Nevertheless, the frequency of Diane's visits to her mother decreased, and she felt guilty. Her other siblings offered to help but were inconsistent in their support. The nurse encouraged Diane to express her feelings about her mother and her siblings and tried to affirm Diane's rights and responsibilities to herself, as well as to her family.

Sexual dysfunction related to alteration in body image. Allsup-Jackson (1981) notes that most stroke patients report decreased sexual contact with their spouses, to a degree inconsistent with the physiological alterations secondary to the CVA. Since sexual function is controlled bilaterally, an infarction in one hemisphere does not have overwhelming physiological impact. The sensory and motor dysfunctions that do occur secondary to stroke might require sexual adaptation, but not abstinence. However, 60% of the males and 70% of the females studied (Allsup-Jackson, 1981, p. 163) reported decreased sexual activity after a stroke. Moreover, 60% of them found this change very disturbing. They attributed it to a loss of sexual attractiveness; in contrast, the unaffected spouses saw it as a protective maneuver to avoid any additional medical problems.

Despite their concern about the matter, stroke patients and their families rarely ask questions about sexual activity (Binder, 1984, p. 175). One man noted, "We grew up in a time when talking about sex was taboo; we don't even know the words to use when talking to a doctor. All we know is the street language. And, we would never ever talk to a woman about it." However, when he said this, he was talking to a woman. Most people are relieved to discuss their sexual problems when given the opportunity.

Six weeks after the stroke, John and Diane were asked, "Many people who have had a stroke report a decrease in sexual activity afterwards; how is it with you?" They verbalized interest in resuming this relationship but also expressed fear about the relationship between stroke and sexual activity. They were reassured to learn that the association is rare. In addition, alternative coital positions were discussed. They decided to try the side-lying position, which they had not used before. The next week they thanked the nurse for her encouragement.

Evaluation

Ten months later, when the nurse saw John and Diane at a stroke club meeting, they appeared to have adapted successfully to the crisis and had coped with the carotid endarterectomy without undue stress. John had been elected president of the stroke club, and Diane had assumed responsibility for planning the social activities. They reported making a lot of friends at the club. John's relationship with his daughter had improved as a result of their increased contact. Diane's relationship with her mother remained strained, but Diane had accepted the situation. She and John seemed closer than they had been in years.

For the Dufours, coping with a life-threatening illness allowed renegotiation of relationships and movement to another stage of the family life cycle. This "regenesis" (Hansen and Johnson, 1979, p. 584) was perceived as a positive experience, albeit one that they would not want to live through again, by both John and Diane. They were fortunate in that they had a great many resources to draw upon during the crisis and perceived the crisis as one which, with help, they could manage. The family cohesiveness they had lacked had finally begun to develop.

CONCLUSIONS

"Stroke," writes Holbrook (1982, p. 100), "is a family matter," in that it disrupts the family's entire life. A family's response to the life-threatening illness is similar to that of any individual or group experiencing object loss; in families of stroke patients, this is commonly compounded by losses due to physiologic aging and other health problems. According to Holbrook (1982), family adjustment to stroke is a four-stage process:
• *Crisis.* Response is characterized by shock, confusion, and high anxiety levels.
• *Treatment.* Families commonly deny the permanence of disability and continue to hold high expectations for recovery. This tends to motivate participation in the rehabilitation program. However, optimism is tempered by periods of grief and fear for the future.
• *Discharge.* Families are forced to face the reality of the disability, resulting in anger and depression.
• *Adjustment.* While most families of stroke victims learn to adjust to their losses, Holbrook contends they need considerable support both in the crisis stage and for many years afterward.

Because of the heterogeneity of stroke families and their lengthy life experiences, providing adequate support can be a challenge to the health care team. The use of the Double ABCX Model (McCubbin and Patterson, 1982) helps the nurse predict an individual family's response to the stress. In addition to recognizing the hardship related to the stroke, the nurse must consider the stressors associated with efforts to cope with the new situation. For example, if the spouse does not drive, going to the hospital every day may constitute a hardship. In addition, the nurse needs to acknowledge the stressors associated with normal aging family development. The second determinant of the family's crisis response is access to resources, both tangible and intangible. Obviously, freedom from economic worry reduces family stress. However, the knowledge that the family has coped well with a past crisis is also important.

Any assessment of resources must consider environmental demands that affect resource allocation. A stroke patient and his wife may be able to live successfully in a small apartment but unable to maintain a two-story house.

Finally, the family's perception of the illness affects its response. For some families, a minor stroke may be viewed as a concomitant of aging and cause little stress. For others, it may remind them of their mortality and be considered a crisis. In order to preserve unity, enhance the family system, and promote individual relatives' growth, all of these variables need to be considered in care planning and implementation.

According to Litman (1974, p. 495), "the family constitutes perhaps the most important social context within which illness occurs and is resolved." The pivotal nature of this relationship is acknowledged in proper nursing actions. Such actions recognize the family as the basic unit of health care and, in doing so, facilitate the aging family's adaptation to stroke.

REFERENCES

Aldous, J. *Family Careers: Developmental Change in Families.* New York: John Wiley & Sons, 1978.

Allsup-Jackson, G. "Sexual Dysfunction of Stroke Patients," *Sexuality and Disability* 4(3):161–68, 1981.

American Heart Association, *Heart Facts.* Dallas: American Heart Association, 1985.

Ballard, N.R. "Nursing Role in Management: Stroke Client," in *Medical-Surgical Nursing: Assessment and Management of Clinical Problems.* Edited by Lewis, S.M., and Collier, I.C. New York: McGraw-Hill Book Co., 1983.

Binder, L.M. "Emotional Problems after Stroke," Stroke 15(1):174–77, 1984.

Broderick, C., and Smith, J. "The General Systems Approach to the Family," in *Contemporary Theories about the Family: Vol. 2. General Theories/Theoretical Orientations.* Edited by Burr, W.R., et al. New York: Free Press, 1979.

Carpenito, L.J. *Nursing Diagnosis: Application to Clinical Practice.* Philadelphia: J.B. Lippincott Co., 1983.

Clough, D.H., and Maurin, J.T. "ROM versus NRx," *Journal of Gerontological Nursing* 9:278–86, 1983.

Dimond, M., and Jones, S.L. *Chronic Illness Across the Life Span.* East Norwalk, Conn.: Appleton-Century-Crofts, 1983.

Duvall, E.M. *Marriage and Family Development,* 5th ed. Philadelphia: J.B. Lippincott Co., 1977.

Fowler, R.S., and Fordyce, W.E. *Stroke: Why Do They Behave That Way?* Dallas: American Heart Association, 1974.

Goodstein, R.K. "Overview: Cerebrovascular Accident and the Hospitalized Elderly—A Multidimensional Problem," *American Journal of Psychiatry* 140(2): 141–47, 1983.

Hansen, D.E., and Johnson, V.A. "Rethinking Family Stress Theory: Definitional Aspects," in *Contemporary Theories about the Family: Vol. 1. Research-Based Theories.* Edited by Burr, W.R., et al. New York: Free Press, 1979.

Hickey, J.V. *The Clinical Practice of Neurological and Neurosurgical Nursing.* Philadelphia: J.B. Lippincott Co., 1981.

Holbrook, M. "Stroke: Social and Emotional Outcome," *Journal of the Royal College of Physicians* 16(2):100–04, 1982.

Litman, T.J. "The Family as a Basic Unit in Health and Medical Care: A Social-Science Overview," *Social Science and Medicine* 8:495–519, 1974.

Mathis, M. "Personal Needs of Family Members of Critically Ill Patients with and without Acute Brain Injury," *Journal of Neurosurgical Nursing* 16(1): 36–44, 1984.

McCubbin, H.I., and Patterson, J.M. "Family Adaptation to Crisis," in *Family Stress, Coping, and Social Support.* Edited by McCubbin, H.I., et al. Chicago: Charles C. Thomas, 1982.

McDowell, F.M. "Rehabilitating Patients with Stroke," *Postgraduate Medicine* 59(3):145–56, 1976.

O'Brien, M.T., and Pallett, P.J. *Total Care of the Stroke Patient.* Boston: Little, Brown & Co., 1978.

Pallett, P.J., and O'Brien, M.T. *Textbook of Neurological Nursing.* Boston: Little, Brown & Co., 1985.

Rodgers, R.H. *Family Interaction and Transaction: The Developmental Approach.* Englewood Cliffs, N.J.: Prentice-Hall, 1973.

Rudy, E.B. *Advanced Neurological and Neurosurgical Nursing.* St. Louis: C.V. Mosby Co., 1984.

Snyder, M., ed. *A Guide to Neurological and Neurosurgical Nursing.* New York: John Wiley & Sons, 1983.

Stonnington, H.H. "Rehabilitation in Cerebrovascular Diseases," *Primary Care* 7(1):87–106, 1980.

Stroker, R. "Impact of Disability on Families of Stroke Clients," *Journal of Neurosurgical Nursing* 15(6):360–65, 1983.

Taylor, J.W. "Nursing Management of Stroke: Acute Care—Part 1," *Cardiovascular Nursing* 21:1–5, 1985.

Taylor, J.W. "Nursing Management of Stroke: Acute Care—Part 2," *Cardiovascular Nursing* 21:7–11, 1985.

Toole, J.F. *Diagnosis and Management of Stroke.* Dallas: American Heart Association, 1979.

Wright, L.M., and Leahey, M. *Nurses and Families: A Guide to Family Assessment and Intervention.* Philadelphia: F.A. Davis Co., 1984.

22 Intervening with gay and lesbian couples and cancer

Judith M. Saunders, DNSc, FAAN
Assistant Research Scientist
Department of Nursing Education and Research
City of Hope National Medical Center
Duarte, California

OVERVIEW

Nurses working with gay couples facing life-threatening illness need to know not only about the health condition, but also about gay and lesbian life-styles and their own attitudes toward homosexuality. Since, in most areas, same-sex couples fall outside the legal definition of family, the nurse may need to adapt existing resources and consult with services in the gay and lesbian community in order to effectively care for clients through the living-dying interval and bereavement. Interventions negotiated between nurse and family and spelled out in a treatment contract are particularly effective since patient and family can remain in control of their situation. Homophobia should not be part of any aspect of nursing the gay man or woman.

CASE STUDY

Anna, age 34, has been diagnosed as having malignant melanoma with extensive metastasis. Her lover-partner, Deb, is 32 years old and has a daughter, Tricia, age 12. The three of them live in a three-bedroom house in the suburbs of a northwestern city. They bought the house jointly 5 years ago and are well accepted by their neighbors, although their community interactions are fairly superficial. Anna and Deb both have master's degrees in education and work as schoolteachers. Neither openly identifies herself as a lesbian at work for fear of losing her job; the issue has never arisen in the neighborhood. Anna has an older brother, Dave, who disapproves of her lesbianism. Their contacts have been infrequent and strained over the years. Deb's sister Amy, on the other hand, is very supportive of her and of her relationship with Anna. Deb's former husband, John, has remarried and lives in a nearby state. Tricia usually visits him and his wife for 2 weeks during the summer. John knows that Anna and Deb are a lesbian couple but has promised not to challenge Deb's custody of Tricia as long as the relationship remains "low-key," without major difficulties or adverse publicity. He considers homosexuality wrong but admits that Deb is doing a good job of raising their daughter. Tricia attends a private, liberal school in the city where she is an above-average student. She knows her mother is a lesbian and has occasionally been placed in awkward situations by classmates who wonder why she lives in a home with two adult women. The child has a few friends in the neighborhood, but most of her friends are from school and live closer to the city than she does. Both Anna and Deb are active in their professional community, as well as in selected gay/lesbian organizations where they can both enjoy their friends and protect their identities. Neither woman is religiously active, but both have Protestant backgrounds and occasionally attend services at the gay and lesbian Metropolitan Community Church. Tricia attends Sunday School in the neighborhood.

Household tasks are divided; generally, Anna does the cooking and shopping, while Deb does more housecleaning. Unpopular tasks, such as taking out the garbage, are allocated each week by a "loser's lottery." Both positive and negative emotions are expressed fairly openly, although Tricia seems more emotionally constrained than either Anna or Deb.

Deb was the first to notice a "funny-looking mole" on Anna's back. Since Anna was due for her annual school physical, she asked the physician about it at that time. The physician referred her to a surgeon, who recommended removal, just to be on the safe side. Although the mole was found to be a malignant melanoma, the physician was confident that it was localized and that the surgery had removed the entire tumor. Anna did not worry much about it, since she had heard about skin cancers and how little threat they pose.

About a year later, in April, Anna found another suspicious mole. This time the physician was more subdued and cautious, and Anna and Deb both became concerned. The concern was justified, as the melanoma was found to have already invaded adjacent tissue, including lymph nodes.

Family assessment was initiated by the nurse at the cancer center. A series of interviews with the total family and individual members was conducted. No formal assessment tools were used. Anna decided to die at home, and the nurse conducted a site visit to ensure that she could be made comfortable in that setting. Assessment and intervention were considered to be an ongoing team function coordinated by the nurse.

NURSING PROCESS

Assessment

The health problem: Malignant melanoma. Malignant melanoma arises within pigment-producing cells called melanocytes. Usually, the primary tumor is found in the skin, although the disease can invade almost any bodily organ. While melanoma accounts for less than 2% of all cancers, its incidence and mortality are increasing so rapidly that it has been referred to as an epidemic; only lung cancer's mortality rate is increasing faster. In the United States alone, about 1 in every 150 people will develop a malignant melanoma in his lifetime, a rate that is expected to increase to 1 in 100 by the year 2000 (Friedman et al., 1985). Moreover, this higher incidence is a *true* increase, unrelated to improved detection and certification (unlike, for instance, the apparent increase in cervical cancer following development of the Pap smear).

Melanoma's etiology appears to be both genetic and environmental, involving insufficient skin pigmentation and exposure to sunlight, respectively.

Although no internationally accepted cancer classification system yet exists, there is increasing reliance on the so-called "TNM approach." In this system, "T" refers to specific characteristics of the primary tumor, "N" to the degree of lymph node involvement, and "M" to the degree of metastasis. Information about all three is needed to determine prognosis and guide the selection of appropriate interventions.

The lymphatic system is the common metastatic pathway, and the pattern of lymph node involvement depends upon the primary tumor site and its lymphatic drainage. About one third of patients with metastatic melanoma have multiple skin lesions; common metastatic sites include the lungs, liver, lymph nodes, kidneys, heart, gastrointestinal organs, and central nervous system (Gutterman and Scher, 1982). Symptoms vary with the metastatic site. Most metastatic melanoma lesions are painless, yet bone lesions can be excruciating.

Localized melanoma is usually treated by excision of the tumor and a fair amount of surrounding tissue. Metastasized disease, however, cannot be surgically removed and has proven resistant to both systemic chemo- and radiation therapies. Prognosis has been correlated with tumor thickness. Breslow (1970) found that patients whose tumors were less than 0.7 mm thick responded better to treatment.

Gay and lesbian families. A homosexual is a man or woman whose sexual and affectional orientation is toward people of his or her own sex. The fact that one is homosexual says something about the tendency and capacity to love others of the same sex, but nothing about attitudes toward the opposite gender. While widely studied and disputed, homosexual etiology is no better understood than that of heterosexuality. Most homosexuals are not open about their sexual orientation, since social disapproval remains fairly extensive; therefore, only estimates can be used to calculate the number of gays or lesbians today. Most often, the figures identified by The Institute of Sex Research are used; it estimates that 10% of the U.S. population (13% of the men and 5% of the women) is homosexual.

Only recently has homosexuality gained acceptance as a variant lifestyle, rather than a manifestation of sickness or immorality. A milestone in the formal removal of homosexuality from the categorization of illness was created by the American Psychiatric Association, which removed the entry from its *Diagnostic and Statistical Manual* of mental illness (Bayer, 1981). Despite this formal action, most people continue to express unfavorable opinions and attitudes about homosexuals (Herek, 1984; Kite, 1984; Millham et al., 1976).

Bozett (1981, p. 552) points out that gay fathers have to meld two identities "that are at the opposite extremes of social acceptance: homosexuality at the negative extreme and fatherhood at the positive." Although many people do not realize that gay people may also be parents, the two roles are not mutually exclusive. Hoeffer cites Davies (1981, p. 536), who estimated that "1.5 million lesbian mothers reside with their children as a family unit in the United States." Accurate statistics on how many children have parents who are gay simply do not exist.

The information collected during nursing assessment derives partly from traditional concepts and norms that shape the definition of family—and is limited by them. Likewise, health care and social welfare policies are shaped by the beliefs that a family is composed of a husband with a wife and children, and that the father works and the mother stays home to raise the children (Moroney, 1980). Moroney suggested that contemporary definitions of family were generated to meet the needs of the bureaucrat or the professional. While valid and somewhat useful, such definitions have not always been relevant to social reality. Nevertheless, they are used to include or exclude families from services and benefits (Moroney, 1980).

The couple relationships, with or without children, that are formed by gay men and lesbians fall outside most definitions of family, although many agencies informally extend their definitions and practices in order to offer services to that population. Moroney (1980) advocates moving away from the tendency toward concrete definitions of family in favor of an approach recognizing variant family forms and thus strengthening the many such styles that exist. This approach would shift the emphasis of family from structural parameters to functional parameters, and it would at least create the possibility that any group functioning as a family could be treated as such by health and social service agencies. As it is, many agencies list every unmarried patient as single and may interact with that man or woman without ever determining whether the person is gay, has a lover-partner, or is truly single.

Most nursing staff, having had only limited contact with gay men and lesbians, know little about their life-styles. It is not surprising, then, that most of their concepts about homosexuality match the stereo-types of the masculine woman who hates men and the feminine man who hates women. In truth, gay men and women are as diverse in appearance, values, life-styles, religious beliefs, and other traits as heterosexuals.

Recent studies have begun to shed light on the characteristics of gay men, lesbians, and the couple relationships they form (Bell and Weinberg, 1978; Blumstein and Schwartz, 1983; Caldwell and Peplau, 1984; McWhirter and Mattison, 1984; Mendola, 1980; Tuller, 1978).

Gay men and lesbians display many characteristics and represent diverse life-styles. Educational, occupational, and income levels vary. Very few gay men or lesbians match the stereotypes of extreme masculinity (lesbian) or femininity (gay men).

Both gay men and lesbians value equal power distribution within a relationship. They are likely to divide household tasks according to likes and dislikes rather than any predetermined pattern. Neither gay women nor men use "role play" in their relationships; that is, neither tend to have one partner assume the role and duties of "wife" or "husband" (Tuller, 1978).

Both spend much of their leisure time together with their partners, which implies a friendship component of the relationship (Blumstein and Schwartz, 1983). In fact, studies have found that friendship is critical to the formation and maintenance of lesbian relationships. Often friendship relationships endure when couple relationships have ended (Vetere, 1983; Wolf, 1980). Gay men and women are more likely to have close friendships than are heterosexuals (Bell and Weinberg, 1978).

Both gay men and lesbians form long-term loving relationships. While the general impression is that lesbian couple relationships last longer than relationships between gay men, recent information challenges that belief (Blumstein and Schwartz, 1983; McWhirter and Mattison, 1984). In truth, the length of relationships is as varied as it is for heterosexual couples. Expectations that gay men and women hold for their partners do not differ appreciably from those of heterosexual men or women (Laner, 1977).

While most gay couples will not have children as part of their household, some will. The children may be from one partner's former marriage, or both partners' children may be living with their parents. In recent years, gay men have sought to adopt children; gay women have chosen to become pregnant and bear their own children (Tuller, 1978).

Traditionally, lesbians have established monogamous relationships that do not include the option of outside sex. Traditional gay relationships, however, did include the option of outside sex; this pattern is now being altered by the AIDS epidemic and the adaptations in sexual practice necessary to reduce the risk of contracting or spreading this illness (Tuller, 1978; "Gays Change," 1985).

Gay men and women who establish couple relationships have the same issues to contend with as their heterosexual counterparts: earning a living; maintaining a household; working out the intricacies of an intimate relationship; providing community service; and, sometimes, raising children.

Children in gay households. Few studies have examined the effects on growing children of living in a gay household. Those that have report generally healthy and well-adjusted children and describe gay households that compare favorably with heterosexual ones (Miller et al., 1981). Generally, comparative studies have established no differences in gender development, psychological pathology, or sex role behavior between children of lesbian and heterosexual mothers (Hoeffer, 1981; Kirkpatrick et al., 1981). Children living with a gay parent/lover pair encounter the same difficulties as other children with a stepparent. Children of lesbians, living with their mother and her lover, reported both problems and specific gains when they talked of learning about their mother's homosexuality and accepting her lover into the household (Lewis, 1980). Many gay and lesbian parents hide their homosexuality from their children because they fear rejection or court action to deny them access to their offspring. Learning of a parent's gay orientation is likely to be traumatic, but gradually children can accept this as they do other difficult news. The child's age influences what can be absorbed and adapted to. Lewis (1980) found many children of lesbians proud of their mothers for challenging society's rules. The child often becomes very attached to the lover-partner and accepts this person as a new parent. In such cases, facing the death of this person is both frightening and sad, especially when the child is a preadolescent whose understanding of death has progressed to accepting it as universal and personal (Gonda and Ruark, 1984; Swain, 1979).

Gay families and life-threatening illness. Typically, tasks for a family with preadolescent children revolve around providing a stable environment—a secure base from which children can begin to explore and thus increase their independence from the family, and from which the family itself can pursue change and growth. Life-threatening illness in one of the parents is a major threat to this stability. When the family consists of closeted lesbian parents, additional strains may be presented by the desire to cope with the illness without exposing sexual preferences.

Legal issues. The family that a nurse caring for a gay patient must assess, support, and mobilize often differs dramatically from the family as it is defined legally and by the community. The implications of this difference were apparent in a recent case in which a lesbian woman was paralyzed in a car accident. Nearly a year after the incident, the woman's parents obtained a court order to move her closer to their home, which was 150 miles away from the woman who had been living with their daughter for 4 years prior to the accident and visiting her daily since. The parents tried unsuccessfully to bar the lover from visiting their daughter ("Lover Sues Family," 1985). This type of conflict is not uncommon, and the legal definition of family offers the lover no rights, regardless of how long a couple have been together. Stanley Saul discovered this when he was threatened with the loss of the cooperative apartment he had shared with his lover for 11 years. The city of New York claimed that Stanley and his lover did not constitute a family, and therefore Stanley was not eligible to continue co-ownership after his lover died ("Gay Widows," 1980). Gay men and lesbians do not have the option of marriage by either license or common-law arrangement, and they are therefore vulnerable when "legal" family members assert their rights against the lover/partner's rights.

Nurses' attitudes. Health professionals' fears and misconceptions about homosexuality and how they are manifested in dealings with gay clients can constitute a real barrier to adequate health care for homosexuals. Cohn (1978) observed that she has "seen unnecessary frustration and anger in nurses dealing with 'uncooperative' patients and families when what was needed was not a change in the client, but a change in the way the nurse viewed him and the family."

Homophobia is the term applied to the fear of homosexuality (Weinberg, 1973). In a sense, most of the public can be thought of as being homophobic, in that most people are at least uneasy about homosexuality, and many are totally disapproving. Herek (1984) points out that one person can hold several attitudes toward gay men and lesbians, and those attitudes themselves may serve different functions. They may have formed from experience with gay men and lesbians and then become generalized to others; if the experiences were positive, the attitudes will be also. Another attitude may emerge as a defensive function and be linked with individual sexual security. This defensiveness is strongly linked with the homophobia; it implies that a person of insecure sexuality is threatened by homosexuality. The nurse who wishes to provide effective care and advocacy for the gay or lesbian family will need to recognize and confront any negative attitudes that might interfere with nursing practice.

The dying patient is also stigmatized, according to Epley and McCaghy (1977–78). While many writers through the 1970s (Brim et al., 1970; Glaser and Strauss, 1965; Quint, 1967) pointed out how staff and family avoided the person who was dying, a more current perspective is that avoidance and shame are no longer cornerstone characteristics of the dying process (Saunders and McCorkle, 1985).

Planning

Family considerations. Effective family intervention stems from ongoing assessment and planning; it is a partnership between nurse, patient, and family. Assessment includes identifying family strengths as well as potential problem areas and requires assistance from other sources. If the family is viewed as an interactive system, then assessment will include information about both individual members and the unit as a whole. The nurse must also determine the appropriate level of assessment. Some tools—for instance, the Family APGAR (Adaptation, Partnership, Growth, Affection, and Resolve)—are directed toward screening (Smilkstein, 1978) and are not meant to be used for comprehensive assessment. Recently, the Clinical Rating Scale for the Circumplex Model of Marital and Family Systems (Olson and Killorin, 1985) was designed for clinical assessment of family (couples or families with children) cohesion, adaptation, and communication. Its formal assessment tools, specially developed and already in existence, were designed for basically traditional families and would need to be evaluated before use with gay or lesbian couples and their children.

Patient and family assessment must be systematic and should consider the following areas (Benoliel, 1985):
• patient and family goals
• knowledge about the illness and treatment
• available support systems
• perceived relationships with health care providers
• environmental supports and barriers in the home
• patient physical status
• effects of disease and treatments on activities of daily living
• family accommodation to the illness.

When planning care in terminal cancer, the nurse must also consider the nature of the family, the role of stigma, the pattern of dying within the living-dying interval, and the symptoms associated with the expected metastasis.

Individuals should be asked about their own, as well as familywide, perceptions and needs. In the case study family, for example, Anna and Deb were each asked about their own goals and what they believed a family goal might be with regard to coping with Anna's illness. This identification of mutually agreed upon goals formed the base of planning the nursing interventions necessary to help this family cope with existing problems. The family's goal of being fully informed about the illness and its progression, for instance, led the nurse to plan patient education.

The impact of health care delivery changes. Despite recent technological advances and trends toward specialization that make a hospital the accepted place for death, it has once again become common to choose death at home. In response, there is a health care trend toward terminal care that blends humanism and technology and is provided by a partnership of families and experts (Saunders and McCorkle, 1985). This trend has been encouraged by advances in cancer care that allow patients longer lives. Two other factors have also been instrumental in increasing the amount of home care: increased medical costs and the movement toward prospective payments to finance them. A by-product of prospective payment is shorter hospital stays for acute care.

In Anna and Deb's case, personal reasons were instrumental in the decision to care for Anna at home. Neither woman had ever felt comfortable in hospitals, and they feared that they would not be able to maintain the personal environment they could at home. Both were also concerned about negative staff attitudes toward their lesbianism.

The nurse planning home care needed to consider available resources for physical care and devise strategies to coordinate personal and community resources that would meet needs without duplicating effort. Physically, the home environment needed evaluation to ensure that it could be modified as Anna's needs changed. Health care staff needed to be willing to support the family's strengths and autonomy and to work from educative and consultative roles more than as direct care providers. The nurse also initiated assessment of care providers' attitudes toward and knowledge about homosexuality to avoid unnecessary barriers to home care.

Intervention

Indications and contraindications for family intervention. Before intervening with a family caring for a terminally ill person, the nurse must be sure intervention is actually needed and is provided at a level appropriate to both problem and family. For example, if the home care patient becomes unable to meet personal hygiene needs, the nurse can arrange for someone such as a home health aide to provide bed baths. But first the nurse should determine if the family can provide similar care with its own resources or support network. In the latter case, the appropriate intervention might be to teach the family what it needs to know about bathing someone who is bedridden.

A second requirement of family intervention is that the intervention be consistent with the family's coping style, not superimposed from the health care provider's value system. For example, Deb had obtained permission to spend the night after surgery in her lover's hospital room, but the night nurse made her leave because "You aren't family."

The example cited above leads to the major contraindication for nursing intervention with gay families: negative attitudes toward homosexuality or toward gay men and women. Patients and families need their energy to cope with a terminal illness, not hostile staff; they need care from sensitive and responsive personnel.

Intervening at diagnosis. Types of intervention used to help Anna and her family cope with her diagnosis included:
• using communication skills to facilitate information processing and emotional response management
• determining who should be present when Anna was told of her diagnosis and its implications
• developing trust within the helping relationship
• monitoring ongoing emotional response
• providing adequate information to help the patient choose among diagnostic and treatment alternatives
• helping Anna learn to maintain family integrity during interactions with health care personnel.

Unlike the climate of a few years ago, there is today no question of whether or not to tell the patient that an illness is potentially terminal. The question now is how much to tell, to whom, and in what order. Anna and Deb were together when the physician told them that the second tumor was malignant and deeply embedded, and that Anna also had some lymph node involvement. She also told them together that although the condition was serious, she could not be sure what it meant without further information. The physician arranged for further tests and arranged to see both women again in a few days.

Anna and Deb had made it clear to the physician that both wanted and expected full information. Other gay or lesbian couples might handle information differently, and their preference should be determined before explanations are offered. The identified patient has the right to full information from the health care staff and may or may not choose to share it with a lover-partner. Information processing styles vary as much among gay couples as they do among heterosexuals.

The initial shock of learning about a terminal illness can result in memory distortion or even complete amnesia regarding certain parts of the interview. Once the health care provider has determined whether to break the news about the diagnosis to the patient alone or to include the lover-partner, the question of how much to say remains to be dealt with. The person—physician or nurse—breaking the news should use simple language, explain all technical terms, and provide opportunities for the patient to clarify what he or she is hearing. Adequate time is critical. Communication skills must be used both to facilitate information processing and manage emotional response if the nurse is to ensure effective intervention during these early encounters (Gonda and Ruark, 1984).

If the patient has included the lover in the interview, then the health provider must ensure that both are hearing the necessary information and that both are allowed to react openly and receive support. A health professional who is judgmental about homosexuality will find it difficult to offer adequate support at this time, to answer questions, if possible, to help the couple plan for the next few days' diagnostic activities and decision making about further treatment, and, perhaps most importantly, to convey hope. One key to balancing hope and realism is to focus on the short term and the achievement of immediate goals (Gonda and Ruark, 1984). If the couple have children, the nurse might also help them determine how to break the news.

The diagnostic impact continues beyond the initial breaking of the news; typical initial responses of shock and emotional numbness often yield to distinct, strong emotions that were not so apparent while shock prevailed. While no specific set of emotions is sure to apppear, fear, anger, helplessness, and sadness are all common responses. Often, the health professional can help by reassuring clients that their responses are normal. If any of these negative feelings become misdirected toward the partner, direct intervention can help the client express feelings without alienating the person whose support is needed. The nurse dealing with a gay family must be particularly perceptive, since clients' distrust of the established health care system and its representatives might lead them to hide their reactions.

Gaining trust during the impact stage is a critical task for the health professional, but it may take more care and planning with the gay or lesbian client than is customary with clients who are not gay men or women. Any evidence of negative attitudes or homophobia will block the relationship; staff holding such views must acknowledge them openly and either alter their attitudes or refer the gay patient to a colleague.

While still grappling with the initial impact of the diagnosis, clients will also probably have to decide about treatments or further diagnostic work requiring hospitalization. It is important to reinforce to gay men and women, as early as possible, that their relationship has no legal sanction and to help them identify available, desirable protection. For example, if Anna had required surgery and been unable to give consent, Deb could not legally have taken responsibility; the nurse would have had to contact Anna's brother, Dave. While the attending physician and other health staff might be willing to acknowledge informally Anna and Deb's relationship, they must remain aware that Dave is legally responsible. The nurse might advise legal consultation to help gay couples avoid complications in the particular jurisdiction. Common options for lesbian couples to consider are power of attorney, guardianship, or durable power of attorney.

Intervening at the metastatic phase. The types of interventions used to help Anna and her family adapt to metastasis crisis and the knowledge of terminality included:
• educating the staff; helping reduce negative attitudes and stereotypes
• helping Anna and her family formulate goals
• establishing a care contract with Anna and her family
• supporting family strengths and facilitating Anna's control of her situation
• coordinating information flow and interpretation
• screening community resources and making appropriate referrals
• monitoring symptoms, interpreting them to Anna, and planning interventions for symptom control
• facilitating family communication
• helping the family anticipate and plan for role adjustments
• seeking information about appropriate resources within the gay/lesbian community.

Most terminally ill patients have time to adapt to living with their chronic illness, its treatments, and the adaptations of daily routine associated with chronic care. Anna really did not have this time. About 3 weeks after the melanoma was diagnosed as life threatening, she learned that no direct treatment was likely to stop its growth. Diagnostic tests indicated metastasis, and another melanoma—pinpoint sized—had appeared on her leg. While the physician had made Anna aware from the outset that her illness was life threatening, this was her first confrontation with certain terminality.

The physician offered little hope for reversing the disease process but believed effective treatment could retard its progress. Anna began a series of appointments at a specialized cancer center, where findings had supported her oncologist's conclusions and recommendations. While surgery had not been completely ruled out, the team of specialists seemed more inclined toward a combination of still-experimental drugs.

During these early weeks, as Anna began to realize that she was going to die from her illness, Deb continued to talk of finding some way to overcome it. Tricia had become quieter and seemed less involved in the family than usual. Anna and Deb finished teaching and had the summer off. Tricia's school was finished for the year as well. Toward the end of May, both Anna and Deb began to understand that they did not have much time to spend together and began struggling with how they wanted to use the weeks they had left. Meeting with the nurse at the cancer center, they set the following goals:
• Anna should keep functioning and enjoying life as much as possible.
• Anna and Deb should remain informed about expected symptoms and problems so they could make informed treatment decisions.

- Tricia should be included in whatever happened and not feel shut out (as she had so far).
- The family should remain close, facing things together.
- Anna should receive care and die at home, not in the hospital.

The nurse agreed with these goals and arranged to help meet them by assessing the family unit's information needs. The family agreed to identify areas of confusion as they arose and allow the nurse to clarify. Several staff-family sessions were scheduled to help assess information processing and decision making and identify useful communication strategies. An important intervention during these sessions was to help family members progress at their own rates and assimilate information in their own most effective fashions. Tricia and Anna arranged time together for reading, shopping, and other pastimes. In order to maintain their level of closeness, Anna and Deb needed information about what sexual practices they could safely continue, but they did not feel comfortable discussing these concerns with the cancer center staff. Therefore, the nurse called the local Gay and Lesbian Community Support Center for referral. This willingness to admit knowledge and skill limitations and to refer to the appropriate resources was a critical step valuable in establishing nurse-patient trust. The nurse suggested Anna and Deb see the team social worker for assessment of personal support and community resources.

Past studies have shown that, while many nurses and other health care providers do hold negative attitudes toward homosexuality, those attitudes are amenable to change with appropriate education (Anderson, 1982). One laboratory technician and nurse demonstrated negative attitudes and some fear when providing home services to Anna, a fact that Deb reported to the nurse coordinator. The nurse recognized that staff members had very limited experience with gay men and women, so she asked the nursing education department to arrange classes in which staff could explore their attitudes and learn about gay and lesbian life-styles.

It soon became clear that Anna's energy level was decreasing and that the illness was progressing at a faster rate than expected. While Deb and Anna continued to explore the possibility of chemotherapy, several weeks elapsed without initiation. During that time, Anna developed new symptoms: appetite disturbance, headaches, depression, and generalized discomfort and malaise. Several more melanomas appeared. A health staff team meeting confirmed the unusually rapid disease progression; subsequent patient and family meetings yielded a renewed contract emphasizing symptom management to facilitate maintenance of independent functioning; agreement on areas in which the core family and personal support network members would assume new responsibilities; and staff support of Anna's decision to die at home rather than in the hospital. These goals necessitated planning for the variety of measures that might be needed, training family and support persons, and adapting the home environment for Anna.

Several excellent community groups exist to help patients and families cope with a terminal illness. Unfortunately, however, few are designed to receive gay men or lesbians, and those communities with such support groups generally have not developed any focusing on terminal illness. Before referring gay families to existing community groups for assistance, the nurse must check the groups' composition and experience with and attitudes concerning homosexuality. These are not the proper circumstances for gay men or women to have to educate others about their life-styles.

Intervening at the terminal phase of the illness. The interventions used to help Anna and her family cope with the terminal phase of the illness included:
• revising the contract to incorporate new problems
• assessing and adapting the home care environment
• identifying personal support network resources for help with home care
• teaching nursing care skills to involved family and support persons
• helping the family maintain privacy and intimacy
• monitoring symptoms and initiating measures to control them
• keeping the family informed
• coordinating care among health care workers and the personal support network
• facilitating expression of existential and spiritual concerns
• helping Anna and her family plan for death, the memorial service, and so forth.

In July, at home, Anna had two grand mal seizures. Too nauseated to take medication orally, she required brief hospitalization until the seizures could be controlled. Tests indicated further, extensive metastasis to many vital organs, including the brain, and that death was probably near. Anna agreed to a limited course of radiation therapy to try to control the seizure activity. While the revised diagnosis changed few of the contracted goals, new activities were necessary to meet them successfully. Goals for the terminal phase follow:
• Return Anna home and continue necessary care from there.
• Arrange care to preserve some family routines and allow Deb some respite.
• Keep the family sufficiently informed.
• Control symptoms to allow Anna as much independent functioning as possible.

- Begin confronting the details of dying: make out a will, arrange a memorial service program.
- Stay involved in the present; do not constantly try to outguess the future.

Only a few physical changes were necessary for Anna to be cared for at home. A bedroom and a bathroom were already located on ground level; the nursing staff had already taught Deb to give injections and suppositories when vomiting prevented oral medication. Necessary assistance was available from willing friends, who met with the nurse to help coordinate their direct care activities. Deb's sister, Amy, came to stay and help, immediately assuming responsibility for telephone messages. The nurse's role as coordinator became progressively more complex as she needed to synchronize the health care team, family, and friends. The additional assistance also threatened to disrupt family routines and privacy, so efforts were made to preserve time for core family activities. Cancer center educational materials provided useful information about burial options, memorial services, funerals, and so on, but the information about wills did not address the particular needs of the gay family. Fortunately, friends were able to identify helpful resources within the lesbian community. The nurse planned frequent contacts with the family so she could monitor potentially problematic symptoms and develop early and flexible interventions. Professional assistance was accessible around the clock, if needed.

Home routines were preserved: Anna, Deb, and Tricia tried to share at least one meal a day, although Anna was not always able to be at the table. Anna continued to be involved in daily decision making, and friends were encouraged to continue visiting and interacting as they always had; this involved a lot of touching and hugging that Anna enjoyed even more as her own movements became more constrained. These friends immediately established a visiting schedule and also arranged to spend time with Tricia, which allowed Anna and Deb privacy.

Anna, Deb, and Tricia were provided opportunities to privately share individual questions and concerns with the nurse. During one such session, Anna talked about her lack of readiness for dying and her spiritual concerns. The nurse explored this area and discovered that Anna and Deb had occasionally attended Metropolitan Community Church activities, and she encouraged Anna to ask one of its ministers to come talk with her.

Anna lapsed into a coma during the first week of August and died three days later. Friends helped Deb make the necessary notifications and arrange for a memorial service.

Intervening during the bereavement process. The nurse helped Deb and Tricia through the bereavement process by:
• monitoring mood, practical problems, and access to physical comforting
• guiding them through painful memories and affect, as well as helping them appreciate successes
• teaching about bereavement
• being alert to such problems as substance abuse, depression/suicide, or stalled grief
• helping the family maintain open communication and encouraging different expressions of grief
• helping them use their personal support networks
• helping them find new meaning in life and shift back to a single identity.

Deb became fairly depressed after Anna's death. She resumed teaching in September but engaged in few activities outside of work. Friends continued to call and visit. Deb said her life had lost all meaning and joy, and while she knew she needed to offer more to Tricia, she did not have the energy to do more than meet daily requirements.

The cancer center's primary bereavement resource was a support social worker, but Deb did not feel comfortable attending meetings at the center. The center did have a follow-up service through which staff called at intervals to see how families were doing and to refer them for assistance if needed.

Marris (1974, p. 33) discussed the loss of meaning that bereaved persons experience: "To say that life has lost its meaning is not . . . just a way of expressing apathy. It describes a situation where someone is bereft of purpose, and so feels helpless." Within a few weeks after Anna's death, Deb's friends began to urge her to put the summer behind her and start becoming involved in current activities. Deb felt awkward with her friends. Being with other couples was painful, and sometimes she resented that they were still alive to enjoy each other, while she was alone. She began to avoid her friends and refused most invitations.

The nurse who called Deb at the 6 weeks' telephone check-in was concerned enough to arrange a second call at 3 months. From those two conversations, it was apparent that Deb needed help with her grief, and she was referred to a clinical specialist. The following goals were established during the appointment:
• Deb would go on without Anna and find some meaning in life.
• Deb would find the energy to meet her responsibilities and to be available for Tricia.

- Deb's sadness would pass; she and Tricia would begin doing things together again.
- Deb would settle the details left after Anna's death (such as disposing of personal belongings and transferring the deed to the house).

Fortunately, Deb and Anna had bought the house together, so Deb's claim to the house was not vulnerable to challenge; other arrangements, made with an attorney early in Anna's illness, further simplified the rearrangement of property rights. Because of her depression, Deb had very little energy, most of which was expended just getting through the workday. The clinician arranged periodic meetings with Deb and Tricia to explore feelings and help them plan and find support. Deb also needed help establishing her identity as a single person (Saunders, 1981) and maintaining connections with her personal support network (Siegal and Hoefer, 1981). This support was even more critical since Deb was not open about her lesbianism at work and therefore lacked colleague support in the loss of her lover-partner.

Saunders (1986) identifies these important nursing interventions for use with bereaved gays and lesbians:
- monitoring the client's mood (confronting practical problems and having access to physical touch can be important factors)
- providing counseling to help guide clients through painful memories and affect and help them identify successes
- teaching the client about bereavement.

Successful bereavement resolution often cannot be confirmed for up to 2 years after a spouse's death. There are many problem areas the nurse should be wary of, including substance abuse, depression/suicide, and stalled grief. The gay and lesbian communities are beginning to develop resources to assist with bereavement because of the AIDS epidemic, but these resources are still scarce and unevenly distributed.

Holidays, birthdays, and anniversaries are particularly difficult for bereaved families. The nurse should help members anticipate and plan for such events. Deb and Tricia needed to face the family holidays of Thanksgiving and Christmas soon after Anna's death and had to decide whether to spend them together at home, with friends, or separately, with Tricia visiting her father.

Bereavement progress is slow and often painful. A critical factor is the ability to reassess and reassign meanings to relationships and events (Saunders, 1986; Marris, 1974). Ultimately, Marris (1974) tells us, "grief is mastered, not by ceasing to care for the dead, but by abstracting what was fundamentally important in the relationship and rehabilitating it."

Evaluation

Goals developed mutually by nurse and family are the keys to determining effectiveness of nursing interventions with gay families facing life-threatening illness. Appropriate and comprehensive goals provide a major judgment standard for individual and family nursing alike. Benoliel (1985) also indicates that risk factors identified within the specific situation, along with the interventions nurses use to offset those factors, provide another set of criteria to use in judging care effectiveness.

Care should be evaluated several times during treatment and for at least a year after the patient dies. Appropriate intervals might be immediately after death and 6 and 13 months afterward (the latter to determine how the family has weathered the anniversary of the death). This allows adjustment if goals are not being attained or risks not managed.

No reported research has dealt specifically with gay families who are struggling to deal with a life-threatening illness, or about the interventions that are used to help them through this stressful process.

CONCLUSIONS

Gay men and women form enduring attachments and can rightfully be called "couples" and "families." When a life-threatening illness affects gay or lesbian families, nonhomophobic assistance is necessary to help them through the death and bereavement processes. Staff can learn about gay and lesbian life-styles and mobilize appropriate community resources to help the family through the illness. Since legal definitions of family block gay couples' access to standard resources, the nurse must be alert to ways to modify existing support or find alternative resources.

REFERENCES

Anderson, C.L. "The Effect of a Workshop on Attitudes of Female Nursing Students Toward Male Homosexuality," *Journal of Homosexuality* 7(1):57-59, 1982.

Bayer, R. *Homosexuality and American Psychiatry: The Politics of Diagnosis.* New York: Basic Books, 1981.

Bell, A.P., and Weinberg, M.S. *Homosexualities: A Study of Diversity among Men and Women.* New York: Simon & Schuster, 1978.

Benoliel, J.Q. "Loss and Terminal Illness," *Nursing Clinics of North America* 20(2):439–48, June 1985.

Blumstein, P., and Schwartz, P. *American Couples.* New York: William Morrow & Co., 1983.

Bozett, F.W. "Gay Fathers: Evolution of the Gay-Father Identity," *American Journal of Orthopsychiatry* 51(3):552–59, 1981.

Breslow, A. "Thickness, Cross-Sectional Areas, and Depth of Invasion in the Diagnosis of Cutaneous Melanoma," *Annals of Surgery* 1272:902–08, 1970.

Brim, O.G., et al., eds. *The Dying Patient.* New York: Russell Sage Foundation, 1970.

Caldwell, M.A., and Peplau, L.A. "The Balance of Power in Lesbian Relationships," *Journal of Homosexuality* 10(7/8):587–99, 1984.

Cohn, L. "Barriers and Values in the Nurse/Client Relationship," *ARN* 3–8, 1978.

Epley, R.J., and McCaghy, C.H. "The Stigma of Dying: Attitudes Toward the Terminally Ill," *Omega* 8(4):379–93, 1977–78.

Friedman, R.J., et al. "Early Detection of Malignant Melanoma: The Role of Physician Examination and Self-Examination of the Skin," *Ca-A Cancer Journal for Clinicians* 35(3):130–51, 1985.

"Gays Change Sex Practice to Avoid AIDS," *Seattle Times,* October 20, 1985.

"Gay Widows," *Christopher Street* 19–24, February 1980.

Glaser, B., and Strauss, A. *Awareness of Dying.* Chicago: Aldine Publishing Co., 1965.

Gonda, T.A., and Ruark, J.E. *Dying Dignified: The Health Professional's Guide to Care.* Menlo Park, Calif.: Addison Wesley Publishing Co., 1984.

Gutterman, J.U., and Scher, H.I. "Melanoma," in *Cancer Medicine.* Edited by Holland, J., and Frei, E. Philadelphia: Lea & Febiger, 1982.

Herek, G.M. "Beyond Homophobia: A Social Psychological Perspective on Attitudes Toward Lesbians and Gay Men," *Journal of Homosexuality* 9(1):1–21, 1984.

Hoeffer, B. "Children's Acquisition of Sex-Role Behavior in Lesbian-Mother Families," *American Journal of Orthopsychiatry* 5(3):536–44, 1981.

Kane, R.A., and Kane, R.L. *Assessing the Elderly: A Practical Guide to Measurement.* Lexington, Mass.: Lexington Books, 1981.

Kirkpatrick, M., et al. "Lesbian Mothers and Their Children: A Comparative Survey," *American Journal of Orthopsychiatry* 5(3):545–51, 1981.

Kite, M.E. "Sex Differences in Attitudes Toward Homosexuals: A Metaanalytic Review," *Journal of Homosexuality* 9(1):69–81, 1984.

Laner, M.R. "Permanent Partner Priorities: Gay and Straight," *Journal of Homosexuality* 3(1):21–39, 1977.

Lewis, K.G. "Children of Lesbians: Their Point of View," *Social Work* 198–203, 1980.

Marris, P. *Loss and Change.* New York: Pantheon Books, 1974.

McWhirter, D.P., and Mattison, A.M. *The Male Couple: How Relationships Develop.* Englewood Cliffs, N.J.: Prentice-Hall, 1984.

Mendola, M. *The Mendola Report: A New Look at Gay Couples.* New York: Crown Publishing, 1980.

Miller, J.A., et al. "The Child's Home Environment for Lesbian vs. Heterosexual Mothers: A Neglected Area of Research," *Journal of Homosexuality* 7(1):49–56, 1981.

Millham, J., et al. "A Factor-Analytic Conceptualization of Attitudes Toward Male and Female Homosexuals," *Journal of Homosexuality* 2(1):3–10, 1976.

Moroney, R.M. *Families, Social Services, and Social Policy: The Issue of Shared Responsibility.* Rockville, Md.: U.S. Department of Health and Human Services, National Institutes of Mental Health, 1980.

"Lover Sues Family," *Off Our Backs,* June 1985.

Olson, D.H., and Killorin, E. "Clinical Rating Scale for the Circumplex Model of Marital and Family Systems," St. Paul: Department of Family Social Science, University of Minnesota, 1985.

Quint, J.C. "The Dying Patient: A Difficult Nursing Problem," *Nursing Clinics of North America* (2):763–73, 1967.

Saunders, J.M. "A Process of Bereavement Resolution: Uncoupled Identity," *Western Journal of Nursing Research* 3(4):319–32, 1981.

Saunders, J.M. "Gay and Lesbian Widowhood," in *Helping Your Gay and Lesbian Client: A Psychosocial Approach from Gay and Lesbian Perspectives.* Edited by Kus, B. Boston: Alyson Publications, 1986.

Saunders, J.M., and McCorkle, R. "Models of Care for Persons with Progressive Cancer," *Nursing Clinics of North America* 20(2):365–77, June 1985.

Siegal, R.L., and Hoefer, D.D. "Bereavement Counseling for Gay Individuals," *American Journal of Psychotherapy* 35(4):517–25, 1981.

Smilkstein, G. "A Proposal for a Family Function Test and Its Use by Physicians," *Journal of Family Practice* 6:1231–39, 1978.

Swain, H.L. "Childhood View of Death," *Death Education* 2:341–58, 1979.

Tuller, N.R. "Couples: The Hidden Segment of the Gay World," *Journal of Homosexuality* 3(4):331–43, 1978.

Vetere, V.A. "The Role of Friendship in the Development and Maintenance of Lesbian Love Relationships," *Journal of Homosexuality* 8(2):51–65, 1983.

Weinberg, G. *Society and the Healthy Homosexual.* Garden City, N.Y.: Anchor Books, 1973.

Wolf, D.G. *The Lesbian Community.* Berkeley, Calif.: University of California Press, 1980.

23 Intervening with single-parent families and multiple trauma

Carol Dashiff, RN, CS, MN, PhD
Associate Professor of Mental Health Nursing
Chair, Department of Mental Health and
    Organizational Behavior
School of Nursing
Vanderbilt University
Nashville, Tennessee

OVERVIEW

This chapter focuses on the special characteristics of single-parent families and the issues they face when a life-threatening situation arises early in the family life cycle. The characteristics of single parenting, multiple trauma, and families with young children are reviewed and provide the context within which assessment, planning, intervention, and evaluation are discussed. Special emphasis is given to strength assessment and recognition. Intervention is discussed from both critical care and outpatient perspectives.

CASE STUDY

Ms. Rangely, age 26, was admitted to the intensive care unit (ICU) following an auto accident—a head-on collision with a drunk driver whose car had crossed the median—during her drive to work. She suffered skull injuries, severe facial trauma, tendon and nerve lacerations of her right wrist, laceration of the globe of her left eye, and a fractured mandible. A tracheostomy was done to prevent respiratory distress from tissue damage and fractures.

Two days after admission, the patient was referred to the liaison nurse specialist by the head ICU nurse. The primary nurse was concerned about Ms. Rangely's extreme wariness of hospital procedures and equipment, her absence of family visitors, and her insistence on pushing herself to physical limits to perform self-care.

Assessment
Because of Ms. Rangely's limited communication and high potential for fatigue, the initial interview centered around three priority areas: client understanding of detailed events from the time of the accident to the present, the accident's family context, and any immediate preoccupations and concerns that would affect treatment or recovery. In addition, permission was obtained to contact a female friend, who visited the patient daily.

Oral communication with Ms. Rangely was impossible and written communication was limited (she was right-handed); limited visual function left her reliant on hearing and touch for stimulation. The interviewing nurse used closed questions, so Ms. Rangely could respond by signaling with her left hand. She indicated on a map where various family members lived. The genogram in Figure 23.1 illustrates her family structure.

Ms. Rangely had no contact with her former husband, whom she had divorced 2 years previously after he deserted the family. His location was unknown and he provided no financial support. Her two children were currently staying with the friend who had visited her. The patient herself was the youngest of three children; her mother and sister lived in nearby cities. Her unmarried brother was in the air force, stationed in England.

Figure 23.1 Genogram—The Rangely Family

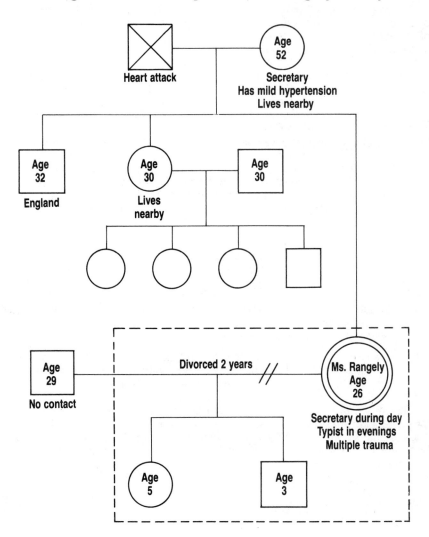

Ms. Rangely's mother had resumed work as a secretary 2 years previously to support herself following her husband's sudden death from a heart attack. She had recently been diagnosed as mildly hypertensive. The patient's sister was married and had recently had her fourth child.

The patient's friend reported that Ms. Rangely worked very hard to support her two children, holding a secretarial job by day and typing at home in the evenings. She had been reluctant to contact her family for financial or emotional support during the past 2 years because she had not wanted to impose additional burdens. She thought her family members, particularly the women, were stressed enough. At the same time, she was the person her siblings and mother called first when they were having difficulties. She was an attractive woman who took great pride in her appearance. Her friend was a major source of day-to-day emotional and instrumental support. (Ms. Rangely later corroborated the above information.)

Ms. Rangely remembered nothing about the accident or her time in the emergency room. She expressed the following concerns: fear about the impact of her appearance and limitations on her children, whom she had not seen since the accident; worry about her mother's emotional response and health should she be told about the extent of the injuries; and uncertainty about possible limitation of her future functioning. She was relieved to be alive and she felt relatively well, but her inner strength did not match her physical capacity; she had not yet been able to look at herself.

Planning and Intervention

Intervention for Ms. Rangely was aimed, initially, at helping her mobilize her family supports in anticipation of a prolonged (several-month) recovery. The liaison nurse met with the patient and her friend, who, at the patient's request, served as her initial spokesperson with the family. At first, in an effort to conserve resources, the patient wanted to put off approaching the family members, anticipating that she would need their help more after leaving the hospital. She also feared her condition would be too stressful for family members to tolerate.

Together, the patient, friend, and primary nurse devised and discussed various interventions and strategies for accurately informing family members. The patient decided to contact her brother (through her friend) first, thinking him the least reactive and therefore best able to convey information to the others calmly. In addition, he had no family responsibilities, was in good health, and, though at considerable distance, had been readily available during previous family crises.

Because of the patient's need to maintain self-control at this time, the nurse decided to teach her about typical responses to life-threatening health crises and about adaptation phases. This was done to help Ms. Rangely help her family members; it was anticipated that she would later use this information to recognize her own responses. Her brother and friend were both included in these teaching sessions. The patient was encouraged to validate her ideas about the family with her brother, working toward the goals of identifying members' strengths and formulating specific requests she might make of them in meeting the current crisis.

The nurse, Ms. Rangely, and Ms. Rangely's friend visited with all family members on the seventh day of hospitalization in order to introduce everyone involved to the reality of the situation. The family members were told what to expect when they saw Ms. Rangely; after 30 minutes with the primary nurse, they were joined by the physician, who answered questions. Later in the day, the liaison nurse met with family members and the patient, encouraging each to talk about his reactions to the patient's injuries and about his thoughts and feelings about the accident's effect on the family. The patient took this opportunity to share her wish that family members could help in different ways, at different times, to relieve the burden on any one relative.

With assistance, Ms. Rangely could communicate with her children. Her friend took pictures of her, the hospital room, and the medical equipment; Ms. Rangely wrote brief descriptive and personal notes to each child on the backs. The friend gave these to the children and answered their questions. The children also took photographs and sent them to their mother. As extended family members arrived, they were invited to take part in both aspects of this process, facilitating direct communication with the children. The liaison nurse also made a home visit to assess how the children were doing and to reinforce the reality of their mother's situation and eventual return home.

Evaluation

Once the initial interventions were implemented, the family appeared to engage in ongoing direct communication and joint problem solving without direct nursing assistance. Nevertheless, at the end of the third week of hospitalization, after the children had visited their mother, the liaison nurse arranged a session to determine family progress in understanding the traumatic event and injury and to help members put the accident into perspective. Ms. Rangely could talk at this meeting.

All family members were able to verbalize what this crisis had meant to them, identify positive aspects of the experience, and attend to what the others had to say. The family appeared to be handling the life-threatening event positively.

In a follow-up meeting 5 months after the accident, the patient was ambulating unassisted and using her energy primarily for care of herself and her children. Altered visual perception disturbed Ms. Rangely's sense of balance, and she had to relearn to walk. Housework was being done by a home health aide, and Ms. Rangely's mother and sister visited on alternate weekends. She reported that the experience of dealing with her family members and requesting their help had led her to a new appreciation of them; moreover, for the first time, she heard them acknowledge directly their own appreciation of her.

Ms. Rangely wished that she had been helped more directly to talk—when she could—about her anger at being a victim, but she felt that dealing with this initially would have made her feel too vulnerable. She was still learning to cope and had been reluctant to go outside before receiving an artificial eye, but support and encouragement from her family allowed her to gradually resume previous social relationships. The hardest thing, she said, was "being young and living life slow and having to learn all over again to do things I had taken for granted."

NURSING PROCESS

Assessment

The health problem: Traumatic injury. More than 68 million persons
annually are affected by traumatic injury (Boyd, 1982); indeed, trauma
is one of the most common causes of death in the United States, sur-
passed only by cancer and cardiovascular disease. Most severe trauma
results from motor vehicle or automobile/pedestrian accidents, both
of which inflict multisystem injuries that are difficult to manage and
have high mortality rates (Fought and Throwe, 1984). Physical assault
resulting in multiple trauma can also occur in certain occupational
settings where heavy equipment may crush or sever body parts, explo-
sive accidents may occur, or workers might fall from great heights.
The most common type of trauma is "blunt" trauma, in which the critical damage is covert. Even when loss of life, bodily function, and
work hours alone is considered, the financial and emotional costs of
trauma are great. Added to this are the costs of highly complex technological intervention, medical and nursing care, and patient rehabilitation.

Single-parent families
Prevalence and economic implications. In 1980, there were 8.5 million
single-parent families in the United States; they represented 17.5% of
all families (Hoeker, 1983), a 79% increase since 1970. Approximately
80% of these families were headed by a female (Duffy, 1982).

In 1979, 73% of working female household heads held low-paying
clerical or service jobs with inadequate benefits and few opportunities
for mobility (Morawetz and Walker, 1984). In 1980, single-parent,
female-headed families accounted for 50% of all poor families (Francke,
1983). Single women and their children are expected to constitute all
of the nation's poor by the year 2000 (National Advisory Council on
Economic Opportunity, 1983).

In 1980, the overall median family income was $21,020 and the
median for male single-parent families was $17,519. In comparison,
female single parents earned $10,400. Single mothers with children
under 6 are even harder pressed financially, with an average 1979
income of only $4,500 (Duffy, 1982).

Most single mothers receive little or no financial help from the absent
father. Child support is awarded to only 59% of women bringing up
children alone, and only 35% actually receive it. The average payment
amounts to $1,800/year, not enough to offset the drop in living stan-
dards experienced by most divorced mothers (Morawetz and Walker,
1984).

Social status. Social reaction to the single parent can be affected by the circumstances that resulted in the parent's being alone. Death of a spouse is generally viewed as uncontrollable and tends to generate sympathy. Divorce is considered a more controllable situation and implies failure (Duffy, 1982); it is viewed as more traumatic to children because, unlike death, separation is not final or definitive (Collison and Futrell, 1982). Moreover, in divorce, children are more likely to be viewed as negative remnants of the marriage (Collison and Futrell, 1982). Adams et al. (1984), however, cite findings that a woman with sufficient economic resources to head a household can avoid many of the negative corollaries often associated with father absence. Research also indicates that divorce can actually benefit the child who has been living in a home characterized by marital strife.

Single-parent families headed by never-married females are likely to experience the severest financial difficulties and to stand the lowest in social esteem. Nevertheless, the numbers of such families are increasing, with out-of-wedlock birthrates rising much faster among whites than among blacks (Godenne, 1977). In contrast to white women, fewer black women marry to legitimize their babies and more keep their babies after birth. Yet black women more often maintain ties with the child's father after the birth (Pope, 1969).

The extended kinship system found in many single-parent black families, however, may not function as a support system. According to Pattison (1979), a chronic lack of reciprocity of affective and instrumental functions within such families may indicate the need to mobilize community systems.

Regardless of the etiology of single motherhood, the single-parent family is regarded and is tolerated in American society as only a temporary state. Popular literature describing "broken homes" and "latch key children" continues despite the increasing presence of the single parent.

Parent-child relationships. According to Eiduson (1983), the stresses common in single-parent families relate primarily to isolation and to a lack of satisfying social interaction. These households are characterized by more frequent change than any other type of family. Single-parent families, though not necessarily experiencing the greatest amount of external stress, appear most vulnerable to its effect.

While single parents are clearly at risk for stress, pathological outcomes for children are neither inevitable nor characteristic. Indeed, single mothers' potential to overcome major economic and social obstacles and incorporate these positive developments into their self-views is attested to by those who work with them (Miller, 1982; Wortman, 1981). Moreover, numerous design errors have been identified in studies that have reported increased risk among children with one parent (Blechman, 1982). For nurses, the message is clear: assess each family's strengths.

While research indicates that children of single parents do not differ significantly in the security of their attachments from either other children of nontraditional families or those of traditional two-parent families (Eiduson, 1983), there are indications that the single parent's child relationships are more intense (Weiss, 1985; Morawetz and Walker, 1984). The absence of a spouse or partner can easily make raising children the single parent's most important goal. Single parents seem particularly alert to their children's emotional status. "They want their children to have lives no less secure, no less protected, and no less gratifying than those of other children. And since they feel their children may have been exposed to special stress, they monitor their children's responses" (Weiss, 1985, p. 489). The nurse needs to recognize the feelings and ideas of single parents and develop a thorough understanding of their family characteristics in order not to label certain adaptive parent-child behaviors as deviant. These families should never be judged according to traditional family standards and operations.

Authority structure. The single-parent family also tends to differ structurally from the traditional family unit. Most two-parent families operate under an "echelon structure," an arrangement in which there is an implicit partnership agreement among those on the superordinate level that gives them authority over those on a lower level. Without a second parent the echelon structure collapses and a new relationship system develops in which children have responsibilities and rights similar to those of parents.

> The parents are often unaware of how the structure of their household has changed. They may recognize that they are closer to their children and rely more on them than they had when they were married, but they are less likely to recognize that their family is no longer hierarchical, and that they have shared with their children some of their decision-making responsibilities as well as responsibilities for specific chores. They may, therefore, be uncertain how to respond to others who say they overindulge their children, that they are too permissive, and that their children are not deferential enough (Weiss, 1985, p. 498).

This is a particular problem when members of the extended family and network systems have had no experience with single parenting (Table 23.1).

Table 23.1   Problems of Single-Parent Families

Common problems (Morawetz and Walker, 1984)	• Perception of the child as a reminder of the absent parent • Parental overattachment to the child • Perception of child care as an overwhelming burden • Lost perspective leading to magnification of minor developmental problems • Feelings of guilt impeding normal function • Parental attempts to deal with the anxiety of reentering social life through the child • Parental overdependence on the family of origin
Problems requiring long-term work and/or support	• Emotional cutoffs from the family of origin • Failure of family members to support the single parent emotionally in the face of frequent support of family members by the single parent • Major changes in the life of the parent in the preceding year • Active, ongoing conflict with the ex-spouse or -partner • A pattern of isolation from the community and from social relationships • The labeling by the family of a child who accepts the dysfunctional, ill, or impaired role so that the family focus is maintained primarily on the child, and symptoms are reinforced.

Reprinted with permission. Morawetz, A., and Walker, G. *Brief Therapy with Single-Parent Families.* New York: Brunner-Mazel Publishers, 1984.

Even young children in the single-parent family are expected to contribute to the household if the mother is working. Children are likely to become self-reliant and "adult" in manner. Consequently, parents may be surprised, or even alarmed, when their child acts older than his age.

Temporary role reversals occur often in single-parent families. Children are often more sensitive to their parent's emotional state; even in very young children, this is not a matter for concern unless the parent's distress is chronic and prolonged and/or there is a shift in their relationship from parent-child complementary to husband-wife complementary (in which the parent is able to return to or maintain the role accustomed to in marriage).

The need for single parents to delegate responsibility to elder children might lead to leadership rivalries among siblings. And since the absence of the other parent releases the custodial parent from the obligation to hold to a particular line, children of the single parent may attempt to negotiate every request made of them. To outsiders, this atmosphere of shared decision making might be negatively interpreted as parental inconsistency.

In order to maintain a cooperative rather than adversarial relationship with the children, and because no other adult is present to review parental decisions, single parents may overlook objectionable behavior or allow privileges against their better judgment. In the early years, when firm enforcement of limits is so important to childhood development, this "peace at any price" can be problematic.

Implications of serious illness. Life-threatening illness in the single-parent family is a major threat to all members. Children whose custodial parent is divorced or widowed have already experienced a major loss and dramatic role changes and will be especially sensitive to possibly losing the parent. The absence of a positive, supporting parent will be keenly and dramatically felt; if significant others are not available to provide continuity during the parent's absence, necessary progress toward mastering separation and expanding the social world can be hampered. Moreover, if child care is taken on by someone who does not appreciate the special dynamics of the single-parent family, discontinuity will be maximized and the child subjected to further stress. Traumatic, accidental injury may also increase feelings of vulnerability and loss of control within a low-income single-parent family that already resides in a community where crime and violence are common (Wortman, 1981). Temporary or prolonged insularity can result, further isolating the family from the community and magnifying the intensity of family relationships and anxiety about potential loss.

Once the critical period is past, the single parent may out of concern for the children return too quickly to the parental role, compromising recovery and short circuiting the opportunity for all family members, including the parent, to express affect arising from the crisis. Finally, the anxiety that pulls the family together to take over parenting may continue to operate when the threat is past, thus interfering with members' needs for separateness, autonomy, and differentiation.

Theories and models. Several theories and models have been proposed for work with single-parent families. By examining the presenting symptom in terms of the cycle of interaction supporting it and overall family organization, structural theorists (Minuchin et al., 1967) elucidated the influence on family issues of such concepts as hierarchy, generational boundaries and subsystems, coalitions, and power allocation. They described a brief, problem-focused approach to restore healthy family organization: parental authority, adherence to generational and subsystem boundaries, and clear expectations. The structural model has been a major force in contemporary work with poor, disorganized (and many times single-parent) families.

Murray Bowen (1978) emphasizes the importance of involving the extended family in resolving problems of single-parent families, but only if the problem serves a balancing function in the larger system. Bowen's model conceptualizes the family as a system of interconnecting triangles. Disturbance in one triangle counterbalances disturbance in another, with the second triangle representing another generation. Optimal intervention then is aimed at coaching a willing member of the presenting symptomatic triangle to make a behavior change that will affect some other key relationship from a different perspective.

A third useful framework was devised by the Milan Associates (Selvini-Palazzoli et al., 1978). Based on the premise that family symptomatology reflects an organization shift following a transitional event, the model's major intervention involves constructing a therapeutic bind that forces the family to establish a new organization.

Regrettably, Bowen and Milan Associates frameworks have not been widely applied to single-parent families except by Morawetz and Walker (1984).

Planning

Careful assessment of the single-parent family (nuclear and extended) helps the nurse determine whether required intervention should be short- or long-term. Because of the immediacy of the family crisis and the need to conserve resources, the nurse should attempt to accomplish short-term goals in five to six sessions, paced according to the number and immediacy of the problems identified. Family input—from primary support persons and children as well as from the single parent—is another important aspect of care planning. If the single parent is unconscious or otherwise unable to participate, family members who have the best knowledge and understanding of the patient should be encouraged to articulate what they believe the parent's wishes would be and engage in mutual problem solving.

Intervention

Single parents who have accessible, strong, and well-formed support systems, including quickly mobilized and synchronized community ties, will probably not require family interventions beyond those important to all families of intensive care patients. These include:
- reliving the critical event leading to the patient's admission (Rasie, 1980; Gardner and Stewart, 1978; Daley, 1984)
- ventilating feelings
- understanding the patient's status and medical equipment
- being involved in care planning
- being prepared for the initial visit
- receiving support and assistance with environmental needs
- interacting with the physician (Gardner and Stewart, 1978)
- visiting the family member frequently (Molter, 1979; Stillwell, 1984).

A program was designed at University Hospitals in Columbus, Ohio, to help families meet these needs; an assessment tool, the Family Assessment Sheet, was devised by the coordinators (with staff feedback) (Hudovanic et al., 1984).

Family meetings. The intrusion of life-threatening illness into a family's routine often precipitates a crisis. The more central the member is to the family and the more dependent others are upon him to meet biopsychosocial needs, the more disrupted the family will be. Family members who have had experience with life-threatening situations and loss will be better able to assign meaning to the predicament. The initial focus of family intervention in severe trauma is clarifying the current situation to all members, preferably in a setting where each can hear the other's questions and observations. The meaning of the traumatic event and its aftermath may be different for each member, depending upon previous experience and developmental stage.

To master the trauma of an uncontrollable life-threatening event, relatives may need, and most will request, details of the traumatic event—information the nurse should help them obtain if they desire it. Often this involves mobilizing family members as well as informing them. Information can be obtained most readily from the single parent or, if the parent is unable to participate at this stage, the first available family member(s). Directing family members to contact as many significant persons (family and others) as possible gives a valuable sense of focus when anxiety is high and information is likely to be sparse. Probing (for example, asking questions such as, "What about [the patient's] grandparents?" or "What about close personal or family friends?") may be needed to facilitate the family's thinking.

Note the manner in which family members enlist support from other relatives and friends. For example, does one family member minimize the situation so as not to burden others, or assume that relatives will not be able to come, or report the situation to others with intense affect? Does the relative initiating the contact indicate any personal desire for others to be present? This will indicate family patterns of help seeking and emotional expression.

At this time, a nurse must help the single parent take an observational stance. Sudden, unexpected events can precipitate a variety of loss-related fears; these feelings are, initially, difficult to articulate, but generally relate to functional, cosmetic, social, and sexual loss, and, ultimately, possible death. The patient needs to channel the vigilance that accompanies being a victim into observing and confirming observations of the family. During this initial impact stage three things may happen: usual family roles may become less clear, habitual communication sequences are likely to be misunderstood, and a gravely serious atmosphere may pervade family functioning. Relatives may attempt to keep things as they were before the injuries. Casting the patient—and all family members—as observers during this stage allows them to distance themselves from the initial impact. This approach promotes thinking, decreases anxiety, and sets the stage for acknowledging and realizing the true extent of trauma and loss.

As they begin to integrate the traumatic experience, family members will theorize about it and attempt to find meaning in a seemingly meaningless event. Sharing these interpretations can lead to mutual appreciation and respect, as well as to role modification. The ability to explore, compromise, consolidate, and joke are hallmarks of this stage (Anthony, 1973) and should be encouraged. When family members settle on a set of explanations for the event, they will have reached a period of stabilization and will be less open to intervention. It is important, therefore, to bring the family together before the meaning of the event is consolidated so that new learning and new interaction patterns can occur.

Family education. Whether a nurse provides information to help the family come to grips with the trauma or simply provides home care instruction, certain principles are vital for her success. She should speak directly and avoid medical terminology whenever possible. She should also arrange meetings between the primary nurse, physician, and family—with the single parent included unless physically unable. This will promote the patient's executive functioning through direct negotiation with family members about performing vacated functions.

Address children's needs. Teaching the family about young children's developmental needs and possible reactions to parental absence is essential. Relatives should be encouraged to help children continue their usual routine; it will diminish stress. By maintaining the established home base, a temporary caretaker can help preserve the injured parent's executive role, promote generational demarcations, and preserve nuclear family boundaries. Finally, it is important to find ways for children to interact with the ill parent if the parent can. Actual contact will validate the parent's continued existence. Other interactional modes are also useful: notes, letters, photographs, tape recordings, and phone conversations, for instance.

A traumatically injured parent, uninformed about a child's developmental level and fearful about his reaction to the parent's changed appearance, may wish to rely on false reassurance, half-truths, and evasion when speaking to the child. This is most likely to happen when the parent feels well and thinks that denial of the condition's seriousness would be appropriate. However, continued parent-child separation will only preserve this denial; in the long run, denial is more costly to the child developmentally than full awareness of what has happened.

Parents need to know that children's stress diminishes when they know what is going on around them. Therefore, when the child arrives, the nurse should encourage conversation about the parent's current disability. That opens the topic for further discussion if the child—or parent or caretaker—wants to return to it later. Inquiring about the children and their reactions to their parent's accident, or about whether the parent or caretaking adult would like help coping with the child's needs, is a useful preliminary approach to the subject (Cancer Care, Inc., and The National Cancer Foundation, 1973).

Promote affective expression. Verbalization and sharing of feelings should be encouraged. As the family continues to relive the traumatic event in order to gain some control over feelings of vulnerability, questions and comments that facilitate the connection between current events and feelings (for example, "What were you thinking about just then?" when a grandparent becomes tearful; "What feelings did you have about that?" when a brother begins focusing on the cost of hospitalization) are particularly helpful. Cohesion, connection, and support among family members should be promoted by asking, "Who else in the family feels this way?" By the same token, asking, "Who is least likely to feel as you do?" can promote antonomy. Creative materials—finger paints, crayons, clay, dolls, and small cars—should be made available to young children to promote affective expression.

Deal with parental anxiety. Many victims of multiple trauma experience a great deal of anxiety and frustration related to their home responsibilities, communication difficulties, and greatly decreased mobility. The feelings of helplessness related to these functional deficits can lead to negative thinking processes and depression. The patient's actual and perceived physical status affect both psychological and socioemotional functioning. It is useful to reflect the patient's feelings, to help the patient validate negative emotion, and to help the patient understand that such feelings are shared by others in similar situations.

Family members may, in some cases, react more intensely to the patient's emotional changes than to the actual physical trauma; they will probably require teaching about useful patient and family interactions. Helping everyone concerned vent frustrations verbally can prevent the evolution of a rising cycle of family conflict and emotionality, or the triangulation of staff members and nursing care issues as a way of shifting anxiety.

Recognize family strengths. The single parent's strengths need to be respectfully acknowledged. This will facilitate the joining process, reinforce functional capabilities, and support the patient's executive authority at a time when certain parental tasks will be assumed by others. Such reinforcement can also facilitate reintegration of the recuperating single parent back into previous family roles and prevent chronic, dysfunctional role reversals, which can permanently damage the family's power structure. If the family's trauma-related anxiety remains high, there is a real risk that the injured parent may begin to construct a dysfunctional self-image based on the reflected appraisals of others and personal feelings of vulnerability. Support should not overemphasize strengths to an extent that prevents either patient recognition of current difficulties or patient and family verbalization of distress.

Both patient and family must acclimate to the illness first, then later, to the return of wellness. Anthony (1973) contends that most families overreact to the passive, dependent nature of illness by being more supportive, sympathetic, and indulgent than is necessary or useful. He describes a cycle in which "both the sick and the well become immersed in a common pool of suffering" (p. 137).

Provide support during role changes. Any role change reverberates throughout a family by establishing new interactional sequences. The single parent who has been relieved through illness or injury of many tangible role activities may return home expecting to resume previous parental authority immediately. Likewise, the temporary caretaker may expect instant relief from child care functions. However, the children may have difficulty recognizing the parent's authority at first. In fact, in an attempt to help the recovering parent a child may be overly solicitous or may spontaneously perform new chores; the parent, in turn, may react with increased authoritarianism. The family's significant adults need to be aware of this transition stage and the importance of supporting the parent's executive authority with the children. Collaboration is essential. The parent must inform the helping adult when she is ready to resume additional activities and point out areas where assistance will be needed (especially child care and discipline). If the helping adult learned how to provide physical assistance and care to the parent during hospitalization, both persons' role transitions during the recuperative period will be eased.

Use direct interventions. Direct intervention approaches are suitable for most client families, especially right after the initial trauma, when anxiety is high. Indirect approaches can be reserved for those families in which the children have displayed long-standing behavior problems or the parent has demonstrated problematic functioning prior to the multiple trauma. These families should be referred to mental health professionals.

Evaluation

Evaluation of nursing care for single-parent families with multiple trauma requires attention to the cognitive, affective, and behavioral domains (Wright and Leahey, 1984). Are you able to consider the family's particular dilemmas in a social context? Can you identify with feelings conveyed? Do your behaviors help facilitate useful patterns of family energy expenditure and a balance of distance-closeness? What feedback does the family give you about what has taken place? If you are viewed as central to the change process, question in your mind whether you have been triangulated into the family as a new executive authority for a present or absent parent.

CONCLUSIONS

Single-parent families are likely to experience major and multiple physical traumas to family members more intensely than other types of families. The quality of the support available to them is an important determinant of their crisis response. Their structure facilitates certain perceptions and dynamics that might at first appear to be but are not necessarily maladaptive. Recognition of strengths is therefore a priority component of assessment, planning, intervention, and evaluation.

REFERENCES

Adams, P., et al. *Fatherless Children.* New York: John Wiley & Sons, 1984.

Anthony, E.J. "The Mutative Impact of Serious Mental and Physical Illness in a Parent on Family Life," in *The Child in His Family: Vol. 2. The Impact of Disease and Death.* Edited by Anthony, E.J., and Koupernik, C. New York: John Wiley & Sons, 1973.

Blechman, E.A. "Are Children with One Parent at Psychological Risk? A Methodological Review," *Journal of Marriage and the Family* 44:179–95, 1982.

Bowen, M. *Family Therapy in Clinical Practice.* New York: Jason Aronson, 1978.

Boyd, D. "Comprehensive Regional Trauma and Emergency Medical Service Delivery Systems: A Goal of the 1980's," *Critical Care Quarterly* 5:4, 1982.

Cancer Care, Inc., and the National Cancer Foundation. *The Impact and Consequences of Catastrophic Illness on Patients and Families.* New York: Cancer Care, Inc., and The National Cancer Foundation, 1973.

Carter, E.A., and McGoldrick, M. "The Family Life Cycle and Family Therapy," in *The Family Life Cycle.* Edited by Carter, E.A., and McGoldrick, M. New York: Gardner Press, 1980.

Collison, C.R., and Futrell, J. "Family Therapy for the Single-Parent Family System," *Journal of Psychiatric Nursing and Mental Health Services* 20:16–20, 1982.

Daley, L. "The Perceived Immediate Needs of Families with Relatives in the Intensive Care Setting," *Heart & Lung* 13:231–37, 1984.

Duffy, M.E. "When a Woman Heads a Household," *Nursing Outlook* 30:468–73, 1982.

Dunbar, S.B. "Women's Health and Nursing Research," *Advances in Nursing Science* 3:1–16, 1981.

Eiduson, B.T. "Conflict and Stress in Nontraditional Families: Impact on Children," *American Journal of Orthopsychiatry* 53:426–35, 1983.

Fought, S.G., and Throwe, A.N. *Psychosocial Nursing Care of the Emergency Patient.* New York: John Wiley & Sons, 1984.

Francke, L.B. *Growing Up Divorced.* New York: Linden Press, 1983.

Gardner, D., and Stewart, N. "Staff Involvement with Patients in Critical-Care Units," *Heart & Lung* 7:105–10, 1978.

Godenne, G. "Unwed Mothers," *International Encyclopedia of Psychiatry, Psychology, Psychoanalysis and Neurology,* vol. 2. New York: Aesculopius Pubs., 1977.

Hudovanic, B.H., et al. "Family Crisis Intervention Program in the Medical Intensive Care Unit," *Heart & Lung* 13:243–49, 1984.

Hoeker, A., ed. *U/S: A Statistical Portrait of the American People.* New York: Penguin Books, 1983.

Lindblad-Goldberg, M., and Dukes, J.L. "Social Support in Black, Low-Income, Single Parent Families: Normative and Dysfunctional Patterns," *American Journal of Orthopsychiatry* 55:43–58, 1985.

Mahler, M.S., et al. "Stages in the Infant's Separation from the Mother," in *The Psychosocial Interior of the Family.* Edited by Handel, G. New York: Aldine Publishing Co., 1985.

McDermott, J.F. "Parental Divorce in Early Childhood," *American Journal of Psychiatry* 124:1424–32, 1968.

Miller, J.B. "Psychological Recovery in Low-Income Single Parents," *American Journal of Orthopsychiatry* 52:346–52, 1982.

Minuchin, S., et al. *Families of the Slums: An Exploration of Their Structure and Treatment.* New York: Basic Books, 1967.

Molter, N.C. "Needs of Relatives of Critically Ill Patients: A Descriptive Study," *Heart & Lung* 8:332–39, 1979.

Morawetz, A., and Walker, G. *Brief Therapy with Single-Parent Families.* New York: Brunner-Mazel, 1984.

National Advisory Council on Economic Opportunity. "No, Poverty Has Not Disappeared," *Social Policy* 25–28, January/February 1983.

Pattison, E., et al. "Social Network Mediation of Anxiety," *Psychiatric Annals* 9:56–67, 1979.

Pope, H. "Negro-White Differences in Decisions Regarding Illegitimate Children," *Journal of Marriage and the Family* 31(4):756–64, 1969.

Rasie, S. "Meeting Families' Needs Helps You Meet ICU Patients' Needs," *Nursing* 10(7):32–35, 1980.

Selvini-Palazzoli, M., et al. *Paradox and Counterparadox.* New York: Jason Aronson, 1978.

Stillwell, S.B. "Importance of Visiting Needs as Perceived by Family Members of Patients in the Intensive Care Unit," *Heart & Lung* 13:238–42, 1984.

Weiss, R. "A Different Kind of Parenting," in *The Psychosocial Interior of the Family.* Edited by Handel, G. New York: Aldine Publishing Co., 1985.

Wortman, R.A. "Depression, Danger, Dependency and Denial: Work with Poor, Black, Single Parents," *American Journal of Psychiatry* 51:662–71, 1981.

Wright, L.M., and Leahey, M. *Nurses and Families: A Guide to Family Assessment and Intervention.* Philadelphia: F.A. Davis Co., 1984.

INDEX